Method of
Urology

Method of Urology

ARTHUR W. WYKER, Jr., M.D.
Professor

JAY Y. GILLENWATER, M.D.
Professor and Chairman
Department of Urology, University of Virginia
School of Medicine, Charlottesville, Virginia

with contributions by

E. DARRACOTT VAUGHAN, Jr., M.D.
Assistant Professor
Both of the Department of Urology

STUART S. HOWARDS, M.D.
Associate Professor

THE WILLIAMS & WILKINS COMPANY

Copyright ©, 1975
The Williams & Wilkins Company
428 E. Preston Street
Baltimore, Md. 21202, U.S.A.

Made in the United States of America

Library of Congress Cataloging in Publication Data

Wyker, Arthur W.
      Method of urology.
      Bibliography: p.
      1. Urology. I. Gillenwater, Jay Y., joint author. II. Title. [DNLM: 1. Urologic diseases.
WJ100 W981m] RC871.W94   616.6   75-8588
ISBN 0-683-09300-2

Composed and printed at the
Waverly Press, Inc.
Mt. Royal and Guilford Aves.
Baltimore, Md. 21202, U.S.A.

This book is dedicated to our wives—
Yvie, Shirley, Anne, and Carter.

Preface

This book is written primarily for medical students and residents, but it may also be useful to others who wish to gain insight into the fundamentals of urology. It is in large part an outgrowth of the teaching program at the University of Virginia, where for 10 years the senior staff members have had daily tutorials with one or two students to discuss various topics in urology. The students are expected to review the subject prior to the sessions. Then utilizing an informal question and answer technique, we attempt to synthesize the material and give them a clear, updated version of the subject. To prepare for these meetings, the students must choose between reading the large, standard textbooks of urology which are often too lengthy and detailed for their purposes or the smaller, condensed versions which often only enumerate information without giving emphasis to either basic pathophysiological principles or the most reliable diagnostic and therapeutic modalities for a specific entity. We trust that this volume will fill the gap between the definitive reference books and the simplified manuals. A special effort has been made to emphasize pathophysiologic mechanisms.

The entire spectrum of urology is presented in this work, from adrenal physiology and disease to a review of male sexual inadequacy. The first chapter comprehensively discusses the common signs and symptoms of urology which must be mastered to properly identify and treat urologic disorders. With this foundation, the student can initiate an appropriate investigative program which should lead to a diagnosis. In order to keep the book reasonably compact, only a modest number of illustrations are included. At the end of each chapter, there is a selected list of references and suggested further reading.

We would like to thank Miss Betsy Byrd and Mrs. Sallie Feild for their invaluable secretarial help and for their patience and cheerfulness. We would also like to express our appreciation to Mr. William Fairweather for his fine illustrations.

Arthur W. Wyker, Jr., M.D.

Contents

1

Signs and Symptoms of Urological Disorders with Differential Diagnoses

ARTHUR W. WYKER, JR.

PAIN

Mechanism

The chief cause of pain in the urinary tract is *distention*. The severity of the pain is *not* related to the degree of distention but to the rapidity with which it develops. Sudden distention of the ureter, renal pelvis, or calyces causes severe pain whereas gradual distention of the same structures causes little or no pain (Fig. 1).

1. In case A, with acute distention of the left ureter and renal pelvis above an obstructing calculus, the patient experienced severe pain requiring morphine for relief, yet the ureter was only slightly dilated.

2. In case B, the ureter was greatly dilated, yet the patient experienced no pain since dilation took place over many months.

There are two other less important causes of pain in the urinary tract.

1. *Distention of the renal capsule* causes a mild aching pain in the costo-vertebral angle (CVA) region only.

A. This most commonly occurs with swelling of the renal parenchyma secondary to acute pyelonephritis or obstructive hydronephrosis, but it may also occur with subcapsular hematoma secondary to renal trauma.

2. *Renal ischemia* may produce mild to moderate pain in the CVA region only.

A. This usually occurs with embolus or thrombus of the main renal artery or one of its branches.

Type and Location of Pain

Pain due to distention of the renal capsule or to renal ischemia is *steady* and limited to the CVA region. Pain due to distention of the ureter and renal pelvis may also be steady, but about 50% of the time it is spasmodic. This spasmodic type of pain is called *colic* and it is produced by intermittent contractions of the ureteral smooth muscles. With each peristaltic wave, more urine is pumped into the partially obstructed segment of ureter with a resultant increase in the hydrostatic pressure

1

A. ACUTE OBSTRUCTION   **B. CHRONIC OBSTRUCTION**

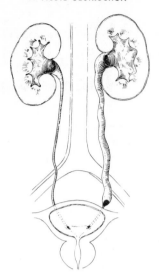
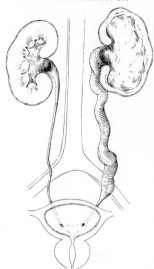

Fig. 1.

and in the intensity of the pain. With colic, the pain is variable in intensity, but it does not usually disappear completely. The most common cause of renal colic is an *obstructing calculus in the lower ureter*.

The distribution of urinary tract pain has been carefully mapped out by distending the renal pelvis and various portions of the ureter with small balloon catheters. The location of renal and ureteral pain is shown in Figure 2.

1. Notice that urinary tract pain does not occur in the central portion of the abdomen but is *lateralized* to the outer abdomen, flank, and CVA region.

2. Localization of pain with distention of the ureter.

   A. Distention of the ureterovesical junction causes pain in the *suprapubic region*.

   B. Distention of the midureter (15 cm above the ureterovesical junction) causes pain *adjacent to mid-Poupart's ligament*.

   C. Distention of the ureteropelvic junction causes pain *adjacent to the anterior superior iliac spine*.

3. Distention of the renal pelvis causes pain in the CVA region.

Pain Pathways and Referred Pain

Pain impulses arising within the abdominal and thoracic cavities reach the central nervous system (CNS) by three pathways.

1. Parasympathetic nerves.
2. Sympathetic nerves.
3. Somatic nerves innervating the body wall and diaphragm.

Kidney and ureter pain impulses are carried in *visceral afferent fibers*

Primary pain sites   Referred pain sites

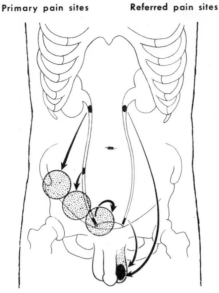

Fig. 2.

that accompany the *sympathetics* whereas bladder pain impulses are carried chiefly in the *parasympathetics*. Sympathectomy from T7 to L3 abolishes renal and ureteral pain but has no significant effect on bladder pain.

With distention of the ureter, the afferent visceral fibers accompanying the sympathetics carry the pain impulses to the appropriate segment of the spinal cord, and, if the impulses proceed *unmodified* to the brain, *true visceral pain* results. True visceral pain is usually deep, diffuse, and aching in nature.

Referred Pain

Referred pain is pain projected to an area distant from the point of stimulation, and it is frequently present in urinary tract disorders.

The exact mechanism of referred pain is unknown! In the pain sensory pathway, the visceral afferent fibers are in close proximity to the somatic neurons, and the ureteral pain impulse may be diverted to the somatic neuron so that the brain interprets the pain as having come from the skin segment. The skin and ureter share a *common segmental innervation* so that the location of referred pain depends upon the spinal cord segment involved.

Spinal cord segments T11 to 12 receive sensory fibers from both the upper ureter and testis, so that the distention of the upper ureter may cause *referred pain to the testis*. In like fashion, distention of the lower ureter may cause *referred pain to the scrotum*.

Pain in the Lower Urinary Tract

1. Bladder distention causes fullness initially, then pain in the suprapubic region associated with an intense desire to urinate.
A. Normal bladder mucosa is sensitive to stimuli, and this sensivity is greatly increased by inflammation.
2. Stimulation of the trigone, ureteral orifice, and anterior urethra causes referred pain to the end of the penis.
3. The posterior urethra is relatively unresponsive to stimuli.

FREQUENT URINATION (FREQUENCY)

Urinary frequency is the *most common* urological symptom. When it occurs at night (nocturia), it is particularly disturbing and often is the reason for medical consultation.

To evaluate frequency, it is essential to know the normal voiding pattern. The normal adult voids four to five times during his waking period and has zero to one time nocturia. The volume per voiding is usually *over* 200 ml, often around 300 ml.

The relationship among age, urinary frequency, and average 24-hour urine volume is shown in Table 1.

The average volume per voiding of children aged 4 to 10 is *100 to 200 ml.*

Etiology

There are two primary causes of urinary frequency.
1. Decreased bladder capacity with resultant decrease in the volume of urine per voiding.
2. Increased urine volume (polyuria) with resultant normal volume of urine per voiding.

Differential Diagnosis

1. Decreased bladder capacity with decreased urine volume per voiding.
   A. Infravesical obstruction.
     1) Early.

TABLE 1

Age	Frequency of Voiding	Urine Volume
	times/24 hr	*ml/24 hr*
1-2 days	2–6	30–60
3-6 months	16–20	300–400
6-12 months	12–16	400–500
1-2 years	10–12	500–600
2-3 years	8–10	500–600
3-4 years	6–8	600–700
4-10 years	5–6	650–1000
> 10 years	4–5	800–1400

a. Initially the bladder musculature hypertrophies because of the increased effort necessary to empty the bladder. This hypertrophied muscle has a *higher resting tonus* so that smaller than normal volumes of urine initiate the desire to void.

b. Patients will often note a decrease in the size and force of their urinary stream.

2) Late.

a. Bladder musculature, initially able to compensate for obstruction by more forceful contraction, eventually becomes fatigued and is unable to empty the bladder. The bladder is now decompensated and the *resultant residual urine decreases the functional capacity of the bladder* with resultant frequency.

b. Bedwetting or stress incontinence in a man over 50 years of age suggests this diagnosis. With high residual urine, coughing, sneezing, or bending may raise the intravesical pressure sufficiently to overcome the urethral resistance with resultant urinary incontinence (overflow).

3) Causes of infravesical obstruction.

a. Benign prostatic hyperplasia (BPH) is the most common one, accounting for over *90% of all cases.*

b. Carcinoma of the prostate.

c. Urethral stricture.

d. Contracture of the bladder neck.

e. Stenosis of the urethral meatus.

f. Posterior urethral valves in boys.

g. Neurogenic bladder.

B. Inflammation of the bladder.

1) Normal bladder mucosa is pain-sensitive, and, when it is inflamed, its *pain threshold is markedly decreased* so that it takes fewer stimuli to initiate the desire to void.

2) Causes.

a. Acute bacterial cystitis, primary or secondary to inflammatory process in adjacent bowel or vagina.

b. Bladder calculus.

c. Bladder tumor.

3) Patients usually complain of painful urination and urgency, and urinalysis may reveal pyuria, hematuria, and bacteriuria.

C. Extravesical lesions pressing upon the bladder.

1) Mass may mechanically interfere with normal bladder expansion, or it may cause an irritable focus in the bladder wall.

2) Causes.

a. Pregnant uterus.

b. Fibroids.

c. Ovarian tumor.

3) Patients may note that their urinary frequency disappears when

they are lying down but recurs when they stand up.

D. Psychogenic frequency due to anxiety.

1) These patients, usually women, characteristically have marked daytime frequency but *no nocturia*.

2. Increased volume (polyuria) with resultant normal urine volume per voiding.

A. Due to increased solute per nephron.

1) Diabetes mellitus—unreabsorbed glucose is an *osmotic diuretic*.

2) Chronic renal insufficiency—with a diminished nephron population the remaining nephrons are subject to severe *osmotic diuresis due to increased filtration rate per nephron*.

B. Due to decreased circulating antidiuretic hormone (ADH).

1) Decreased production of ADH due to disease of the supraopticohypophyseal system—diabetes insipidus.

2) Decreased need to secrete ADH because of high fluid intake—*compulsive water drinker.*

3) The mean plasma osmolality in diabetes insipidus—295 ± 15 mOsm/kg—is significantly higher than in normal subjects (280 ± 6 mOsm/kg), whereas in compulsive water drinking it is significantly lower—269 ± 14 mOsm/kg (de Wardener).

a. In patients with diabetes insipidus, the initial disturbance is polyuria and the excessive drinking is a normal response to the contraction and concentration of body fluids.

b. In compulsive water drinkers, the initial disturbance is excessive drinking and the polyuria is the normal response to expansion and dilution of body fluids.

4) If you administer ADH (pitressin), urine flow decreases in normal people, compulsive water drinkers, and patients with diabetes insipidus. In the compulsive water drinkers, thirst continues unabated, intake of water exceeds output, and overhydration develops.

C. Due to failure of kidney to respond to normal amounts of circulating ADH.

1) Nephrogenic diabetes insipidus.

2) Hypokalemia.

3) Hypercalcemia.

Program of Investigation

1. Determine urine volume per voiding, 24-hour urine output, and whether there are any additional urinary symptoms.

A. If polyuria is the cause of urinary frequency, there will be no additional urinary symptoms; urine volume per voiding will be in the normal range but the 24-hour urine output will be increased.

B. If a decreased bladder capacity is the cause of urinary frequency, additional urinary symptoms are usually present, urine volume per voiding is usually decreased, and the 24-hour urine output is normal.

2. If a decreased bladder capacity is noted, determine whether this is secondary to infravesical obstruction, inflammation of the bladder, or extravesical pressure upon the bladder.

A. Infravesical obstruction.

1) Check urethral meatus for stenosis, palpate urethra for stricture, and examine prostate for BPH and carcinoma.

2) Observe the patient voiding when his bladder is comfortably full.

3) Determine residual urine.

4) Give neurological examination to rule out neurogenic bladder.

5) Perform cystourethrogram.

B. Inflammation of the bladder.

1) Palpate urethra and bladder for tenderness.

2) Examine fresh urinary sediment for bacteria, white blood cells (WBC), red blood cells (RBC), and trichomonads.

C. Extravesical lesions compressing the bladder.

1) With bladder empty, palpate lower abdomen and pelvic region for abnormal masses.

3. If polyuria is noted, initial studies should include the following.

A. Blood—osmolality, creatinine, glucose, potassium, calcium.

B. Urine—osmolality, glucose.

4. Urinalysis is often diagnostic.

A. Glycosuria indicates diabetes mellitus.

B. Bacteria ± WBC indicates acute bacterial cystitis.

C. Urine specific gravity.

1) Less than 1.005—diabetes insipidus, compulsive water drinker.

2) 1.010 consistently—chronic renal insufficiency.

URINARY INCONTINENCE

Involuntary loss of urine is a common and distressing symptom.

Causes of Urinary Incontinence

1. Urgency.
2. Stress.
3. Overflow.
4. Neurogenic (true).
5. Ectopic ureter in female.
6. Injury to lower urinary tract with resultant damage to the urinary sphincters or formation of a urinary fistula.

Urgency Incontinence

1. The patient has a sudden, strong desire to urinate but is unable to reach the bathroom in time.

A. The desire to void *precedes urinary leakage*, and the patient is very aware of loss of urine.

2. This occurs most commonly with acute bacterial cystitis in women but may also occur with infiltrative bladder tumors and with tumors adacent to the bladder.

Stress Incontinence

1. A squirt of urine occurs *only after a sudden increase in intravesical pressure* (IVP).

    A. Usual causes of increased intravesical pressure.

        1) Coughing and sneezing.

        2) Bending and lifting.

        3) Laughing and walking up or down stairs.

        4) Intercourse and defecation.

    B. When leakage occurs, it does so in *jet fashion*, often in sizable quantities.

    C. Lying down decreases the intravesical pressure significantly (50% of standing pressure) so that patients are *usually continent* at night as well as between episodes of stress.

2. Stress incontinence occurs chiefly in women who have had *multiple pregnancies or difficult labors*.

    A. The musculoelastic support of the urethrovesical region is damaged with resultant incontinence.

Overflow Incontinence

1. Urine leakage is triggered by a rise in intravesical pressure not unlike stress incontinence, but the mechanism of incontinence is entirely different.

    A. In stress incontinence, residual urine is insignificant and the primary defect is loss of muscular support in the urethrovesical region.

    B. In overflow incontinence, long standing infravesical obstruction has caused bladder decompensation with resultant chronically high residual urine, usually over 1000 ml.

        1) The intravesical pressure is *consistently elevated* so that slight increases in intra-abdominal pressure may raise the intravesical pressure sufficiently to overcome the urethral resistance with escape of urine.

        2) The first sign of overflow incontinence is often *bedwetting*.

Neurogenic Incontinence

1. The urinary leakage associated with neurogenic bladder is not the leaky faucet type but rather an *active type of incontinence*.

    A. Urinary sphincter tone is often hypertonic, and this increased resistance results in irregular and unsuccessful attempts of the bladder to empty its contents.

    B. Urinary leakage is usually *intermittent and unpredictable*, but occasionally it is almost a constant dribble.

2. This is often called "true incontinence" because the urine is usually lost without any warning.

3. The nature of the neurological disorder responsible is usually apparent after a careful history and physical and neurological examination.

Ectopic Ureter in Females

1. Despite a completely normal voiding pattern, these little girls are constantly wet (leaky faucet type of incontinence).

2. The cause of urinary leakage is an ectopic ureter opening *beyond the urinary sphincters*, most commonly in the distal urethra or in the vestibule adjacent to the urethral meatus.

   A. Less common openings—vagina, cervix, uterine cavity.

   B. If a ureterocele is present in the urethra, incontinence often occurs, primarily because of the mass interfering with the normal closing mechanism of the female urethra.

3. The ectopic ureter is usually associated with complete ureteral duplication with the ectopic ureter going to the upper segment of the kidney.

   A. The function of this renal segment is usually poor, so that little or no function may be evident on intravenous urogram.

4. Urinary incontinence does not occur in males with ectopic ureters, because all possible Wolffian duct derivatives—posterior urethra, vas deferens, epididymis, and seminal vesicles—are proximal to the external urinary sphincter.

   A. Because of its Wolffian duct origin, the ectopic ureter must open somewhere along the course of the Wolffian duct.

Injury to the Lower Urinary Tract with Resultant Urinary Incontinence

1. The urinary sphincters may be damaged during a prostatectomy.

   A. Often these patients can remain continent as long as they contract the external urinary sphincter, but as soon as this muscle becomes fatigued, urine leakage occurs.

2. Pelvic surgery sometimes results in a urinary-vaginal fistula due to injury to a ureter or the bladder.

   A. The mechanism of urinary incontinence here is readily apparent (see Table 2).

3. External nonsurgical trauma may also produce incontinence either by damaging the urinary sphincters or by creating a urinary fistula.

ENURESIS

Enuresis is *repeated*, *unintentional*, and *unconscious* voiding of urine usually with a full, steady stream. It usually occurs at night, and so it is commonly called *bedwetting*. Bedwetting is normal in infancy, but between age 2 to 4 most children stop. Enuresis is a major problem for pediatricians since 10 to 15% of all children aged 4 to 12 wet the bed virtually every night.

TABLE 2
Differential Diagnosis of Urinary Incontinence

	Sex	Neurological Abnormality	Residual Urine	Nature of Urine Leakage	Precipitating Factor
Urgency	F	No	No	Intermittent	Modest filling of bladder
Stress	F	No	No	Intermittent	Increase IVP, cough, sneeze
Overflow	M	No	Yes (>1000 ml)	Intermittent	Increase IVP, cough, sneeze
Neurogenic	=	Yes	Yes (modest)	Variable	None
Ectopic ureter	F	No	No	Continuous	None
Injury	=	No	No	Continuous	None

Etiology

If all enuretics were studied urologically, including a voiding cystoure-throgram and cystoendoscopy, probably around *10%* would have obstructive lesions in the lower urinary tract. These lesions include narrowing of the urethral meatus, urethral stricture, bladder neck contracture, and posterior urethral valves seen only in boys. With infravesical obstruction, the bladder muscle hypertrophies because of the increased effort necessary to empty the bladder. This thickened bladder muscle has a higher resting tonus so that smaller than normal volumes of urine may trigger the voiding mechanism. These children often have other urological symptoms such as urinary frequency and urgency, and some may have had urinary infections. The force and caliber of the urinary stream may be less than normal, but the child is usually unaware of this since his stream—big or little—has been that way all his life. If you are able to observe him voiding when his bladder is comfortably full, you may detect an abnormal urinary stream.

The large majority of enuretics, around 90%, have no structural abnormalities of the urinary tract, but they tend to have the following three features in common.
1. Decreased bladder capacity.
   A. To go through the night without wetting the bed or getting up to void, the functional bladder capacity must be around 300 ml.
   1) Normal children reach this bladder capacity by age 4 to 5, whereas enuretic children usually reach it by age 9 to 10.
   B. Esperanca and Gerrard obtained the data shown in Table 3.
2. Urinary frequency.
   A. Normal children over 4 years of age usually void 5 to 6 times a day whereas enuretics usually void 9 to 10 times per day.
   B. Esperanca and Gerrard obtained the data shown in Table 4.

TABLE 3
Physiological Maximal Bladder Capacity in Children

Age	Normal	Enuretics	
yrs	ml		
4	296	180	
5	301	238	<300 ml necessary
6	359	279	to go through the
7	394	217	night
8	428	272	
9	457	281	
10	473	353	

Reprinted from Esperanca, M. and Gerrard, J. W.: Nocturnal enuresis in bladder function in normal children and enuretics. Can. Med. Assoc. J. 101: 326, 1969.

TABLE 4
Frequency of Micturition in 24 Hours

Age	Normal	Enuretics
yrs		
4	5.3	11.9
5	5.7	11.0
6	6.4	10.0
7	5.5	8.4
8	5.3	9.7
10	4.6	10.7

Reprinted from Esperanca, M. and Gerrard, J. W.: Nocturnal enuresis in bladder function in normal children and enuretics. Can Med. Assoc. J. 101: 326, 1969.

3. Unusually heavy sleepers.

A. Enuretics are usually very difficult to arouse, and they rarely wake up after wetting the bed.

There are other possible causes of enuresis.

1. Emotional or behavioral problem.

A. When enuresis is not continuous from infancy but reappears after a period of continence, this may be the cause.

B. This is suggested by the presence of thumb sucking, nail biting, speech impediment, or temper tantrums.

2. Brain dysfunction.

A. Most enuretics sleep more deeply than normal children, but not all deep sleepers wet the bed.

B. Some enuretics have an abnormal sleeping electroencephalogram, suggesting that their enuresis may be a manifestation of focal epilepsy.

1) Dilantin may eliminate this form of enuresis.

3. Environmental factors.

A. Enuresis occurs more commonly in poor families, particularly large families.

1) Toilet facilities and space are often inadequate so that toilet training and cleanliness are virtually ignored.

Management

It is important to allay the anxiety of the child and the parents. If the child is 6 or older, structural abnormalities may be ruled out by performing an intravenous urogram with a voiding cystourethrogram. The voiding film is the most important one and is best obtained after a short waiting period during which time the child is allowed to drink water or Coca Cola. This produces a comfortably full bladder, facilitating voiding without undue dilution of the contrast medium in the bladder.

To counteract the small bladder capacity usually found in enuretics, children should be encouraged to hold their urine until they are uncomfortable. Anticholinergic drugs may also aid in increasing the functional bladder capacity.

Tofranil, a drug that works primarily on the central nervous system, has successfully eliminated enuresis in many cases, although the mechanism of action is not clearly defined as yet.

PAIN ON URINATION

Pain on urination is usually secondary to inflammation of the lower urinary tract! The patient may localize this discomfort to the suprapubic area or to the end of the penis or urethra. Milder degrees of pain are often described as a burning sensation. The usual cause is a *nonspecific bacterial infection.* Other less common causes include the following.

1. Specific infections.
   A. Tuberculosis.
   B. Viral.
   C. Fungal (candidal).
   D. Parasitic (schistosomal).
2. Stone or foreign body in the bladder or urethra.
3. Infiltrating carcinoma.
4. Interstitial cystitis.
5. Drug (cytoxan).
6. Excess phosphates in the urine.

It is important to determine when pain or burning is noted during urination. If it begins with the onset and stops abruptly at the end, the primary pathology is probably in the urethra. When the bladder is primarily involved, as in acute bacterial cystitis, patients experience some discomfort during urination but often the most severe pain occurs after voiding has ceased.

URGENCY OF URINATION

Urgency of urination is a sudden, strong desire to urinate. When this sensation cannot be resisted, involuntary voiding occurs, and this is called urgency incontinence. As with pain on urination, the usual cause is an inflammatory lesion of the lower urinary tract. There are several additional causes which are of clinical interest.

1. Stone in the lower ureter—urgency of urination and defecation often accompany a stone near the ureterovesical junction.

2. Uninhibited neurogenic bladder.

HEMATURIA

The passage of blood-stained urine may be the first sign of serious disease in the urinary tract, and a single episode of hematuria warrants a thorough urological investigation.

The presence of blood is established by finding an *abnormal number of RBC in the urinary sediment*. A normal individual usually excretes about 30,000 RBC/hour but may excrete up to 100,000 RBC/hour, or about 1,600 RBC/min. If the urine output is 50 ml/hour (1,200 ml/day), up to 2000 RBC/ml may be excreted (100,000/50 ml), and this concentration of RBC gives urinary findings of zero-to-one RBC/HPF. *Greater than 2 RBC/HPF may be considered microscopic hematuria.*

There are two clinical situations where hematuria may be present yet the urinary sediment shows no RBC (see Table 5).

1. Hypotonic urine—urine specific gravity less than 1.008.

2. Alkaline urine—urine pH greater than 7.0.

Under these conditions, RBC are lysed with release of hemoglobin and this may be detected with a dipstick test for hemoglobin. These impregnated cellulose strips are designed to detect free hemoglobin or hemoglobin contained in RBC.

TABLE 5

Osmotic Rupture of RBC by Hypotonic Urine

Urine containing 100,000 RBC/ml with urinary sediment finding of 30 RBC/HPF was used as the standard.

Urine Specific Gravity	RBC/HPF	Dipstick	Lysis
			%
1.001	0	++++	100
1.005	0	++++	100
1.007	0	++++	100
1.010	30	+	0
1.015	30	+	0
1.020	30	+	0
1.025	30	+	0
1.028	30	+	0

1. Notice that the dipstick test is positive in *all* cases of hematuria regardless of urine specific gravity.
2. Osmotic lysis of RBC may occur whenever the urine specific gravity is 1.007 or less.
3. In evaluation of hematuria, examine fresh urinary sediment for RBC and also test the supernatant with dipstick.

Pseudohematuria (Red Urine Not Due to Blood)

Certain urinary pigments may impart a pink to red color to the urine mimicking hematuria, but the urinary sediment shows no RBC and the dipstick test is negative.

Causes of Red Urine

1. Anthocyanins in beets and berries (beeturia).
2. Phenolphthalein in alkaline urine—present in some laxatives.
3. Pyridium—drug often prescribed for relief of burning on urination; it tends to make the urine an orange-red color.
4. Heavy concentration of urates.
5. Porphyria—*rare* disorder of porphyrin pigment metabolism; red color may appear only after urine has been exposed to sunlight.
6. Vegetable dyes coloring food.
7. Serratia marcescens infection in infants (red diaper syndrome)—diapers turn red after standing for a period of time.

Classification of Hematuria

It is helpful to classify hematuria in two ways—first as to quantity and second as to the time of its appearance during voiding.

Quantitatively, it is called gross or macroscopic hematuria if it is evident to the naked eye, and microscopic if it is demonstrable only under the microscope.

Blood noted chiefly at the beginning of urination is called *initial hematuria*, and it indicates pathology in the urethra. Blood noted chiefly at the end of urination is called *terminal hematuria*, and it indicates pathology near the bladder neck or in the posterior urethra. Uniformly bloody urine, *total hematuria*, indicates pathology in the bladder, ureters, or kidneys. Blood stains noted on underclothing or pajamas with clear urine indicates pathology at the urethral meatus.

Source of Hematuria

1. The longer blood stays in contact with urine, the more the blood changes from bright red to a rusty brown color owing to formation of acid hematin.

A. Upper urinary tract bleeding usually produces dark brown urine, whereas lower urinary tract bleeding usually produces pink-red urine.
2. Renal source is suggested by the following.

A. Flank or CVA pain or tenderness.

B. Passage of wormlike clots in the urine.

C. Significant proteinuria, many casts.

3. Ureteral source is suggested by the following.

A. Pain along course of the ureter or in scrotum, particularly if severe and colicky in nature.

B. Urgency of urination and defecation without any accompanying dysuria.

See data contained in Tables 6–9.

Hematuria and Tumors of the Urinary Tract

Gross hematuria, usually painless, is often the first manifestation of a urinary tract tumor, particularly bladder tumor. The episodic nature of the bleeding may lull both patient and physician into a false sense of security, so that urological investigation is often recommended only after multiple episodes of hematuria.

In one review, of 1,000 cases presenting with gross hematuria, tumors were found in *21.5%* and two-thirds of these were bladder tumors.

In another evaluation of 500 cases of *asymptomatic microscopic hematuria*, tumors were found in 2.2%. Therefore, with gross hematuria the probability of a tumor is about 20%, whereas with asymptomatic microscopic hematuria, the probability of a tumor is about 2%.

Hematuria in childhood is *rarely secondary to a tumor*, but a Wilms' tumor of the kidney occasionally bleeds.

Although tumor will be at the bottom of your list in the differential diagnosis of hematuria in children, it would be at the top of your list in

TABLE 6

Most Common Causes of Hematuria for Different Age Groups

0 to 20 Years

1. Acute glomerulonephritis
2. Acute urinary tract infection
3. Congenital urinary tract anomalies with obstruction

20 to 40 Years

1. Acute urinary tract infection
2. Calculus in ureter or kidney
3. Bladder tumor

40 to 60 Years (*Males*)	*40 to 60 Years* (*Females*)
1. Bladder tumor	1. Acute urinary tract infection
2. Calculus in kidney or ureter	2. Calculus in kidney or ureter
3. Acute urinary tract infection	3. Bladder tumor
Over 60 Years (*Males*)	*Over 60 Years* (*Females*)
1. Prostatism; benign hypertrophy or carcinoma	1. Bladder tumor
2. Bladder tumor	2. Acute urinary tract infection
3. Acute urinary tract infection	

TABLE 7

Classification of Causes of Hematuria Based on the Presence or Absence of Urinary and Nonurinary Symptoms

Hematuria only	Hematuria + urinary symptoms	Hermaturia + nonurinary symptoms
	Relatively Common Causes	
Calculus (20%)	Calculus (80%)	
Bladder tumor (75%)	Bladder tumor (25%)	
Kidney tumor	Kidney tumor	Kidney tumor
	Acute urinary tract infection	
		Acute glomerulonephritis
	Congenital anomalies	
Trauma		
Tuberculosis (5%)	Tuberculosis (95%)	
	Benign prostatic hypertrophy	
	Uncommon Causes	
Sickle cell trait		Sickle cell anemia
Renal artery aneurysm		
Renal A-V fistula or malformation		
Hemangioma		
Calycovenous connections		
Hereditary hemorrhagic telangiectasia		
Exercise		
Unexplained		
	Renal infarction	
		Renal vein thrombosis
		Polyarteritis nodosa
		Systemic lupus erythematosus
		Henoch-Schoenlein purpura
		Leukemia
		Coagulation and platelet dysfunction

middle-aged men. A man of 50 with gross hematuria has about a 50% chance of having a bladder tumor.

The Diagnostic Approach to Hematuria

A careful, detailed history is the important first step in evaluation of hematuria! This usually reveals whether the hematuria is initial, terminal, or total; whether it is the only symptom or is accompanied by urinary or nonurinary symptoms; whether bleeding followed trauma or strenuous exercise; and whether bleeding has occurred from other sites.

On physical examination, look for the following.

TABLE 8

Hematuria Only—Age and Sex Incidence

Disorder	Peak incidence age	Sex
	yrs	
Calculi	20–50	M/F = 3/1
Bladder tumor	40–70	M > F
Trauma		M > F
Tuberculosis	20–60	M > F
Sickle cell trait	18–40 (blacks)	M = F
Renal artery aneurysm		M = F
Renal A-V fistula	> 20	M = F
Hemangioma		M = F
Calycovenous connections	20–60	M = F
Hereditary hemorrhagic telangiectasia	15–40	M = F
Exercise		M > F
Unexplained		M = F

1. Mass in flank or pelvis.
2. Skin abnormalities—evidence of trauma, purpura, edema, hemangiomas, telangiectases.
3. Tenderness in flank or CVA region, along course of ureter, suprapubic area (bladder).
4. Hypertension, arrhythmias.

The fundamental means of diagnosis are examination of the urine, cystoscopy during the bleeding episode, and intravenous urography.

Urinalysis

Urine should be *fresh*, well mixed, and if possible acid and concentrated, for formed elements are best preserved under these conditions. Examination of the urine should be performed *by the physician*, for it often gives a clue to the source of the bleeding into the urinary tract and it may enable one to make the diagnosis.

Upper tract bleeding is suggested by the findings of smoky brown urine, wormlike clots, proteinuria, or an excessive number of casts. Lower tract bleeding is suggested by bright red urine and irregularly shaped clots.

Diagnostic Findings on Urinalysis

1. Persistent proteinuria indicates renal parenchymal disease.
2. An abnormal number of casts indicates renal parenchymal disease.

A. RBC casts indicate active glomerulitis, most commonly seen in acute glomerulonephritis but also present in systemic lupus erythematosus and polyarteritis nodosa.

B. WBC casts may occasionally be present in active glomerulitis but are more commonly seen in acute pyelonephritis.

TABLE 9

Hematuria and Urinary Symptoms—Age and Sex Incidence

Disorder	Peak incidence age	Sex	Associated symptoms
	yrs		
Calculi	20–50	M/F = 3/1	Pain in flank or along course of ureter
Bladder tumor	40–70	M > F	Urgency, dysuria
Kidney tumor	40–60	M > F	Flank pain, mass
Acute urinary infection		M > F	Frequency, burning and urgency of urination
Congenital anomalies	0–20	M = F	Mass in flank or supra-pubic area
Tuberculosis	20–60	M > F	Frequency, burning, and urgency of urination
Benign prostatic hypertrophy	> 50	M	Urinary frequency, de-crease in size and force of urinary stream
Renal infarction	> 40	M = F	Flank pain

Hematuria and Nonurinary Symptoms

Acute glomerulone-phritis	3–20	M = F	Edema, hypertension
Kidney tumor	40–60	M > F	Fever, metastatic bone pain
Sickle cell anemia	18–40 (blacks)	M = F	Weakness
Renal vein thrombosis	0–2	M = F	Dehydration, flank mass
Polyarteritis nodosa	30–70	M/F = 4/1	Fever, arthralgia, neuritis
Systemic lupus erythematosus	17–34	M/F = 1/9	Fever, arthralgia, skin rash
Leukemia			
Henoch-Schoenlein purpura	> 20	M/F = 1.6/1	Rash, arthralgia
Coagulation + platelet deficiencies			Bleeding, other sites

3. Significant bacteriuria (over 10 rodlike bacteria per HPF in fresh urinary sediment) indicates urinary tract infection.

A. If urine pH is greater than 7, Proteus infection probably is present, and this is often associated with formation of calculi.

4. Cystine crystals in the urine indicate cystinuria and the probable presence of cystine calculus.

A. Other crystals are usually not diagnostic, for they may be found in normal urine.

5. Pyuria (leukocyturia) may accompany hematuria in the following clinical situations.

A. Infections, including tuberculosis.

B. Glomerulitis—proteinuria and many casts often present.

C. Calculi.

D. Tumors of bladder or kidney.

6. Malignant cells may be found, indicating urinary tract tumor, most commonly a bladder tumor.

Cystoendoscopy

This procedure is extremely informative if performed while the patient is experiencing hematuria, for it may be the only chance to discover the source of bleeding! Later x-ray studies may be inconclusive, particularly when the bleeding is due to a small lesion in one kidney. Knowing the source of the hematuria facilitates further investigative study.

Retrograde studies are particularly useful in evaluation of possible small tumors in the renal pelvis or calyceal system, and they should be performed when hematuria has ceased so that retained blood clots will not obscure the diagnosis.

Cystoendoscopy is not usually indicated in children with hematuria, in the presence of urinary infection, or after major trauma.

Intravenous Urogram

An intravenous urogram is indicated in all cases not clearly due to acute glomerulonephritis. If bleeding has ceased, this study should precede cystoendoscopy.

After these fundamental studies have been completed, the diagnosis will be apparent in about 75% of cases. For the remaining 25% with unexplained hematuria, additional studies may be indicated in selected cases.

1. Sickle cell preparation and hemoglobin electrophoresis.

A. Hematuria may occur in all three varieties of sickle cell disease —sickle cell trait (SA), sickle cell hemoglobin-C disease (SC), and sickle cell anemia (SS).

B. Sickle cell trait is the most important one clinically.

1) Common—10% of all American blacks have sickle cell trait, and this is 50 times more common than sickle cell anemia.

2) Asymptomatic except for hematuria.

2. Renal angiography.

A. This is particularly helpful in detecting renal tumors or renal vascular lesions and in assessing extent of renal trauma.

3. Renal biopsy.

A. This is primarily indicated when renal insufficiency occurs in the presence of apparent renal parenchymal disease.

4. Laboratory studies to detect hemorrhagic disorders.

A. Complete blood count and platelet estimate on the differential smear.

1) Platelet count is done if number appears decreased on smear.

B. Bleeding time.

C. Partial thromboplastin time.

D. Prothrombin time.

Although hematuria *cannot occur without a cause*, in 5 to 10% of cases no definite cause can be found.

PYURIA

Pyuria is an increased number of WBC in the urine. Clinically this is usually determined by counting the number of WBC in the urinary sediment, but this may be misleading for the concentration of WBC per urine volume is being determined—not the actual rate of excretion of WBC, the more significant factor. Prescott, using a special stain that enabled him to differentiate WBC from renal tubular cells, noted *wide variation* in the WBC excretion rates in normal individuals (see Table 10).

For practical purposes, *400,000 WBC/hour may be considered the upper limit* of normal WBC excretion. Since urine flow rate averages 50 ml/hour (1,200 ml/day), the upper limit of WBC concentration is 8,000 WBC/ml, giving urinary sediment findings of 4 to 5 WBC/HPF (6,000 WBC/ml is equivalent to urinary sediment finding of 4 WBC/HPF). *Pyuria is present when the urinary sediment shows greater than 5 WBC/HPF.*

Factors of Importance in Assessing Pyuria

1. Urine volume per unit time (Table 11).

A. Despite identical urinary sediment findings of 4 WBC/HPF, the WBC excretion rates are 50,000, 100,000, 500,000, and 1,000,000 per hour.

B. To determine whether an abnormal number of WBC are being

TABLE 10

Clean Catch Urines (Prescott)

	Mean WBC Excretion Rate	Upper Limit of Normal
	cells/hr	
Males	28,700	95,000
Females	107,800	470,000

Reprinted from Prescott, L. F.: The normal urinary excretion rate of renal tubular cells, leucocytes and red blood cells. Clin. Sci. 31:428, 1966.

TABLE 11

Urine Volume	WBC/HPF	WBC excreted in 12 Hours
ml/12 hr		
100	4	600,000
200	4	1,200,000
1,000	4	6,000,000
2,000	4	12,000,000

excreted into the urinary tract, one must know the *volume of the specimen* and the *period of time over which it was collected.*

2. pH of urine.

A. In acid urine WBC survive remarkably well, but alkaline urine destroys WBC and converts them into unrecognizable debris.

1) WBC may be lysed in strongly alkaline urine or in mildly alkaline urine if sufficient time elapses.

B. Stansfeld did serial WBC counts on urine adjusted to various pH levels and noted the results shown in Table 12.

C. Clinically WBC in alkaline urine most commonly occur in patients on prolonged catheter drainage. Urea-splitting organisms such as *Proteus* create an alkaline urine so that the urinary sediment shows no WBC.

Significance of Pyuria

Pyuria is the body's *response* to *inflammation* of the urinary tract. Bacteria, calculi, and tumors are the most common causes of inflammation and resultant pyuria. If the body's response mechanism is impaired, as in renal transplant patients on immunosuppressants, a bacterial infection may result in urinary sediment findings of many bacteria but *no WBC.*

Pyuria and Urinary Infection

1. Pyuria is *not* synonymous with urinary infection, although infection is the most common cause of pyuria, accounting for about 75 to 85% of cases.

A. Presence of pyuria should suggest the *possibility* of urinary infection.

2. Pyuria is absent in 50% of documented urinary infections.

A. Bacteria are responsible for the infection so are always present, whereas pyuria is a reaction to the presence of bacteria and is present *only half the time.*

B. The diagnosis of urinary infection may be made by finding over 10 rodlike bacteria/HPF in *fresh urinary sediment.*

1) This indicates significant bacteriuria, and urine cultures will

TABLE 12

pH	WBC Persisting
	%
5.6	100
6.0	100
6.4	100
6.8	100
7.4	80
7.8	60
8.4	40

Reprinted from Stansfeld, J. M.: The measurement and meaning of pyuria. Arch. Dis. Child. 37:258, 1962.

usually show greater than 100,000 colonies/ml of urine.

3. Tuberculosis often produces pyuria, frequently accompanied by hematuria.

A. Special stains and special culture media are necessary to detect tubercle bacilli, so that on routine studies no bacteria may be seen in the urinary sediment and urine cultures on conventional media may show no growth.

4. WBC casts originate in the kidney and are virtually diagnostic of pyelonephritis.

Noninfectious Causes of Pyuria

Nonbacterial inflammatory lesions account for 20 to 25% of cases of pyuria. The most important ones are *calculi* and *tumors of the urinary tract*. It is not uncommon to see a patient with a calculus or tumor who has been treated for long periods of time with various antibiotics for a supposed infection. These patients may have associated hematuria, but bacteriuria is absent and urine cultures are negative.

If fresh urinary sediment shows pyuria but no bacteriuria, keep in mind the possilibity of *tumor, calculus*, or *tuberculosis*.

PNEUMATURIA

Pneumaturia is the passage of gas in the urine. Gas within the bladder resides above the urine, since it is much lighter (1/700 as heavy) and consequently it is passed at the end of urination. Normally there is no gas in the urinary tract.

Causes of Pneumaturia

1. Fistula between gas-containing portion of the intestinal tract and the urinary tract.

A. The most common communication is a sigmoidovesical fistula secondary to diverticulitis of the sigmoid colon.

B. Less commonly.

1) Ileovesical or colovesical fistula secondary to granulomatous disease of the small and large bowel (Crohn's disease).

2) Rectourethral or rectovesical fistula secondary to an imperforate anus in the male.

3) Carcinoma of the sigmoid colon invading the bladder wall.

2. Gas may be produced by bacteria.

A. Diabetes mellitus is often present, but gas-forming infections also occur in nondiabetics.

1) Glucose in the urine is an important source of energy for the growth of pathogenic bacteria, and the increased levels of tissue and urinary glucose in the diabetic facilitate bacterial fermentation and formation of gas.

B. Responsible bacteria.
  1) *Escherichia coli.*
  2) Clostridial organisms.
  3) Aerobic and anaerobic cocci.
3. Gas may be introduced from the atmosphere.
  A. Cystoscopy or catheterization of the bladder.
  B. Traumatic injury to the bladder.

CHYLURIA (MILKY URINE)

Chyluria is the passage of lymphatic fluid or chyle in the urine due to the presence of an *intrarenal, lymphatic-urinary fistula.* The cause of this fistula is mechanical obstruction of the lymphatics superior to the kidney. This causes an increase in back pressure with eventual rupture of the proximal lymphatics at their weakest point—calyceal fornix—and this abnormal communication allows milky lymph to escape into the urine intermittently.

Etiology

1. Filariasis due to *Wuchereria bancrofti* is the most common cause.
  A. The adult filarial worms invade the suprarenal lymphatics, causing obstruction and severe inflammation.
  B. Most cases occur in patients with known or suspected filariasis.
2. Uncommon causes.
  A. Retroperitoneal tumors.
  B. Tuberculosis.
  C. Trauma.

Clinical Picture

Patients with chyluria usually give a history of living in or visiting a tropical or semitropical country where filariasis is endemic. The passage of milky urine occurs intermittently, varying with the amount of fat ingested and sometimes with the patient's posture.

Diagnosis

1. Urinalysis.
  A. Small amounts of fat produce a cloudy urine whereas large amounts of fat produce the characteristic milky white urine.
    1) The more common causes of cloudy urine—excess crystals and infection with gross pyuria—are easily ruled out.
      a. The suspended white particles *do not* disappear when acid is added or when the urine is heated.
      b. The urine does not contain WBC, and centrifugation causes no visible change in the appearance of the urine.
  B. The presence of fat may be confirmed by the following tests.

1) When chylous urine is mixed with ether and then shaken or centrifuged, there will be a significant reduction in the turbidity of the urine, and the fat present can be seen as a ring between the ether above and the slightly turbid urine below.

2) Fat droplets may easily be identified under the microscope if stained with an appropriate fat dye.

2. Determination of fat content of the urine.

A. Special techniques are available to measure the kind and amount of fat in the urine.

3. Cystoendoscopy establishes which kidney is the site of the lymphatic-urinary fistula.

A. When a high fat diet is administered prior to examination, creamy white efflux can be seen coming from the ureteral orifice on the side of the fistula.

4. Pedal lymphangiography will demonstrate the precise location of the intrarenal lymphatic-urinary fistula—usually at a calyceal fornix.

5. Intravenous urogram and retrograde ureteropyelograms.

A. These studies are usually normal even when performed when the urine is milky white.

B. Occasionally the fistula is demonstrated on retrograde pyeiography.

Most of these patients are managed satisfactorily with a low fat diet and high fluid intake.

PROTEINURIA

Proteinuria literally means the presence of protein in the urine. For the last 150 years, since the teachings of Richard Bright, proteinuria has been thought to represent renal disease. Clinically the term proteinuria usually is used in the context of an abnormal 24-hour urinary excretion of greater than 150 mg of protein. This definition recognizes that normal healthy individuals do excrete small amounts of protein in their urine. The term proteinuria generally has replaced the term albuminuria in recognition of the fact that most plasma proteins have been demonstrated in normal and pathological urines, not just albumin. The current hypothesis is that the glomerular membrane functions as a sieve normally allowing passage of small amounts of protein which is reabsorbed by the tubular cells, so that little protein is detected in the urine. Various disease states alter the permeability in such a way that there are greater amounts of plasma protein filtered through the glomerulus than can be reabsorbed by the tubules, giving an excess excretion of protein in the urine.

Clinically proteinuria is detected by the precipitation of the protein by acid or use of dipsticks which change color with various concentrations of protein. Heat plus the various acids are slightly (1%) more accurate than the colorimetric dipsticks. Tests of urine for proteins with the acids include 5% sulfosalicylic acid added to 0.5 ml of urine, or 1 ml of urine added to 1 ml of concentrated nitric acid; or after heating 5 ml of urine, three drops of 1% acetic acid are added. A negative test consists of no precipitation of protein or turbidity at the urine and acid interface. Trace (0.3 to 0.5 g/liter) is when there is faint turbidity; 1+ (0.5 to 1.0 g/liter), turbidity or ring easily seen; 2+ (1.0 to 3.0 g/liter), particles begin to flocculate; 3+ (3 to 8 g/liter), more flocculent particles; and 4+ (8 to 10 g/liter), a solid, thick opaque ring. Colorimetric testing works because protein in solution causes certain pH indicators to exhibit color altered from that of the same pH in the absence of protein. This protein error of indicators was first described by Sorenson in 1909. A buffer of such pH is employed so that a selected indicator will just barely be on one side of the pH at which it changes color, usually the acid side. With the actual pH held constant by a buffer, the protein error will cause color changes on the other side of the pH range as if it were alkaline. Albustix consists of filter paper impregnated with a solution of tetrabromphenol blue and citrate buffer at pH 3. Trace results indicates less than 30 mg% protein. False positives are reported with highly alkaline urine, penicillin, small amounts of prostatic fluids, gall bladder dye, tolbutamide, and hemoglobin.

Protein of less than 150 mg/24 hours is normally found in urine. With a protein in the glomerular filtrate (GFR) of 20 mg/100 ml (160 liters/day GFR), this represents the active reabsorption of 32 g of protein. Larger amounts of the smaller size protein molecules of myoglobin, β-microglobulin, and Bence-Jones protein are filtered. Smaller amounts are filtered of the intermediate size protein molecules of albumin and IgG. The larger molecules of a_2 macroglobulin and IgM normally are not filtered. Protein in normal urine is usually two-thirds globulin and one-third albumin. Forty milligrams per day of a high molecular weight protein called Tamm-Horsfall mucoprotein are excreted. This protein is not filtered but is excreted by cells of the distal and collecting tubules. Tamm-Horsfall mucoprotein forms the matrix of renal casts.

In renal disease, the predominant protein in the urine is albumin. Globulin excretion exceeds albumin in only a few diseases: multiple myeloma, amyloidosis, macroglobulinemia, Fanconi renal tubular disorder, and occasionally pyelonephritis. Bence-Jones in 1848 described a protein in the urine of patients with myeloma which coagulated on heating from 45 to 55°C and redissolved on boiling. The Bence-Jones protein has been reported in the urine of 50 to 60% of myeloma patients. Bence-Jones protein has been shown to be an abnormal light chain protein of the IgG or IgA myeloma proteins found in the plasma of these patients.

Clinically it is helpful to divide proteinuria into two categories: intermittent and continuous. Postural proteinuria has been reported in 3 to 5% of healthy individuals when they are in the upright position. The mechanism for postural proteinuria is not known but has been postulated as renal vasoconstriction and venous congestion. Total excretion of protein is usually less than 1 g/day in patients with postural proteinuria. The assumption of the upright position, however, may increase protein excretion in many patients with many forms of renal disease. Intermittent protein-uria is also caused by exercise, fever, exposure to heat or cold, and congestive heart failure. These are usually termed as functional proteinuria and the cause is not known. Postural proteinuria is believed usually to have a good prognosis with most patients not having active renal disease. However, renal biopsies show some changes in about one-half of the patients, and a few of the patients will go on to progressive renal disease. Continuous proteinuria usually is evidence of renal disease. Excretion of more than 4 g/day of protein is caused by diseases that increase glomerular membrane permeability. These diseases include lipoid nephrosis, glomeru-lonephritis, lupus erythematous, and intercapillary glomerulosclerosis.

HYPERTENSION

Incidence

Significant elevation of blood pressure occurs in at least 10% of the total population, 20% of the adult population, and an even higher percentage of the black population. Its presence is a leading risk factor in the occurrence of morbid cardiovascular complications. Since treatment has been proven to lower these complications, it is imperative that patients with high blood pressure be identified and treated. Thus the urologist's role is 2-fold: identification of the hypertensive patient and evaluation for specifically treatable forms (surgical hypertension).

Mechanism

Surgically curable forms of hypertension, *i.e.*, coarctation of the aorta, pheochromocytoma, hyperaldosteronism, Cushing's syndrome, renovascular hypertension, and hypertension due to renal parenchymal disease probably account for no more than 5 to 10% of the total hypertension population. The residual large group of patients have essential hypertension. However, recent dramatic advances into the mechanisms of essential hypertension allow more rational treatment and control. There is increasing evidence that high blood pressure is maintained by an inappropriate interaction of volume (sodium) excess and vasoconstriction (angiotensin II-induced). For example, the anephric patient is the prime example of pure volume-induced hypertension while renovascular hypertension is primarily renin (angioten-sin II)-dependent with a lesser volume component. A spectrum of inappro-priate interactions exists in essential hypertension and the hypertension found in patients with coexisting renal disease. These mechanisms will be discussed more specifically in the chapter on hormonal function of the kidney.

Treatment

Treatment is dependent on the primary mechanism that is found. Past

TABLE 13

Disease	Evaluation
1. Coarctation of aorta	Physical examination, chest film
2. Arteriovenous malformation	Physical examination, selective arteriography
3. Hyperthyroidism	History and physical examination, T3, T4
4. Pheochromocytoma	Metanephrine, vanillylmandelic acid (VMA), urine and plasma catecholamines, arteriogram
5. Cushing's syndrome	History and physical examination, skull and bone films, glucose tolerance test (GTT), 24 hr urine for keto and ketogenic steroids, adrenocorticotropin stimulation, dexamethasone suppression, plasma cortisol, adrenal venography
6. Hyperaldosteronism	History, CO_2, K^+ during Na^+ loading, peripheral renin activity in relation to 24-hr sodium excretion with patient on low Na^+ diet, 24-hr urinary aldosterone excretion on Na^+ loading, adrenal scan, adrenal venography
7. Renal disease	History, physical examination, urinalysis, blood urea nitrogen, creatinine clearance, 24-hr urinary protein, collagen profile, renal biopsy, intravenous urogram
8. Renovascular hypertension	History and physical examination, arteriography, peripheral renin activity in relation to 24-hr urinary sodium excretion, differential renal vein to arterial renin analysis

studies would suggest that "curable" forms of hypertension encompass a small portion of the hypertension population. However, when identified, the hypertension can be ablated, thus offering protection against the long term devastating complications and avoiding a lifetime of antihypertensive therapy. Alternatively the determination that a patient has essential hypertension should not be viewed as a diagnostic failure, for identification and more specific treatment are essential to the control of cardiovascular disease which exists in epidemic proportions in this country.

Differential Diagnosis and Evaluation

Exclusion of curable, *i.e.*, specific, forms of hypertension can be determined by a variety of available tests. These forms and the tests utilized are shown in Table 13.

Obviously, all tests are not suggested for all patients found to be hypertensive. The importance of a complete history and physical examination in order to determine the most likely mechanism involved cannot be overemphasized.

REFERENCES AND SUGGESTED FURTHER READING

Pain

1. Bockus, H. L. Abdominal pain—mechanisms and philosophic concepts. Lahey Clin. Found. Bull. 17:77, 1968.
2. Kellgren, J. H. On the distribution of pain arising from deep somatic structures with charts of segmental pain areas. Clin. Sci. 4:35, 1939.
3. Lewis, T. and Kellgren, J. H. Observations relating to referred pain, visceromotor reflexes and other associated phenomena. Clin. Sci. 4:47, 1939.

4. McLellan, A. M. and Goodell, H. Pain from the bladder, ureter and kidney pelvis. Res. Publ. Ass. Nerv. Ment. Dis. 23:252, 1942.
5. Ockerblad, N. F. and Carlson, H. E. The distribution of ureteral pain. J. Urol. 39:745, 1938.
6. Ray, B. S. and Neill, C. L. Abdominal visceral sensation in man. Ann. Surg. 126:709, 1947.
7. Ruch, T. C. Pathophysiology of pain. In *Physiology and Biophysics*, edited by Ruch and Patton, chap. 6. W. B. Saunders, Philadelphia, 1966.
8. Wolff, H. G. and Wolf, S. Pain. American Lecture Series, 1958.

Frequent Urination

1. deWardener, H. E. *The Kidney*. 3rd Ed. Chap. 23 Little, Brown and Company, Boston, 1967.

Enuresis

1. Bakwin, H. Enuresis in children. J. Pediat. 58:806, 1961.
2. Esperanca, M. and Gerrard, J. W. Nocturnal enuresis: studies in bladder function in normal children and enuretics. Can. Med. Ass. J. 101:324, 1969.
3. Fisher, O. D. and Forsythe, W. I. Mic*urating cystourethrography in the investigation of enuresis. Arch. Dis. Child. 29:460, 1954.
4. Hallman, N. On the ability of enuretic children to hold urine. Acta Paediat. 39:87, 1950.

Hematuria

1. Bome, A. W., Haltiwanger, E., and Chambers, R. L. Football hematuria. J.A.M.A. 158:1516, 1955.
2. Brearley, R. Hematuria and allied conditions. Biochem. Clin. 2:183, 1963.
3. Burkholder, G. V., Dotin, L. W., Thomason, W. B., and Beach. P. D. Unexplained hematuria. J.A.M.A. 210:1729, 1969.
4. Cameron, J. S. Glomerulonephritis. Brit. Med. J. 4:285, 1970.
5. Frohnert, P. P. and Sheps, S. G. Long-term follow-up study of periarteritis nodosa. Amer. J. Med. 43:8, 1967.
6. Greene, L. F., O'Shaughnessy, E. J., Jr., and Hendricks, E. D. Study of 500 patients with asymptomatic microhematuria. J.A.M.A. 16¹:610, 1956.
7. Lee, L. W. and Davis, E. D., Jr. Gross urinary hemorrhage: a symptom, not a disease. J.A.M.A. 153:782, 1953.
8. MacMahon, H. E. and Latorraca, R. Essential renal hematuria. J. Urol. 71:667, 1954.
9. Northway, J. D. Hematuria in children. J. Pediat. 78:381, 1971.

Pyuria

1. Addis, T. The number of formed elements in the urinary sediment of normal individuals. J. Clin. Invest. 2:409, 1926.
2. Houghton, B. J. and Pears, M. A. Cell excretions in normal urine. Brit. Med. J. 1:622, 1957.
3. Kunin, C. M. The quantitative significance of bacteria visualized in the unstained urinary sediment. N. Engl. J. Med. 265:589, 1961.
4. Prescott, L. F. The normal urinary excretion rates of renal tubular cells, leucocytes and red blood cells. Clin. Sci. 31:425, 1966.
5. Stansfeld, J. M. The measurement and meaning of pyuria. Arch. Dis. Child. 37:257, 1962.
6. Wright, W. T. Cell counts in urine. A.M.A. Arch. Int. Med. 103:76, 1959.

Proteinuria

1. Strauss, M. B. and Welt, L. G. *Diseases of the Kidney*, Chap. 3. Little, Brown and Company, Boston, 1971.

2

Urological Evaluation–History, Physical and Fundamental Urological Examinations

ARTHUR W. WYKER, JR.

HISTORY

The majority of patients seen by a urologist are *referred* to him for evaluation of a *specific urological complaint*. To arrive at the correct diagnosis he relies primarily on a good history supplemented by a careful physical examination and appropriate laboratory studies.

Obtaining a Good History

1. Establish a satisfactory patient-physician relationship.

A. You must convince your patient by your *actions* that you are interested in him and his problems.

B. When you have this rapport, he will want to confide in you.

2. Allow the patient to talk about his chief complaint in his own words, preferably without interruptions.

3. Clarify terms used by the patient.

A. "I have stomach pains," may indicate a burning or quivering sensation in the epigastrium in one patient, severe, deep visceral pain in the suprapubic region in another.

4. Get the necessary details about each complaint.

A. Avoid the temptation to take a quick, superficial history.

B. An example of the *importance of details* is seen in the assessment of a common presenting complaint—two times nocturia in a 60-year-old man.

　　1) If the patient is in bed 12 hours instead of the usual 8 hours, or if he habitually drinks 2 cans of beer just before going to bed, his nocturia may be *physiological*.

　　2) If the patient has noted that his urine volume per voiding is reduced and his urinary stream is weaker, he may have *prostatic obstruction* due to benign prostatic hyperplasia (BPH) or prostatic carcinoma.

　　3) If the patient is constantly thirsty and voids frequently day and night in normal-to-large quantities, his nocturia may reflect polyuria secondary to *diabetes mellitus* or *renal insufficiency*.

　　4) If the patient has some ankle edema at the end of the day which is absent on awakening in the morning, he may have *congestive heart failure* with the nocturia being secondary to mobilization of fluid from the extremities in the supine position.

5. Use discretion and tact in eliciting information regarding sexual function or the genitalia.

A. Questions of this nature, asked in a straightforward manner without embarrassment, are usually answered in kind.

B. *Conceal* any moral judgments you might have regarding his attitude or behavior.

6. Do not limit your history to the urinary tract.

A. It is dangerous to assume that the referring physician has thoroughly evaluated the patient and ruled out nonurological causes for the patient's symptoms.

7. Do not be unduly influenced by the referring physician's urological diagnosis.

A. Uncritical acceptance of another physician's diagnosis may lead you to take an inadequate history or perform a superficial examination resulting in an incorrect diagnosis.

8. If your patient has a well defined chief complaint such as high blood pressure, you can take a detailed history quickly and easily by visualizing the common causes for this complaint and asking the appropriate questions for each cause.

Causes of Hypertension

1. Essential hypertension.
2. Renal.
   A. Renal artery stenosis (most common form of curable hypertension).
   B. Acute and chronic glomerulonephritis.
   C. Chronic pyelonephritis.
   D. Polycystic kidney disease.
   E. Hydronephrosis.
   F. Periarteritis nodosa.
   G. Radiation nephritis.
3. Adrenal.
   A. Pheochromocytoma.
   B. Primary aldosteronism.
   C. Cushing's syndrome.
4. Coarctation of the aorta.

Questions to Ask

Examples of the appropriate questions for some of the above causes are the following.

1. Essential hypertension—accounts for around 90% of total.
   A. Is there a family history of high blood pressure?
   B. When did you first know that you had high blood pressure? Characteristically it is recognized in the 4th decade.
2. Renal artery stenosis—accounts for around 5% of total.

A. Did you experience any sudden abdominal or back pain or sustain any injury to the abdominal or back region prior to the onset of your high blood pressure? History of abdominal pain or trauma suggests the possibility of renal artery injury.

B. How old are you? This lesion frequently occurs in persons younger than 35 or over 55 years of age.

3. Chronic pyelonephritis.

A. Have you ever had any bladder or kidney infections, flank or costovertebral angle (CVA) pain?

B. Have you ever been told that your urinalysis was abnormal in any way?

4. Pheochromocytoma.

A. Has any member of your family or any close relative had high blood pressure or a pheochromocytoma? These tumors are frequently familial.

B. Have you experienced any sudden attacks or spells with any of the following symptoms—headache, perspiration, palpitation, pallor, nausea, vomiting, nervousness, or anxiety?

5. Primary aldosteronism.

A. Have you noticed any muscle weakness?

B. Are you passing more water than usual requiring you to get up at night to void? Muscle weakness and polyuria with nocturia are both secondary to hypokalemia, a key feature of primary aldosteronism.

In Chapter 1, urological signs and symptoms are discussed in detail and the differential diagnosis for each is presented.

PHYSICAL EXAMINATION

Kidney

Inspection

A kidney must be grossly enlarged or displaced to cause a perceptible bulge in the upper abdomen or flank. If a mass is suspected, careful palpation is helpful in determining its nature and location. If a perinephric abscess is suspected, the patient should be examined in the knee-elbow position. The normal shallow depression below the lowermost rib may be obliterated by fullness and edema secondary to an underlying abscess.

Palpation

Because of their location in the uppermost portion of the abdominal cavity, normal kidneys are *usually not palpable.* An exception is the newborn where both kidneys are palpable during the first 48 hours of life due to the hypotonicity of all muscles. They are not palpable in children and adult males but in 10% of adult women, usually slim ones, the lower pole of the right kidney can be felt. There are two maneuvers which aid palpation.

1. Deep breathing.

A. The normal kidney is movable because it is fixed only by its vascular pedicle; and with deep inspiration, the descending diaphragm pushes the kidney down towards the examiner's fingers.

2. Bimanual examination.

A. The kidney is most easily felt between the fingers of both hands as a firm, smooth mass slipping upwards as expiration starts.

B. The posterior hand lifts up the soft tissues in the CVA and the anterior hand presses deeply into the upper abdomen.

1) A renal mass is characteristically *ballottable*, unlike the liver and spleen which usually can only be palpated with the anterior hand.

Tenderness due to inflammation in or around the kidney is best detected by exerting firm pressure in the CVA region—the angle between the 12th rib and the paraspinal muscles.

Auscultation

In patients with hypertension particularly, it is important to listen over the renal artery areas for the presence of a bruit. These murmurs are best heard anteriorly after complete exhalation.

Transillumination

This examination is used primarily in newborns or small children with large, easily palpable abdominal masses. With the room as dark as possible, manipulate the mass against the abdominal wall with one hand while firmly applying a high intensity light (*e.g.*, fiberoptic light cord) to the mass with the other hand. If the mass is cystic rather than solid, it will transilluminate and you will see a reddish glow.

Ureter

In males the ureter is not palpable, but in females, the *lower ureter can be felt on vaginal examination.* One or two fingers are gently pushed upwards and outwards, and at the limit of your fingertips, the ureter lies close to the bony pelvic wall and lateral to the ovary. From this point, the ureter can be followed to its junction with the bladder by carrying the fingers downwards and inwards. If the ureter is normal, it is usually not identifiable because it is soft and nontender. If a stone is present, *both the stone and the ureter are usually palpable.* The ureter can be felt as a tender, tubular mass proximal to the stone.

Urinary Bladder

The normal empty or near empty bladder is neither palpable nor percussible because of its anatomical location in the pelvis. When it contains around 125 ml, it rises out of the pelvis into the lower abdomen projecting one fingerbreadth above the pubis. With further filling, it rises progressively towards the umbilicus.

Inspection

If the bladder contains over 500 ml, it may be identifiable as a bulge in the midlower abdomen. This swelling rising out of the pelvis is best appreciated by observing from the side with the eyes more or less level with the lower abdomen.

Percussion

Whether or not a mass is visible, the lower abdomen should be percussed from the umbilicus to the pubis. If the patient has a distended bladder, the normally resonant note is replaced by dullness. Percussion over a distended bladder may also cause the patient to experience a desire to void because of the sudden, induced rise in intravesical pressure.

Palpation

The distended bladder may be palpated as a firm, round movable mass rising out of the pelvis into the lower abdomen. On bimanual examination, the mass can often be ballotted between the two hands. For assessing the presence and extent of bladder tumors, bimanual examination is performed under anesthesia with the bladder empty.

Penis

If the patient is uncircumcised, retract the foreskin to rule out phimosis with an obstructing, small aperture. To inspect the urethral meatus, pinch the glans between the thumb and finger placed at the 6 and 12 o'clock positions. If the urethral meatus is not in the normal location, it can be found by following the midline raphe to its end on the undersurface of the penis. The shaft of the penis is palpated, looking particularly for the firm, fibrous plaques of Peyronie's disease. Palpate the floor of the urethra from the corona to the bulb, looking for induration secondary to a stricture.

Scrotum and Testes

After inspecting the scrotal skin and perineum, palpate the testes and epididymides between the thumb and finger. The comma-shaped epididymis is closely attached to the posterolateral side of the testis. You can get your fingers into the groove between the epididymis and testis everywhere except superiorly where the two structures are anatomically joined. In many men, a small ovoid lump—the rudimentary appendix testis, can be felt in or near the groove between the upper pole of the testis and the epididymis. The cord structures at the neck of the scrotum should be sifted through your fingers. The solid cord-like vas is easily identified and followed to its junction with the tail of the epididymis. The other soft, stringy structures in the cord cannot be defined. To rule out the presence of the gravity-dependent varicocele, the cord must also be examined with the patient standing. If a varicocele is present, the intrascrotal varicosities secondary to valvular incompetence of the internal spermatic vein become distended in the upright position and feel like a bag of worms.

Prostate and Seminal Vesicles

The prostate and seminal vesicles are palpated through the anterior rectal wall. Rectal examination may be performed with the patient in a variety of positions. Older patients are best examined in the lithotomy position, whereas younger men may be examined while bending over or in the knee-elbow position.

Two distinct lobes about the size of the distal segment of the thumb are separated by a shallow median furrow. The normal gland is smooth, slightly movable and nontender, and it has a rubbery consistency.

Above the prostate, if your finger is long enough, you may be able to feel the soft, tubular seminal vesicles. Coming off the base of the prostate somewhat obliquely, they are most easily felt when they are distended or tender.

LABORATORY FINDINGS

Urinalysis

A urinalysis is an essential part of any complete examination, but it becomes critically important when a urological disorder is suspected. This key examination should not be relegated to disinterested laboratory personnel but *must be performed by the physician*. For reliable urinalyses, the urine must be collected properly and examined promptly.

Collection of Urine Specimen

Timing

1. The first morning specimen is the best one for detecting formed elements in the urine and for determining if urinary infection is present.

    A. The formed elements—red and white blood cells (RBC, WBC) and casts—are preserved in this characteristically *acid and concentrated urine*, but they may be lysed and disappear in alkaline or dilute urine.

    B. Bacterial colony counts are usually highest in this specimen because the bacteria have had more time to multiply during overnight incubation in the bladder.

2. Whenever qualitative measurements are made on substances in the urine, it is essential to know the *volume of urine passed* and the *time period of its collection*.

    A. Substances such as WBC, RBC, and casts are generally excreted into the urine at a *fairly constant rate*, so the urine concentration of these substances and the related urinary sediment findings vary directly with urine volume.

B. The following examples illustrate the importance of urine volume and the time period of collection.

 1) A male patient is excreting substance X into his urine at the rate of 1X per hour (Table I).

  a) Notice the marked differences in the urine concentration of substance X due to variations in urine volume and in the time period of collection.

  b) If X were WBC, then the first and last specimens would have four times as many WBC/high power field (HPF) in the urinary sediment as the two middle specimens.

Method

The external genitalia, perineum, and urethra of normal males and females have bacteria on their surface. If the urine specimen is to reflect the true bacteriological status of the urinary tract, these contaminating bacteria must be excluded as far as possible from the specimen. This is most commonly accomplished by obtaining a clean-catch, midstream specimen.

1. Clean-catch urine.

 A. The reliability of a urine specimen obtained in this fashion varies directly with the adequacy of the cleansing procedure.

  1) If a female patient cleanses her own perineum in a perfunctory manner, the urine specimen may contain bacteria from both the urethra and genitalia with a resultant reduction in reliability.

  2) However, if the same patient is placed in the lithotomy position, the perineum is thoroughly cleansed by a trained nurse, and with the labia held apart, a midstream specimen is collected in a sterile receptacle, the *reliability approaches 100%.*

 B. In males, almost all specimens are collected in the clean-catch fashion.

  1) A midstream specimen collected after cleansing the glans penis is a very reliable one.

2. Catheterized urine.

 A. This technique, used primarily in women, has a reliability of around 95%, but it has some significant drawbacks.

TABLE I

Effect of Time and Urine Volume on Urine Concentration

Time Period	Urine Volume	Urine Concentration of X
hrs	ml	
2	100	2X/100 = 2X per 100 ml
2	400	2X/400 = 0.5X per 100 ml
2	400	2X/400 = 0.5X per 100 ml
8	400	8X/400 = 2X per 100 ml

1) Passage of a catheter may carry urethral bacteria back into the bladder. This may cause contamination of the urine specimen or, less commonly, an actual urinary infection (2% of patients catheterized).

    a) Counting the number of bacteria present and identifying the organism help you determine whether the bacteria are contaminants. When nonpathogenic bacteria are detected or the number of bacteria is small, contamination is probable.

2) Catheterization evokes some discomfort in all patients and produces urethral edema in a few with resultant voiding difficulty.

B. In males, this technique is reserved for those men who are unable to void.

3. Suprapubic aspiration of the bladder.

A. The reliability of this technique approaches 100%, but it is not practical for routine usage.

B. It is the preferred method in prematures, infants, and some children and is useful in selected adults.

1) In prematures and small children, the bladder is largely an abdominal organ facilitating aspiration.

C. The procedure requires the presence of enough urine within the bladder to push it above the pubis where it can be palpated or percussed.

1) This usually requires over 125 ml in adults.

D. Properly performed, the risk of this procedure is slight but it does cause some discomfort in virtually all patients.

Prompt Examination

For best results, urine should be examined fresh—*i.e.*, within 30 min of collection. If urine is allowed to stand, bacterial growth takes place, rapidly alkalinizing the urine with resultant destruction of RBC, WBC, and casts. If for some reason the urine cannot be examined promptly, it should be refrigerated, for this is the best method of preservation.

Urinary Sediment

When urine stands in a bottle, the formed elements gradually fall to the bottom, so just before taking a sample, mix the urine thoroughly. If your sample is cloudy and alkaline, acidify it to dissolve amorphous phosphates; if it is cloudy and acid, heat it to dissolve urates. Centrifuge 15 ml for 3 to 5 min, pour off supernatant, and examine the sediment under the microscope using reduced light.

A special effort should be made to detect bacteria, for if there are more than five per high power field, infection is usually present. If double refractile fat bodies are suspected, examine the sediment under polarized light looking for the characteristic "maltese crosses."

Other Routine Tests on the Urine

Dipstick tests have greatly simplified urinalyses. The Ames Labstix dipstick is a firm, cellulose strip with five test areas impregnated with chemicals which react with abnormal substances in the urine to produce color changes. Within 1 min, using this single dipstick, you can perform colorimetric determination of urinary pH, ketonuria, proteinuria, glycosuria, and hematuria.

Three-Glass Test

This test is often helpful in *locating the source* of WBC or RBC in men with significant microscopic pyuria or hematuria. When the urinary sediment shows over 20 WBC or RBC/HPF, a diagnostic test can be anticipated.

Method of Performing the Test

1. Cleanse the glans penis and collect the first 10 to 20 ml voided in bottle 1.
2. The patient continues voiding and after approximately 100 ml have been passed, collect another specimen in bottle 2.
3. The patient stops voiding, and after massage of the prostate gland, the subsequent first 10 to 20 ml voided are collected in bottle 3.

Interpretation

1. *All* specimens have stored bladder urine which may contain WBC or RBC dumped into it by the kidney, ureter, or bladder.
   A. Therefore this test does not permit detection of a specific upper urinary tract source.
2. Specimen 1 adds urethral washings to the bladder·urine, and specimen 3 adds prostatic fluid.
   A. When the source of WBC or RBC in the urine is the kidney, ureter, or bladder, all three specimens will have similar urinary sediment findings.
   B. If the urethra is the source of WBC or RBC, specimen 1 will contain significantly more cells in the urinary sediment than specimens 2 and 3.
   C. If the prostate is the source of WBC or RBC, specimen 3 will contain significantly more cells in the urinary sediment than specimens 1 and 2.
3. Sample cases (Table II).

Intravenous Urogram

This is the fundamental x-ray study of the urinary tract! The quality of

TABLE II

Three-Glass Test

Urinary Sediment Findings			Source of WBC or RBC
Specimen 1	Specimen 2	Specimen 3	
30	30	30	Kidney, ureter, or bladder
60	30	40	Urethra
30	30	60	Prostate

an intravenous urogram depends primarily upon the *urine concentration of contrast medium*.

Physiology of Contrast Excretion

1. Contrast agents, are eliminated by glomerular filtration and are neither excreted nor absorbed from the tubules.

A. Water reabsorption along the nephron causes a progressive rise in the urine concentration of contrast.

1) With normal renal function, the urine concentration of contrast is usually 30 to 50 times the plasma concentration.

2) There are three factors which primarily determine the urine concentration of contrast—plasma concentration of contrast, glomerular filtration rate, and the state of hydration of the patient.

A. Plasma concentration of contrast.

1) This varies directly with the amount of contrast administered per body weight.

2) Since the concentration of contrast in the filtrate is identical with that in the plasma, increasing the dose of contrast raises *both* the plasma and urine concentration of contrast.

B. Glomerular filtration rate (GFR).

1) This determines the quantity of contrast that reaches the filtrate.

a) If 50% of the nephrons are destroyed or are nonfunctional, one-half as much contrast reaches the filtrate.

2) If the GFR is reduced, you can compensate for this loss of nephrons by increasing the amount of contrast administered.

a) Using high doses of contrast, adequate visualization of the urinary tract can be achieved in most patients retaining at least 10 to 20% of their normal renal function.

C. State of hydration.

1) The state of hydration determines the activity of ADH on water transfer in the distal tubules and collecting ducts.

a) With dehydration, there is a high level of ADH, and the increased water reabsorption from the distal nephron increases the urine concentration of contrast.

D. Urine concentration of contrast.

1) Increased by:
   a) High doses of contrast per body weight.
   b) Dehydration.

2) Reduced by:
   Low dose of contrast per body weight.
   Renal insufficiency with decreased GFR.
   Hydration and high urine flow.

3. The early nephrogram phase of the intravenous urogram is due to contrast within the lumen of the proximal convoluted tubules.

A. The density of the nephrogram is directly proportional to the dose of contrast administered and is unaffected by the state of hydration.

B. Certain pathological disorders produce abnormally dense nephrograms by slowing the rate of flow and increasing the amount of water reabsorbed from the proximal convoluted tubules.

    1) Urinary tract obstruction.

    2) Hypotension.

4. Effects of renal insufficiency on urography.

A. With loss of nephrons, visualization of the collecting system is impaired owing to the *decreased urine concentration of contrast* secondary to reduced GFR and loss of concentrating ability.

B. Reduced GFR.

    1) When the GFR is lowered, less contrast gets into the filtrate and the urine.

    2) This can be compensated for by raising the level of contrast in the plasma—high dose urography.

    3) Loss of concentrating ability.

        a) Urea-induced osmotic diuresis decreases water reabsorption throughout the nephron.

        b) With loss of nephrons, the remaining normal nephrons hypertrophy with resultant increased filtration rate per nephron. The increased load of water and solute cause an osmotic diuresis per nephron reducing water reabsorption.

        c) With the loss of nephrons, there are fewer loops of Henle, so the osmotic gradient required for urinary concentration cannot be maintained.

CYSTOENDOSCOPY

Superbly made optical instruments are available today, allowing the urologist to make a thorough visual inspection of the urethra and bladder in all individuals, even newborns. The panendoscope is designed for looking almost straight ahead, and so it is particularly useful for inspection of the urethra, bladder neck, and posterior bladder wall. The cystoscope has an angled tip facilitating inspection of the entire bladder wall.

RETROGRADE PYELOGRAM

A retrograde pyelogram is an x-ray study of the upper urinary tract obtained by injecting contrast through a ureteral catheter introduced via cystoscopy. It is primarily performed when the upper urinary tract is not adequately visualized on the intravenous urogram. When minute detail of the collecting system is desired, the ureteral catheter is passed to the renal pelvis and contrast is instilled via gravity. When ureteral pathology or obstruction is suspected, a bulb-tip catheter can be engaged in the ureteral orifice and contrast injected to outline the entire ureter and collecting system.

There are a number of less commonly used diagnostic procedures which are helpful in selected cases. These will not be discussed here. The interested reader is referred to a recently published book, *Kidneys, Ureters and Urinary Bladder*, Volume 6 of the Ciba Collection of Medical Illustrations. In this book, the following procedures are discussed in detail by recognized authorities and are illustrated in color by Dr. Frank Netter.

1. Retroperitoneal pneumography.
2. Nephrotomography.
3. Aortorenal angiography.
4. Radioisotope renography.
5. Renal scintillation scanning.
6. Renal biopsy.
7. Cystourethrography.
8. Retrograde pyelography.
9. Tomography.
10. Intravenous pyelography.
11. Cystometry.

3

Renal Physiology

JAY Y. GILLENWATER

ANATOMY

An understanding of renal anatomy is essential to understanding renal function. The kidneys are paired, 150-g organs lying retroperitoneally in the upper abdomen. They are embedded in fat and surrounded by Gerota's fascia which is derived from the transversalis fascia. The kidneys are protected from injury by the rib cage, the vertebral column, and back muscles (psoas major, quadratus lumborum, sacrospinalis, and tendon of the transversus abdominis).

Blood Supply

Arterial

The kidneys receive 25% of the cardiac output, usually from a single artery on each side of the aorta. However, more than 30% of patients have an aberrant artery which usually goes to one of the poles of the kidneys. No anastomoses are seen in the arterial vessel, so that ligation of a renal vessel or its branches will cause infarction of that region of the kidney. Fortunately for the surgeon, the branching of the renal artery is usually constant allowing him to avoid injury to the arterial vessels. The anterior is the larger of the arterial branches and supplies about two-thirds of the renal mass. The arterial divisions are shown below:

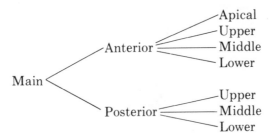

These vessels divide dichotomously into branches called interlobar, arcuate, and intralobar which subdivide into the afferent arterioles.

Figure 1A shows the four surgical segments of the kidney formed by these arterial divisions.

1. Apical.
2. Anterior.
3. Posterior.
4. Basilar.

As shown in Figure 1B, a relatively avascular plane as described by Brodel in 1901 is shown to enter the posterior calices.

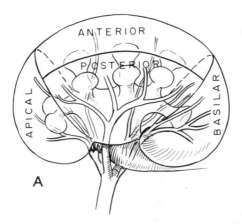

Fig. 1A. Distribution of the major branches of the renal artery looking at the kidney from the posterior view. The larger distribution from the anterior branches is seen. (Reproduced with permission from Boyce, W. H.: Surgery of renal calculi, in *Urologic Surgery*, Chapt. 3 edited by Glenn, J. F. and Boyce, W. H., Paul B. Hoeber, Medical Division, Harper & Row, New York, 1969.)

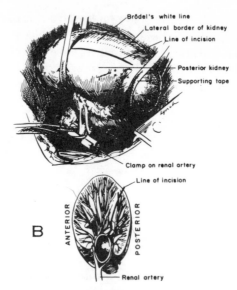

Fig. 1B. Operative approach for a longitudinal nephrotomy. The right kidney is shown after it has been mobilized through a flank incision. The renal artery is clamped to prevent blood loss. The line of incision is between the anterior and posterior branches of the renal arteries. Note that the anterior branches supply about two-thirds of the kidney. *Lower*, operative approach for a longitudinal nephrotomy. The right kidney is shown after it has been mobilized through a flank incision. The renal artery is clamped to prevent blood loss. The line of incision is between the anterior and posterior branches of the renal arteries. Note that the anterior branches supply about two-thirds of the kidney. (Reproduced with permission from Boyce, W. H.: Surgery of renal calculi, in *Urologic Surgery*, Chapt. 3, edited by Glenn, J. F. and Boyce, W. H., Paul B. Hoeber Medical Division, Harper & Row, New York, 1969.)

Venous

The venous drainage parallels the arterial circulation. However, the veins do anastomose, allowing surgical ligation of the branches. Accessory veins are seen in 14% of cases, which is less common than supernumerary arteries. Accessory veins are more common on the right side.

Lymphatics

Renal lymphatics drain into capsular or hilar lymphatic channels. Renal lymph flow varies with urine flow and increases with increased venous or ureteral pressure. The lymphatics play an important role by carrying off protein to maintain the osmotic gradient higher in the vasa recta, so that water can move in this vascular space and be carried off by the venous system. Obstruction to the renal lymphatics interferes with urinary concentrating ability.

Renal Innervation

The kidney receives autonomic nerve supply from the twelfth thoracic to the second lumbar ganglia. The nerve fibers accompany the vessels. Stimulation of the sympathetic nerves will cause renovasoconstriction.

There is little evidence that stimulation of the parasympathetic nerves causes change in renal blood flow. The kidney also contains afferent pain fibers which are stimulated by stretching of the capsule. The nerve fibers are thought to play little role in renal function.

Glomerular Filtration

Glomerular filtration rate (GFR) is defined as the volume of fluid that is filtered across the glomerular capillary membrane per minute. In normal man, the GFR is approximately 125 ml per minute per standard 1.73 m² of body surface area, which is 180 liters/day. The adult female has a normal GFR of 115 ml/min.

Filtration Fraction

As blood passes through the glomerulus, approximately 20% of the serum is filtered (filtration fraction):

$$\text{Filtration fraction} = \frac{\text{GFR}}{\text{RBF}} = \frac{125 \text{ ml/min}}{660 \text{ ml/min}} = 0.19$$

Where RBF = renal blood flow. Glomerular filtration rate is not uniform in all nephrons of the kidney, with higher values in the juxtaglomerular glomeruli than in the cortical glomeruli.

Glomerular Membrane

A schematic of the glomerular membrane is shown in Figure 2. The filtered fluid must pass through three layers.
1. The endothelial cells of the capillary.
2. The basement membrane.
3. The epithelial cells that are derived from the inner lining of Bowman's capsule.

The glomerular membrane becomes progressively more restrictive to the passage of materials with the endothelial layer, allowing passage of molecules as large as 60 to 100 A (angstrom equal 10^{-7} mm), the basement membrane restricting molecules 50 to 60 A, and the epithelial cells (podocytes) retarding the passage of molecules the size of serum albumin and hemoglobin (32 A).

Filtration Pressure

The filtration rate is determined by the net hydrostatic forces acting across the glomerular capillary, the permeability characteristics of the glomerular membrane, and its surface area. The net effective filtration pressure is 15 mm Hg.

Glomerular hydrostatic capillary pressure	60 mm Hg
Plasma protein osmotic pressure	−30 mm Hg
Hydrostatic pressure in Bowman's capsule	−15 mm Hg
Net filtration pressure	15 mm Hg

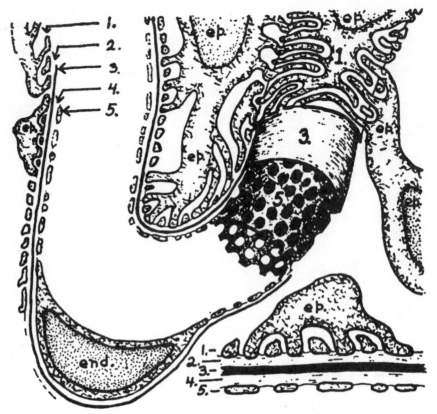

Fig. 2. Schematic illustration of the gomerular capillary. *Upper right*, parts of the three epithelial cells (ep.) are shown with terminal processes interdigitating upon the capillary surface (layer 1). The appearance of these feet in cross section is indicated at the *left*, and in the *inset (lower right)*. The epithelial feet are slightly embedded in a cement layer (layer 2), which in turn rests upon the dense structural portion of the basement membrane (layer 3). An inner cement layer (4) provides a bed for the endothelium (layer 5). The very attenuated endothelial sheet is perforated by closely spaced holes a little over 0.1 μ in diameter, as may be seen in surface view to the *right* of the figure, and in the transverse section to the *left*, and in the *inset*. (Reproduced with permission from Pease, D. C.: J. Histochem. Cytochem. 3:259, 1955; and Gilmore, J.: *Renal Physiology*, The Williams & Wilkins Company, Baltimore, 1972.)

The process of renal filtration thus does not require any local expenditure of metabolic energy. It is derived from the hydrostatic pressure within the glomerular capillary as a result of contraction of the heart. The maintenance of this hydrostatic pressure is greatly facilitated by the interposition of the glomerular capillary between the afferent and efferent arterioles. This unique arrangement lets the glomerular filtration rate be controlled somewhat independently of blood pressure and renal blood flow. Constriction of the afferent arteriole lowers glomerular hydrostatic pressure while dilation permits the glomerular hydrostatic pressure to approach that in the aorta. Constriction in efferent arteriole increases glomerular hydrostatic pressure with dilation giving the opposite effect.

Renal Autoregulation

These properties of constriction and dilation of the renal afferent and efferent arterioles enable it to autoregulate a reasonably constant glomerular filtration rate and renal blood flow over a wide range of arterial perfusion pressures. There are several postulated mechanisms of autoregulation with the myogenic or stretch response most widely accepted. This hypothesis states that an increase in pressure causes stretch of the vascular smooth muscle which responds by contracting, raising afferent arteriolar resistance. Similarly, relaxation of vascular smooth muscle and lowering afferent arteriolar resistance are seen with a decrease in pressure (Fig. 3).

This concept of renal autoregulation is clinically important because the hypertensive patient will not have an increased glomerular filtration rate with the resultant increased reabsorption that would be necessary to maintain body homeostasis. In addition, if one infuses a liter of isotonic fluid into a patient, the excess fluid will not be lost by an increased filtration rate but by changes in the tubular reabsorption of solutes and water. Conversely, when a patient is hypotensive, the glomerular filtration will continue until the systemic arterial pressure is below 45 to 50 mm Hg.

Measurement of Glomerular Filtration Rate

Measurement of glomerular filtration rate is based on the well known concept of "clearance." The renal clearance of a substance is defined as the number of millimeters of plasma completely cleared of that substance in 1

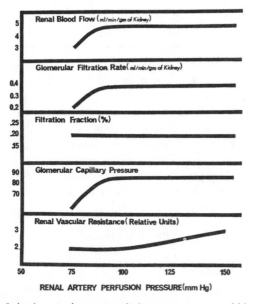

Fig. 3. Influence of altering renal artery perfusion pressure on renal blood flow, glomerular filtration rate, filtration fraction, glomerular capillary pressure, and renal vascular resistance.

min. Inulin is used as a measurement of glomerular filtration rate since it is freely filterable through the glomerular capillary, is not reabsorbed or secreted by the kidney, and not metabolized by the body. The clearance is expressed by the formula UV/P where U equals urine concentration (mg/ml), V equals urine volume (ml/min), and P equals plasma concentration (mg/ml). To measure the GFR with inulin requires the infusion of inulin, waiting for 45 to 60 min for equilibration, and the collection of timed urine specimens. Inulin is also somewhat difficult to measure.

Creatinine Clearance

Creatinine is the anhydride breakdown product of muscle metabolism of creatine phosphate and in man the creatinine synthesis is highly constant; it is only minimally influenced by physical activity, protein intake, or catabolism. Creatinine clearance has been shown to equal inulin clearance

$$H - N -$$
$$C = NH$$
$$N - CH_3$$
$$CH_2 - C \overset{O}{\|}$$

in the rabbit, sheep, seal, and the female dog. In normal man, creatinine is filtered and 5 to 10% of the urinary output is also secreted. Endogenous creatinine clearance is widely used for clinical purposes of measuring GFR and approximates the values of inulin clearance by the cancelling out of two errors. Plasma contains noncreatinine chromogens that react with the color reagent used to measure creatinine giving a "total creatinine chromogen" which is 10 to 20% higher than "true creatinine." In man, 10 to 20% of urinary creatinine comes from tubular secretion. Thus the 10 to 20% errors in the numerator and denominator cancel each other out, and endogenous creatinine clearance approximates inulin clearance and is accurate enough for clinical use. If the laboratory measures "true creatinine" (as is done by some autoanalyzers, the creatinine clearance may exceed the inulin clearance by as much as 50 to 100%. These discrepancies may also be seen in patients with renal failure who will secrete more creatinine. These difficulties are not as great clinically as one would imagine, since clinically it makes little difference in the management of the patient with renal failure whether the GFR is 6 or 10 ml/min.

Serum Creatinine as an Index of GFR

Serum creatinine can be used as an index of glomerular filtration since there is a constant production of creatinine from muscle. Any limitation on urinary excretion from a reduction in renal excretion will cause an increase in serum creatinine until a new steady state is reached (amount excreted equals production). Normal serum creatinine ranges from 0.8 to 1.3 mg/100 ml in males, and 0.6 to 1.0 mg/100 ml in females. Normal creatinine production in man is around 1,500 mg/day or 1 mg/min. If excretion of creatinine equates production, the numerator of our formula for GFR (urine volume x urine creatinine concentration) equals 1 mg/min. Thus if we know the denominator which is the serum creatinine value, and divide it into the assumed 1 mg/min urinary excretion, we can get a fairly close approximation of GFR

$$\frac{1 \text{ mg/min}}{0.01 \text{ mg or } 1 \text{ mg/100 ml}} \quad \text{or} \quad \frac{100}{1} = 100 \text{ ml/min GFR}$$

in the male, dividing the serum creatinine value into 100 will closely approximate the GFR. Likewise in the female, who has a slightly lower creatinine excretion, the GFR can be estimated roughly by dividing the serum concentration per 100 ml into 90, $i.e.$, 90/0.8 mg/100 ml = 115 ml/min GFR.

With any loss in GFR, the serum creatinine will rise, although it may not be measurable or even rise out of the "normal range." For every 50% reduction in GFR, the serum creatinine will double when it has again *reached the steady state.* As shown in Figure 4, small changes in GFR will not raise serum blood urea nitrogen (BUN) or creatinine in the normal patient as much as in the patient with renal failure.

Thus a 50% loss of function in the normal patient will raise the serum

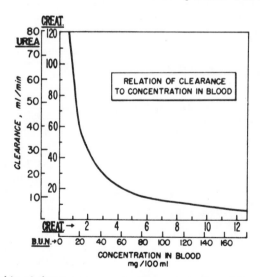

Fig. 4. Relationship of clearance or urea to the concentration of these substances in the blood. A constant excretion of creatinine (1.2 gm/day) and urea nitrogen (11.5 gm/day) is assumed. It can be seen that on the *left side* of the graph in the normal range, a large reduction in clearance causes small changes in blood concentrations. By contrast, on the *right side* of the graph, small changes in the clearance cause large changes in the blood concentrations. (Reproduced with permission from Belman, A. S. and Levinsky, N. G.: *Diseases of the Kidney*, edited by Strauss, M. B. and Welt, L. G., Little, Brown and Company, Boston, 1971.)

creatinine from 1 to 2 mg/100 ml. In the patient with moderate renal failure, a 50% loss of renal function would raise the serum creatinine from 5 to 10 mg/100 ml. Thus it is the relative changes, not the absolute changes, that are important.

Serum BUN as an Index of GFR

Urea is the end product of nitrogen metabolism in man.

$$NH_2 - CO - NH_2$$

Urea

Blood urea concentrations are dependent on the many factors which affect nitrogen metabolism and its renal clearance. Nonrenal factors that alter the blood urea concentrations are protein dietary intake, liver function, protein breakdown from trauma, infection, fever, and breakdown of blood in the tissues or the gastrointestinal tract. The blood urea concentration is usually expressed in terms of BUN, which constitutes approximately half of the weight of urea. Serum BUN normally is 10 to 15 mg/100 ml. Urea is filtered and partially reabsorbed (40 to 60%). Urea reabsorption is passive and is somewhat dependent upon urine flow. At low urine flows, urea concentration in the collecting tubules is high and urea diffuses through the tubule into the interstitium. Antidiuretic hormone increases the permeability of the collecting ducts to both urea and water. With high urine flow rate, there is less equilibration time and less gradient, so less urea is reabsorbed and therefore more is excreted. When fractional tubular reabsorption is constant, the urea clearance is proportionate to GFR. BUN will then vary inversely with GFR, similarly to serum creatinine clearance.

Tubular Reabsorption

Tubular reabsorption requires the major expenditure of the kidneys' metabolic energy. The magnitude of the reabsorptive problem can be readily appreciated by the fact that with a glomerular filtration rate of 125 ml of plasma per min, 180 liters of water, 1,500 g of sodium chloride, 500 g of sodium bicarbonate, and 250 g of glucose are filtered each day. Only about 1% of what is filtered is eventually excreted by the kidney.

Sodium Transport

Sodium transport occurs by active reabsorption along the whole nephron.

Proximal Tubule

In the proximal tubule, approximately 80% of the filtrate is reabsorbed isosmotically, and urine entering the loop of Henle is the isotonic. In the proximal tubule, the epithelium is highly permeable to sodium and there is probably some flux of sodium into and out of the lumen (certainly the net movement of the sodium is toward the peritubular capillary). Sodium absorption is believed to consist of three steps, steps 1 and 3 being passive.

1. Entry of sodium across the luminal membrane into the cell.
2. Exit of sodium from the peritubular membrane into the interstitial space.
3. Entry of sodium from the interstitial space into the peritubular capillary.

Water and ions may cross the epithelium by a noncellular route through the regions of tight junctions and intercellular spaces. This would allow a passive back leak from the peritubular surface to the capillary lumen.

The Loop of Henle

The loop of Henle plays an important role in urinary concentrating mechanism and sodium transport. In the descending limb of Henle's loop, water diffuses out and sodium diffuses in. Sodium is actively transported out of the ascending limb of Henle which must also be relatively impermeable to the outflow of sodium. This allows a buildup of the medullary concentration of sodium which will be discussed further under urinary concentration.

Distal Collecting Tubule

Fluid that enters the distal tubule is hypotonic because of the sodium reabsorption in Henle's loop. There are many differences between the sodium reabsorption in the proximal and distal tubules. Sodium absorption in the distal tubules is active against a concentration gradient, unlike the proximal tubule. The distal tubules transport a smaller fraction of sodium and water, which is rate-limited as opposed to the proximal tubules. Aldosterone causes increased reabsorption of sodium in the distal and collecting tubule. Epithelium of the distal tubule has been shown to be less permeable than the proximal tubule to sodium, water, and urea, thus preventing equilibration and making it possible to maintain the steep concentration gradient for sodium.

Potassium Transport

Forty to 50% of the filtered potassium is reabsorbed in the proximal tubule. Potassium is actively reabsorbed in the loop of Henle, less than 10% of filtered potassium reaching the distal tubule. During conservation of potassium, there is continual reabsorption in the distal nephron. With potassium excretion, there is secretion of potassium in the distal and convoluted tubules. Potassium secretion is probably not a one-to-one exchange of sodium for potassium as once thought. It has been proposed that a reciprocal exchange of hydrogen and potassium at the peritubular membrane is the mechanism of potassium secretion.

Hydrogen Ion

Hydrogen ion secretion and the acidification of tubular fluid take place throughout the nephron. The concentration gradient is established in the distal nephron.

Glucose

Glucose and other substances such as phosphate, sulfate, amino acids, uric acid, and proteins are reabsorbed in the proximal tubule by a T_m-limited mechanism. Glucose is said to have a tubular maximum (T_m) since the transport system is limited. When more glucose is filtered than the transport system can carry, the excess is excreted in the urine.

Tubular Secretion

Transport of materials from the peritubular fluid to tubular lumen involves both active and passive mechanisms.

The active mechanisms are usually divided into T_m-limited mechanisms and gradient-time-limited mechanisms. To calculate tubular secretion, the amount filtered is subtracted from the total amount excreted in the urine per unit time.

T_m-Limited Mechanisms

Organic Acids

Compounds transported include phenol red, penicillin, *para*-aminohippurate (PAH), diodrast, and creatinine. It has been shown that there is competition between the different compounds in the transport system and that the transport system will have greater affinity for certain compounds. Probenecid has been shown to depress penicillin secretion by competitive inhibitions and thus raise the penicillin plasma levels. PAH is actively transported from the peritubular side, accumulating in the proximal tubular cell. There is then a passive diffusion of the PAH from the tubular cell into the lumen of the nephron. At low serum levels (less than 2 mg/100 ml), all the PAH is secreted in each passage of the blood through the kidney. Thus by calculating the PAH clearance (UV/P) one can calculate renal blood flow. At plasma levels above 10 mg/100 ml, PAH is filtered and actively secreted by the proximal tubular cell to a tubular maximum (T_m); that is, above plasma levels of 10 mg/100 ml, the tubular secretory mechanism of PAH is saturated. T_m for PAH in man equals 80 mg/min.

Strong Organic Bases

Compounds transported in this system include guanidine, piperidine, thiamine, choline, and histamine. Like the transport of strong acids, the strong organic base transport system is located in the proximal tubule.

Gradient-Time-Limited Mechanisms

An example of this system is hydrogen ion transport. Hydrogen ions are actively transported from the tubular cell to the tubular lumen. The quantity secreted varies by gradient and time in various portions of the nephron. In the proximal tubules, large quantities of hydrogen ions are secreted against a small gradient. In the distal nephron, small quantities of hydrogen ion are secreted against a large gradient.

Passive Tubular Secretion

This involves transport of substances down an electrochemical gradient. The secretion of weak acids and weak bases results from diffusion down an electrochemical gradient through the tubular cells with trapping of the ionic form in the tubular lumen. Potassium is thought to be actively reabsorbed in the proximal tubule, and the potassium which is excreted in the urine is added by passive secretion in the distal nephron.

Hydrogen Ion Excretion

Hydrogen ions are produced in the body from the metabolism of 1) fat, 2) carbohydrate, and 3) protein. Most of the fat is completely metabolized to carbon dioxide and water. However, some is incompletely oxidized with the production of hydrogen ions.

The normal hydrogen ion production and excretion are shown below.*

Hydrogen Ion Produced	mEq/24 hr/1.73 m² s.a.
From protein	39
From other sources	21
(organic acids)	—
Total	60

Hydrogen Ion Excreted	
Titratable acid	30
Ammonium	31
Bicarbonate	−1
Total	60

The total urinary excretion of hydrogen ion thus is equal to the sum of titratable acid plus ammonium minus bicarbonate.

$$UV_{H^+} = UV_{TA^+} UV_{NH_4^+} - UV_{HCO_3^-}$$

It is important for the student to have a concept of total hydrogen ion turnover as is shown below.*

Total CO$_2$ turnover	24,000 mmoles/24 hr
Total hydrogen ion turnover	60 mEq/24 hr
Total buffer in body	2,100 mEq
Total hydrogen in buffer	105 mEq
Total free H$^+$ in body fluids	0.0021 mEq

* From Elkinton, in *Renal Disease*, edited by D. A. K. Black. F. A. Davis Co., Philadelphia, 1967.

Thus there is little hydrogen ion dissociated at any one time in the body. No net hydrogen ion excretion takes place through the lungs; however, a large amount of CO$_2$ is expired through the lungs. If the pulmonary excretion of CO$_2$ differs from production (hyper or hypoventilation), the concentration of hydrogen ion is altered by changes in the ratio of the buffered pair H$^+ \cdot$HCO$_3^-$/B$^+$HCO$_3$. The lung is important in controlling body fluid pH only in that it controls body fluid, PCO$_2$ and thus H$_2$CO$_3$ concentration. The kidney therefore controls the body fluid hydrogen ion concentration by its ability to secrete hydrogen and control the level of blood bicarbonate. Normally urine is acid (pH 6.5) relative to plasma (pH 7.4).

Bicarbonate Reabsorption

Normally over 99.9% of filtered bicarbonate is reabsorbed (5,000 mEq/24 hr), preventing acidosis by loss of base. The kidney stabilizes the plasma concentration of bicarbonate at a level of 26 to 28 mEq/liter. When an excess of bicarbonate exists, the kidney excretes the excess. Sodium bicarbonate is reabsorbed by the exchange of H ions for the Na ions of sodium bicarbonate into the tubular lumen. The resultant carbonic acid (H$_2$CO$_3$) is rapidly catalyzed by carbonic anhydrase to H$_2$O and CO$_2$. CO$_2$ then diffuses into the cell passively along a concentration gradient to enter the cell and reform carbonic acid. The carbonic acid dissociates and HCO$_3^-$ and Na$^+$ ions are reabsorbed into the peritubular fluid and blood, while the intracellular H$^+$ ion is exchanged in the tubular lumen for Na$^+$ to start the cycle over again.

Excretion of Titratable Acid

Titratable acid is the hydrogen ion that is excreted in combination with urinary buffer (phosphates and sulfates). It is measured by titrating the acid urine with sodium hydroxide to the pH of the glomerular filtration (pH 7.40). This determines the mEq of hydrogen excreted in this form and thus the amount of bicarbonate added to the body. In urines which are already alkaline, there will be no "titratable acid" since no base is required to bring it to 7.40 pH. Normally, disodium phosphate is the major urinary buffer. The exchange of H$^+$ ions for Na$^+$ ions converts the filtered dibasic phosphate to the acid monobasic form.

$$Na_2 HPO_4 \rightarrow Na H_2 PO_4$$

Excretion of Ammonium Ion

Breakdown of amino acids (primarily glutamine) in the renal tubular cell forms ammonia (NH_3). Ammonia readily diffuses across cell membrane into the tubular lumen where it will combine with the secreted hydrogen ion to form NH_4^+. The NH_4^+ is charged, lipid-insoluble, and will not diffuse across the cell wall. Thus the NH_4^+ is "trapped" in the tubular urine and excretes the hydrogen ion. The cellular loss of the trapped hydrogen ion generates HCO_3^- that diffuses from the cell into the blood. Acidosis stimulates the formation of ammonia from the amino acids.

Renal Response to Metabolic Acidosis

The mechanism whereby a normal individual responds to an acid load is shown in Figure 6. During the control days, the subject excreted 130 mEq of chloride, 40 mEq of ammonia, 40 mEq of titratable acid, 125 mEq of sodium, and 78 mEq of potassium per day.

From the 5th to the 10th day, the subject was given an acid load of 290 mEq/day (15 g NH_4Cl). After absorption, the acid is buffered by bicarbonate, CO_2 is expelled by the lungs, and the concentration of bicarbonate in the body fluids decreases. On the 1st day, excretion of sodium and chloride increased sharply with modest increases in ammonia and titratable acid excretion. Thus, on the 1st day, the excess in chloride was balanced mostly by excretion of sodium from the body's reserves. During the next few days, the body was able to excrete more potassium, save more sodium, and significantly increase ammonia production to eliminate most of hydrogen ion. Thus the major response is the increase in the excretion of ammonia. During the recovery phase, the body saved sodium and potassium and continued excretion of ammonia until the acidosis was corrected (Fig. 5).

Urinary Concentration and Dilution

Urinary Concentration

Under conditions of antidiuretic hormone stimulation, greater than 99% of filtered urine is reabsorbed and urine osmolality is raised from 285 to over 1,000 mOsm/kg. This is accomplished through a system of countercurrent multiplication and countercurrent exchange which is familiar to all medical students. This process is summarized in Figure 6.

In this diagram, 100 ml of serum are filtered each minute with a milliosmolality of 300. Eighty percent of the filtrate is reabsorbed isosmotically in the proximal tubule. As the filtrate progresses down the descending limb of Henle, the volume decreases to 15 ml by passage of water out. There is also passage of sodium in from countercurrent exchange. In the ascending limb of Henle, sodium is actively extruded out greatly in excess of water. Thus an isosmotic gradient is created through a countercurrent multiplication to approximately 1,200 mOsm/kg deep in the medulla. The vasa recta

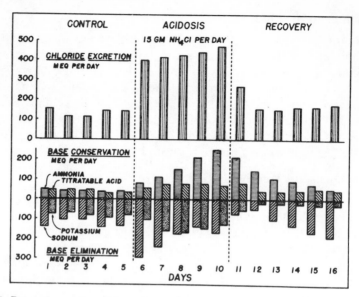

Fig. 5. Rates of excretion of ions prior to, during, and after a period of acidosis induced by the ingestion of ammonium chloride. (Reproduced with permission from Pitts, R. F.: *Physiology of the Kidney and Body Fluids*, Year Book Medical Publishers, Chicago, 1974, and adapted from Sartorius, O. W., Roemmelt, J. C. and Pitts, R. F.: J. Clin. Invest. 28:423, 1949.)

also participates in countercurrent exchange and because of low blood flow does not wash out too much of the sodium. Fluid leaving the ascending limb is thus hypotonic (100 mOsm) and contains the same 15-ml volume as when it entered. Sodium reabsorption continues through the distal tubule. Under the stimulus of antidiuretic hormone, the collecting tubule becomes more permeable to water. Fluid from the collecting tubule then diffuses to the hypertonic medullary interstitium, both concentrating the urine and decreasing the volume of filtrate in our theoretical model to 0.5 ml/min.

Urinary Dilution

In a water diuresis, antidiuretic hormone is not secreted and the epithelium of the distal nephron is no longer permeable to water. Urine is rendered hypotonic by the reabsorption of sodium without water, generating "free water." Filtrate continues to be reabsorbed in the proximal tubule and descending limb of Henle, decreasing the filtrate to 15 ml/min. With the epithelium in the ascending limb of Henle, distal and collecting tubule impermeable to water, the volume of the final urine is large (up to 15 ml/min) and dilute.

Fluid and Electrolytes

Total body fluid and electrolytes are maintained within narrow limits of normal by control mechanisms regulating salt and water excretion.

REABSORPTION AND EXCRETION OF IONS AND WATER

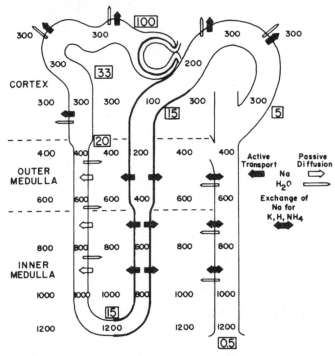

Fig. 6. Summary of countercurrent multiplication and exchange systems in the nephron in the course of elaboration of hypertonic urine. Concentrations of tubular urine and peritubular fluid in mOsm/kg: large, boxed numeral, estimated percentage of glomerular filtrate re maining within the tubule at each level. (Reproduced with permission from Pitts, R. F.: *Physiology of the Kidney and Body Fluids*, Year Book Medical Publishers, Chicago, 1974.)

Body Fluid Compartments

Water constitutes 45 to 75% of body weight. Since adipose tissue has a lower percentage of water (10%) as compared to 75% for muscle, the percentage of total body water will vary from individual to individual. Lean males have about 60% water compared to 52%, in females who in general have more subcutaneous fat tissue. Infants have a very high percentage of water in relation to body weight.

The normal distribution of water into the various body compartments is shown below.

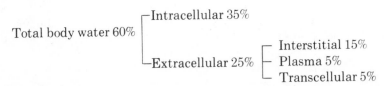

Total body water 60%
  Intracellular 35%
  Extracellular 25%
    Interstitial 15%
    Plasma 5%
    Transcellular 5%

Total Body Water

Total body water constitutes approximately 60% of body weight. This can be measured by injection of antipyrine, deuterium oxide, or tritiated water.

$$\text{Volume} = \frac{\text{quantity injection}}{\text{concentration}}$$

Extracellular Fluid Volume

The extracellular fluid in our theoretical model was 25% and represents that fluid outside the cells. The actual volume depends upon which substance is used to measure it. Substances commonly used are inulin (16% body weight), mannitol, radiosulfate (22% body weight), and radiosodium (30% body weight).

Plasma Volume

The plasma volume usually is around 5% of body weight and the blood volume is 8.3% of body weight. Plasma and blood volumes can be calculated by knowing the hematocrit and measuring the plasma volume with Evans blue or radioiodinated human serum albumin. The volume of red blood cells can be measured by tagging red blood cells with either radioactive phosphorus or chromium.

Intracellular Fluid Volume

Intracellular fluid volume is determined by subtracting the extracellular fluid volume from the total body fluid volume.

Interstitial Fluid Volume

Interstitial fluid volume is determined by subtracting the plasma volume from the extracellular fluid volume.

Control Mechanisms of Body Salt and Water

Sodium Excretion

Sodium excretion is a function of the amount filtered through the glomerulus and reabsorbed in the tubules. In man, the glomerular filtration rate is maintained fairly constant by renal autoregulation, and so the amount filtered usually is directly related to plasma sodium concentration. Under normal conditions, the percentage of sodium reabsorbed in the proximal tubule is constant; this is called the glomerulotubular balance. The mechanism of glomerular tubular balance is unclear, but it is thought to be related to peritubular factors such as oncotic pressure.

1. Aldosterone. In the presence of aldosterone, sodium reabsorption is increased in the distal nephron. An important stimulus to aldosterone

secretion is the renin-angiotensin system. Renin is an enzyme which is released by the kidney and acts on an α-2-globulin made in the liver finally to form angiotensin II. Angiotensin II, in addition to being a potent vasoconstrictor, also stimulates aldosterone secretion. Aldosterone secretion is also stimulated by high plasma potassium and adrenocorticotropic hormone.

2. Third factor. An additional factor besides aldosterone and filtered sodium has been thought to stimulate sodium excretion. In experiments in which large volumes of isotonic saline are infused intravenously, an increase in sodium excretion can be demonstrated despite artificially lowered glomerular filtration rate (and thus filtered sodium) and in the presence of large amounts of aldosterone. The nature of this "third factor" has not been clarified as yet.

Water Excretion

The relationship of intracerebral plasma concentration of solutes to urinary concentration was first shown by Verney in 1947. He administered hypertonic sodium chloride through the carotid artery of an awake dog which was undergoing a water diuresis. Shortly after injection of the hypertonic fluid perfusing the brain, the urine volume decreased and concentration increased similarly to that seen by injection of antidiuretic hormone (ADH). Injection of similar amounts of hypertonic saline into the systemic circulation had no effect on urine flow. He postulated that there are receptors in the brain which cause the release of ADH. It is now believed that ADH is synthesized in the cells of the paraventricular and supraoptic nuclei in the hypothalamus and is diffused along these tracts to the posterior pituitary, where it is stored and released. Thus when the plasma is hypertonic, ADH is released to save water, and when the plasma is hypotonic, ADH is not released, causing a water diuresis.

1. Osmolar and water clearance.

A. Osmolar clearance (C_{osm}) is derived as are other clearances U_{osm} . volume/P_{osm} and represents the milliliter per min of plasma completely cleared of osmotically active solute.

B. Free water (C_{H_2O}) is calculated by subtracting the osmolar clearance from the urine flow $V - C_{osm}$). Free water is the excess water without solute (free) over the solute clearance. It is positive with a water diuresis.

C. Negative free water ($T^c_{H_2O}$) is calculated by subtracting the urine volume from the osmolar clearance ($C_{osm} - V$). Thus if the urine is concentrated, there would be no free water; the volume of water needed to bring the urine back to plasma osmolality is called negative free water.

Importance of Clinical Implementation

When a physician administers fluid to a patient, he has many alternatives to choose from: glucose and water, isotonic saline, or blood and

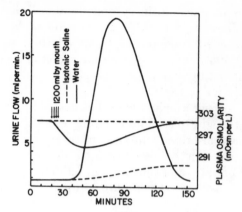

Fig. 7. Differences in the diuresis obtained from the oral ingestion of 1200 ml of water and a similar volume of isotonic saline. (Reproduced with permission from Pitts, R. F.: *Physiology of the Kidney and Body Fluids*, Year Book Medical Publishers, Chicago, 1974.)

plasma. It is important to understand where the administered fluid is distributed and how long it will be available to the body before it is excreted. When a patient is admitted with dehydration, he should receive 5% glucose in water which gives him pure water when the glucose is metabolized. The administered fluid would be distributed over the total body water compartment (60%). If glucose and water is administered to a normally hydrated person, dilution of body fluid occurs, ADH release is inhibited, circulating ADH is metabolized by the liver, and in about 30 to 60 min a diuresis begins. A liter of ingested pure water is eliminated in 2 to 3 hours. Thus if we were administering the glucose in water to a patient seen in shock from blood loss, we would have the disadvantage of the fluid being distributed in the whole body water compartment, 60% versus the 5% plasma compartment where it was lost, and in addition the fluid would be rapidly excreted.

If we had infused isotonic saline, there would be no change in plasma osmolality, so ADH release would not be affected by the osmoreceptors. The fluid would not be excreted before 12 to 14 hours. The mechanisms of excretion would be by inhibition of aldosterone secretion. Isotonic saline would stay in the extracellular compartment (25%). Thus if one is using isotonic saline to replace plasma loss (5% compartment), one must give about 4 to 5 times as much saline to get the same hemodynamic effect as plasma (Fig. 7).

REFERENCES AND SUGGESTED READING

1. Strauss, M. B. and Welt, L. G. (Editors). *Diseases of the Kidney*, Vol. 1 Ed. 2, Little, Brown & Co., Boston, 1971.
2. Pitts, R. F. *Physiology of the Kidney and Body Fluids*. Year Book Medical Publishers, Chicago, 1974.
3. Gilmore, J. P. *Renal Physiology*. The Williams & Wilkins Co., Baltimore, 1972.

4

Obstructive Uropathy

ARTHUR W. WYKER, JR.

E. DARRACOTT VAUGHAN, JR.

INTRODUCTION

Obstruction of urine flow at any level from glomerulus to the penile meatus is of primary importance because of the devastating effects on both nephron function and conduit function necessary for transport of urine from the body. Furthermore, obstruction is frequently associated with infection and stone formation, which accelerate renal deterioration. With its protean etiologies, obstructive uropathy is one of the most common urological problems that confronts clinicians of all disciplines.

CLASSIFICATION

Obstruction of urine flow can be due to either intrinsic or extrinsic mechanical blockage or due to dysfunction without actual anatomical obstruction.

1. With mechanical obstruction, there is anatomical blockade of urine flow which can occur at any level. It may be congenital or due to acquired disease and may be due to abnormalities within the urinary system (intrinsic lesions) or to disease compressing the urinary system (extrinsic disease). Common forms of mechanical obstruction are shown in Table I.

A. Congenital lesions causing mechanical obstruction may produce severe hydronephrosis with renal damage in the neonate, because the effect of the obstruction will have begun at the time of initial urine formation during the 4th fetal month.

B. Mechanical obstruction often occurs at narrow points in the conduit, i.e., the ureteropelvic junction, ureterovesical junction, the bladder neck, or the urethral meatus.

2. Impairment of urine flow without anatomical obstruction, which can also result in hydronephrosis, is termed functional obstruction. Functional disorders involve both the ureter and the bladder and also may induce secondary mechanical obstruction.

Functional obstruction may occur in a number of ways:

A. The generation of adequate peristaltic movement in the ureter is the chief mechanism of urine transport from the renal pelvis to the bladder. When the transmission of these waves is inhibited, a physiological

TABLE I

Common Causes of Mechanical Obstruction of Urine Flow

	Congenital		Acquired	
	Intrinsic	Extrinsic	Intrinsic	Extrinsic
Ureter	Ureteropelvic obstruction[a] Ureterovesical junction obstruction Ureterocele	Ureteropelvic junction obstruction[a] Retrocaval ureter	Calculus[a] Inflammation Injury Papillary necrosis Tumor Uric acid nephropathy	Retroperitoneal fibrosis Aortic aneurysm Pregnant uterus Uterine leiomyoma Injury Carcinoma Retroperitoneal tumor (lymphoma)
Bladder outlet	Bladder neck obstruction Ureterocele	Bowel abnormalities	Adenomatous hyperplasia of prostate[a] Cancer of prostate[a] Bladder neck contracture Cancer of bladder Stone	Cancer of cervix Cancer of colon Injury
Urethra	Posterior urethral valves Stricture Meatal stenosis Anterior urethral valves Phimosis		Stricture[a] Carcinoma Stone Injury Phimosis	Injury

[a] Most common.

obstruction exists. The transmission of peristalsis is dependent on the ability of the ureter to glide within the adventitia. Thus when any portion of the ureter has been immobilized, it loses this gliding function and may become "obstructed." Periureteral adhesions, fibrosis, or tumor can cause fixation of the ureter and loss of peristalsis with functional obstruction despite a patent lumen. Moreover, peristaltic activity is dependent on normal muscular function, and impairment of muscular activity by infection, ischemia, or dilation also can result in functional obstruction.

B. The integrated activity of the bladder-detrusor contraction and external sphincter relaxation is necessary for normal voiding (see Chapter 16 on neurogenic bladder). If this integrated activity is impaired by either congenital lesions or acquired lesions, there may be functional obstruction.

C. The urine itself may play a role in functional obstruction. Hence, if the integrity of the ureterovesical junction is impaired, then with bladder filling and voiding, the high bladder pressure is transmitted up the ureter and effective peristalsis is impaired both by the increased pressure and by reflux of bladder urine up the ureter. Thus ureterovesical reflux causes functional obstruction and may lead to hydronephrosis and renal impairment in the absence of infection (see Chapter 16 on ureterovesical reflux).

NORMAL URODYNAMICS

1. In the normal human, glomerular filtration is the initial step of urine formation, and its magnitude can be appreciated by calculating that at a filtration rate of 125 ml of plasma per minute, 160 liters of ultrafiltrate reach the tubules each day. Recent evidence has shown that effective glomerular filtration pressure is quite low, about 14 cm of water.
2. The change in pressure down the renal tubule, where the vast bulk of ultrafiltrate is reabsorbed, resulting in a normal urine output of 500 to 2,500 ml/day, is also low, being about 7 cm of H_2O in animals studied by micropuncture technique.
3. The normal resting pressure in the renal pelvis is about 5 cm of water. The renal pelvis does not contract like the detrusor muscle of the bladder, nor does it have peristalsis like the ureter. It rhythmically contracts, possibly with some "pacemaker" control, but it only produces low grade pressure fluctuations. The renal pelvis and upper part of the ureter are in open communication and are most efficient when the ureteropelvic junction is dependent and cone-shaped.
4. The ureter functions by forming the urine into elongated boluses and establishing increases of intraluminal pressure behind these boluses to aid in their distal transport. Recent *in vivo* measurements of ureteral tension (contractile force) have provided proof that inherent contractile properties of the ureter are responsible for initiating peristalsis. Thus when the ureteral tension is maintained at baseline pressure, the ureter remains at rest, and the ureteral pressure also remains low. When wall tension increases, the ureteral walls coapt, and the lumen constricts, resulting in ureteral contraction, the formation of urine boluses, and a rise in ureteral pressure to 20 to 30 cm of water. Hence the ability of the ureter to transport urine is dependent on its capacity to increase contractile force (tension) above baseline.
5. For urine to pass from the ureter to the bladder, the ureteral contraction pressure must exceed the intravesical pressure. If the intravesical pressure is elevated, urine will pass into the bladder only at the expense of abnormally high ureteral pressures, possibly resulting in decompensation.
6. The bladder is a low pressure reservoir that maintains a low pressure as the bladder passively fills. The ability of the bladder to fill at a relatively low intravesical pressure has been termed accommodation. However, there is a large increase in tension as the radius of the curvature of the sphere increases.
7. Voiding is initiated at a critical degree of bladder filling by activation of

the voiding reflex (see the chapter on neurogenic bladder). With voiding, the bladder pressure rises to 30 to 80 cm of water while urethral resistance drops because the active detrusor contraction "pulls" open the bladder neck, creating a funnel. Simultaneously, reciprocal innervation between the pelvic and pudendal nerves causes relaxation of the external urinary sphincter.

UNIQUE RESPONSE OF THE KIDNEY AND URETER TO OBSTRUCTION

Unlike most excretory organs which cease to function when their ducts are obstructed, the kidney continues to function, resulting in a unique form of nephron injury called hydronephrosis. Thus, although impaired, glomerular filtration continues and the urine is modified by reabsorption and secretion. To have continued inflow, there must be egress of urine by alternative routes other than the ureter. In fact, radiographic and isotopic studies have demonstrated outflow of urine into both the venous and lymphatic systems (Table II). Hence the urine in an obstructed renal pelvis is constantly changing and is not a static pool. The degree of hydronephrotic nephron damage depends on the following:
1. The level of the obstruction.
2. The degree of obstruction.
3. The duration of obstruction.
4. The anatomy of the renal pelvis.
5. The degree of impairment of nutrient blood supply.
6. The absence or presence of intercurrent infection.

Mechanism of Nephron Damage

Following acute obstruction, there is a transient rise in renal blood flow lasting several hours followed by a progressive fall. The fall in renal blood

TABLE II

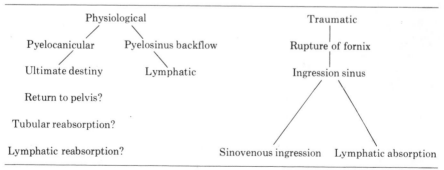

Reprinted from Narath, P. A.: The hydromechanics of the calyx renalis. J. Urol. 43:145, 1940.

flow is due both to the effect of the initially elevated ureteral pressure and to active vasoconstriction. The mechanism of the active vasoconstriction is not well understood, but it would appear to be dominant since the ureteral pressure rapidly falls to levels near normal. Nephron loss occurs owing to ischemic damage and hydrostatic pressure damage. Despite the fact that egress channels open, this compensatory mechanism is never perfect, so that some nephron damage almost always occurs.

Mechanism of Ureteral Damage

Concurrent with the nephron change, there are changes in ureteral urodynamics due to obstruction. Thus, immediately following ureteral obstruction in dogs, there is increase in both baseline and peak ureteral tensions generated. These forceful contractions are capable of producing marked elevations in the amplitude of ureteral pressure waves. However, as the obstruction persists, the ureter utilizes the force it can generate solely to counteract the building pressure within the lumen resulting in a constant high baseline tension without additional elevations. Thus there is no force to generate contractions, and peristalsis ceases. Chronically, the ureteral wall decompensates, resulting in the dilated tortuous ureter that is characteristic of obstruction. With decompensation, there is increased ureteral volume resulting in a low ureteral pressure. This decompensation, coupled with the intrarenal vascular effects of obstruction, explains the often normal intraluminal ureteral pressure found with chronic obstruction. Despite decompensation, the baseline tension remains elevated owing to the increased radius. This ureter may be able to generate contractions, but these are decreased in magnitude from the normal. Thus coaptation of ureteral walls cannot occur, and stasis of urine results, which predisposes to infection and stone formation.

FUNCTIONAL EFFECTS OF OBSTRUCTION

Patterns of Nephron Damage

The nephron damage that occurs with obstruction is characterized both anatomically and functionally as "ascending" damage. Thus distal tubular derangements occur first and glomerular filtration is best preserved. Patients with unilateral hydronephrosis secondary to ureteropelvic junction obstruction have shown impairments in glomerular filtration rate, tubular maxima of p-aminohippurate, concentrating ability, fractional but not absolute sodium reabsorption and acidifying ability. Again there is a variability in the degree of damage with greater damage when there is:

A. High obstruction and less "buffering" by the renal pelvis and ureter.
B. Total obstruction.
C. A long duration of obstruction.
D. Intercurrent infection.

Recovery of Nephron Function

Another unique ability of the kidney is an amazing potential for recovery of renal function following relief of obstruction. This capacity for recovery has been studied best in dogs, where it has been clearly shown that recovery occurs, even in the presence of a hypertrophied opposite kidney, although recovery is enhanced by concurrent contralateral nephrectomy at the time of release of obstruction. The degree of recovery is inversely related to the duration of obstruction. In the dog, there is complete recovery after 7 days of total unilateral obstruction but no recovery after 6 weeks.

CLINICAL MANIFESTATIONS OF OBSTRUCTION

Pain

With acute obstruction of the urinary tract, pain is the most common symptom due to stretching of the ureter, renal pelvis, and renal capsule. The pain may be manifest in the suprapubic region, the lateral abdomen, the flank, or the costovertebral angle (CVA) region. The severity of renal pain is not primarily related to the degree of distension but to the rapidity with which it develops. Thus acute distension by an obstructing stone may cause severe pain, whereas with chronic slow distension a kidney can be totally destroyed with no pain at all. When there is relative obstruction of the urinary tract, the pain may be intermittent and often related to high fluid intake because of the large urine output. This type of obstruction is most commonly found at the ureteropelvic junction.

Voiding Disturbances

If the level of the obstruction is distal to the bladder, the symptom complex is most commonly that of outlet obstruction, as discussed in Chapter 16 on the prostate.

Abnormal Urine Output

While the urine output may be totally normal, there are three patterns which strongly suggest urinary tract obstruction.

1. With total obstruction of nephrons, ureters, bladder outlet, or urethra, there is obviously anuria. If the anuria is due to urinary retention from an intravesical level, the bladder will be distended and palpable, and the patient may complain of lower abdominal pain. If the obstruction is above the bladder, symptoms will usually be referable to the renal areas, and one might suspect that there is only a solitary kidney maintaining renal function.

2. One of the early manifestations of obstructive uropathy is a defect in concentrating ability; therefore polyuria may be a cardinal manifestation of chronic obstructive uropathy. These patients, who have been termed as having "renal" diabetes insipidus, may produce large amounts of urine output relative to their glomerular filtration. Because of the obligate water

loss, these patients often will manifest severe thirst to compensate for the dehydration caused by the excessive urine output.

3. The urine output may alternate between periods of anuria and marked polyuria. This pattern is characteristic of intermittent urinary obstruction due to intrinsic lesions such as stone or pedunculated tumor or extrinsic compression.

Recurrent or Refractory Urinary Infection

Besides the symptoms of obstruction *per se*, one should always consider the presence of obstruction in the patient with symptoms of urinary tract infection. In fact, because of the potential for gram-negative septicemia, all patients with pyelonephritis should have intravenous urography acutely to rule out intercurrent obstruction of the urinary tract, which may be fatal to the patient if not promptly corrected. Moreover, stasis of urine flow with residual urine encourages the persistence of infection and impairs normal defense mechanisms of the urinary collecting system.

Renal Failure

Obstructive uropathy can also lead to chronic renal failure, and a "postrenal" cause for renal failure should always be evaluated in the patient with azotemia. Azotemia due to postrenal obstruction can be insidious in nature and has been termed "silent prostatism." Thus the patient may present with a variety of medical manifestations such as hypertension, congestive heart failure, anemia, or azotemia, without any symptoms of outlet obstruction.

DIAGNOSIS OF URINARY OBSTRUCTION

As with any other entity in medicine, the diagnosis of urinary obstruction should begin with a careful history and physical examination.

History

One should inquire about voiding disturbances, pain, abnormal urine output, symptoms of urinary tract infection, and symptoms which might unveil renal failure. There should also be questions concerning associated systems which might be diseased and cause extrinsic lesions involving the urinary tract. Aside from symptoms directly related to obstruction, the patient should be questioned in detail concerning other urological diseases in the past including stone disease, trauma, or congenital abnormalities.

Physical Examination

The abdomen should be palpated for costovertebral angle tenderness and for renal or pelvic masses; auscultation of the abdomen should be performed for abnormal bowel sounds and vascular bruits. The penis should be inspected for phimosis, meatal stenosis, duplication, or abnormalities of the urethra and induration along the anterior urethra which might indicate stricture. On rectal examination, the prostate can be palpated for either malignancy or benign adenomatous hyperplasia. In addition, on the rectal examination in the male, abnormalities in the bowel or in the rectovesical pouch should be recognized. In examining the female, vaginal and uterine lesions as well as rectal lesions should be identified. In the female, it is sometimes possible to palpate a stone in the lower ureter.

INTRAVENOUS UROGRAM

The radiological hallmark of obstruction is dilation of the urinary conduit proximal to the site of obstruction. Diagnosis of urinary obstruction usually can be made with radiographic techniques if appropriate studies are performed.

The standard initial procedure is the intravenous urogram. During early obstruction, there may be blunting or fullness of all calices, renal pelvis, and visualization of the entire ureter down to the site of obstruction. Late in obstructive uropathy, there is severe dilation of the renal pelvis and calices (hydronephrosis) often accompanied by generalized reduction in thickness of the renal parenchyma. At times, the only clear evidence of contrast material may be visualized at the junction between the functioning medulla and the renal pelvis (crescent sign), or there may be only puddling of contrast material within a massively dilated collecting system. The ureter generally will be dilated and tortuous owing to ureteral decompensation and elongation. It is of utmost importance that delay films be obtained for as long a time period as necessary until the actual site of obstruction is identified. It is not uncommon in cases of severe obstructive uropathy to obtain adequate information only 24 or 48 hours after injection. The bladder should be observed for signs of outlet obstruction such as trabeculation, cellule formation, or diverticula. A postvoiding film should be a routine part of the intravenous urogram so that one can ascertain if there is any post-voiding residual urine.

When there is impairment of renal function, it has been shown that drip infusion urography enhances diagnostic accuracy. In this examination, three or four times the usual volume of contrast material (1 mg/lb) is diluted with an equal volume of 5% dextrose and water and given intravenously in about 10 min. Ensor and Anderson performed more than 1,000 studies utilizing this technique and obtained satisfactory diagnostic findings 75% of the time if the blood urea nitrogen (BUN) was less than 80 mg% and serum creatinine less than 8 mg%, or if the creatinine clearance was greater than 10 ml/min.

Voiding Cystourethrogram

This is a technique whereby the bladder is filled following the passage of a urethral catheter and films are taken while the patient is in the act of voiding. These studies detect lower urinary tract obstruction and are particularly useful to determine the presence of infravesical obstruction. This technique also may be utilized during intravenous urography whereby the bladder is allowed to fill following the early films of the intravenous urogram and a voiding film is obtained. This study is particularly attractive in that total anatomical delineation of the urinary tract, from the renal pelvis down to the urethral meatus, is obtained without the need of urethral instrumentation and the inherent hazard of urinary tract contamination by bacteria.

Cystoscopy

The urologist is in a unique position in that he can directly inspect a large portion of the urinary excretory system. Thus panendoscopy allows direct visualization for abnormalities of the urethra, the prostate, and the bladder. On cystoendoscopy, one may identify both the cause and the site of urinary tract obstruction. The significance of enlargement of the prostate is best ascertained from observation of the bladder for trabeculation and/or decompensation rather than by the size of the prostate itself.

Retrograde Pyelography

During cystoscopy, retrograde ureteropyelograms may be performed when the upper urinary tract is inadequately visualized on drip infusion urography. Cone-tip ureteral catheters can be engaged into the ureteral orifice and contrast material slowly injected, outlining the entire ureter, renal pelvis, and calices. With appropriate flat and oblique immediate and drainout films, the site and degree of obstruction can be accurately determined. Moreover, small ureteral catheters can then be passed up to or through an area of obstruction both for the diagnostic collection of cytology, urine cultures, further radiographic studies and also for therapeutic relief of partial obstruction.

Renal Radioisotopic Studies

Recent advances in renal imaging with radionuclides have proven to be useful primarily in situations where there is severe unilateral or bilateral obstruction, and the question is whether or not relief of obstruction will result in a return of renal function. Thus, if both kidneys are obstructed, a renal dynamic scan utilizing technetium chelate or iron ascorbate followed by delay studies for manifestation of tubular function, may give information as to which kidney is better and therefore could be expected to recover with appropriate relief of obstruction. With further refinement of these techniques, they should hold considerable promise and usefulness in the future.

POSTOBSTRUCTIVE DIURESIS

Following the relief of chronic partial urinary obstruction or total urinary obstruction, there is rarely the occurrence of marked solute and/or water loss. This ensuing diuresis which follows relief of obstruction has been termed "postobstructive" diuresis. It should be emphasized that this entity is rare; however, when it occurs it may be life-threatening and therefore, in any patient who has relief of obstruction, there should be very close observation of the hourly urine output.

1. Postobstructive diuresis appears to occur primarily in patients with a severe degree of urinary tract obstruction, yet with a potential for rapid reversibility of glomerular function while tubular defects persist. The diuresis is often accentuated by significant salt and water retention prior to the time of release of obstruction.

The mechanism of the excessive urine output is best subdivided into two categories.

A. There may be a water diuresis characterized by urine of low specific gravity which may be either physiological due to retained water or pathological due to impairment of concentrating ability by the kidney. The pathological and physiological water diureses can be differentiated by the response to antidiuretic hormone. In the patient with a physiological water overload, the kidneys will respond and lower their urine output when antidiuretic hormone is given intravenously.

B. The second subcategory consists of solute diuresis causing the large urinary output. It has been documented that the solute may be 1) urea, 2) glucose, 3) sodium, or 4) a combination of the above. Postobstructive natriuresis is extremely rare; however, it can lead to the most severe clinical complications.

2. Studies of a significant number of patients with postobstructive phenomena have revealed that, in the majority of these patients, the diuresis is physiological and self-limiting. Thus in these patients, urine output can be monitored closely along with oral intake, body weight, serum electrolytes, and the mental status; and if the patient is alert, he generally can replace his loss with oral intake. Moreover, even if there is persistent abnormality in the concentrating mechanism, the patient can still maintain himself, because as he becomes systemically dehydrated, his thirst mechanism is stimulated, and he can drink. If there is physiological solute loss due to glucose, Na^+, or urea, the diuresis will cease when the serum levels of these compounds return to normal. If there is abnormal sodium loss, however, the patient will become volume-depleted. Replacement with water can induce hyponatremia and neurological manifestations may occur.

Therefore, in the alert patient who continues to have a urinary output of greater than 200 cc/hour over 24 hours, the urine should be examined for sodium, potassium, and osmolality. These same tests are performed initially if the patient is comatose, and fluid replacement has to be via the intravenous route. Following these studies, if there is no inappropriate sodium loss and the patient is awake, generally he can be watched closely on oral intake. If the patient is comatose or if there is inappropriate sodium loss, then approximately one-half the loss can be replaced by the intravenous route with close monitoring of serum and urine electrolytes.

TABLE III
Plan of Management Following Relief of Obstructive Disease[a]

Initial Studies
  Serum creatinine, urea, electrolytes
  Evaluate for fluid retention
Initial orders
  Call physician if urine output is greater than 200 cc/hr
  Accurate weight
  Vital signs with upright blood pressure recordings
  Oral fluids *ad lib*
Patients with postobstructive diuresis (out put > 200 cc/hour x 2 hours)
  Accurate hourly intake and output record
  Hourly vital signs with upright blood pressure
  Weight every 8 hr
  Daily electrolytes, urea, creatinine
  Urine specific gravity (osmolality), sodium, glucose
Low risk patient (no edema, congestive heart failure, azotemia, or confusion)
  IV fluids only if
    Postural hypotension
    Tachycardia
    Low serum sodium
  If diuresis is greater than 24 hr
    Low U_{osm}, try ADH
    High $U_{Na}{}^{+}$, try DOCA
Moderate risk patient (alert, with edema, congestive heart failure, azotemia)
  Therapy is the same as for low risk patient
High risk patient (mental confusion, congestive heart failure, edema, or azotemia)
  Study with ADH, DOCA
  Replace ½ output with ½ normal saline (modify if large salt loss)
  If hypotensive, tachycardia, low central venous pressure, increase IV fluids
  Allow oral intake as soon as possible

[a] Reprinted from Vaughan, E. D., Jr. and Gillenwater, J. Y.: Diagnosis, characterization and management of postobstructive diuresis. J. Urol. 109:286, 1973.

A detailed plan for management is shown in Table III.

REFERENCES AND SUGGESTED FURTHER READING

1. Bricker, N. S. and Klahr, S. Obstructive uropathy. In *Diseases of the Kidney*, edited by M. B. Strauss, Chap. 27. Little, Brown and Co., Boston, 1971.
2. Gillenwater, J. Y., Westervelt, F. B., Jr., Vaughan, E. D., Jr., and Howards, SS. Renal function after release of chronic unilateral hydronephrosis in man. Kidney Int. 7:179, 1975.
3. Hinman, F., Jr. The pathophysiology of urinary obstruction. In *Urology*, edited by M. F. Campbell, and J. H. Harrison, W. B. Saunders Co., Philadelphia, 1970.
4. Howards, S. S. and Wright, F. S. Obstructive injury. In *The Kidney*, edited by B. M. Brenner, and F. C. Rector. W. B. Saunders Co., Philadelphia, in press.
5. Rose, J. G. and Gillenwater, J. Y. Pathophysiology of ureteral obstruction. Am. J. Physiol. 225:830, 1973.
6. Vaughan, E. D., Jr. and Gillenwater, J. Y. Diagnosis, characterization and management of postobstructive diuresis. J. Urol. 109:286, 1973.
7. Vaughan, E. D., Jr., Shenasky, J. H., II, and Gillenwater, J. Y. Mechanism of acute hemodynamic response to ureteral occlusion. Invest. Urol. 9:109, 1971.
8. Vaughan, E. D., Jr., Sorenson, E. J., and Gillenwater, J. Y. The renal hemodynamic response to chronic unilateral complete ureteral occlusion. Invest. Urol. 8:78, 1970.

5

Reflux

ARTHUR W. WYKER, JR.

Urine is normally transported unidirectionally from the kidney to the urethral meatus. When urine is regurgitated from the bladder to the ureter, it is called vesicoureteral reflux. Reflux is *never normal*, and surveys of apparently normal prematures and children and clinical experience with adults reveal the incidence to be close to zero.

URETEROVESICAL VALVE

A properly constructed valve permits movement of fluid in one direction only or temporarily closes a passage or orifice. This is usually accomplished by membranous folds within the lumen (*e.g.*, venous valves) or muscular sphincters around the lumen (*e.g.*, pyloric sphincter). The intravesical ureter has no membranous folds within its lumen and no circular muscle fibers around its lumen. *Its valvelike action appears to be chiefly passive with the intravesical ureter being compressed against its underlying bladder muscle by the intravesical pressure.* This valvelike action does not require the presence of active neuromuscular function, for reflux cannot be produced in excised or intact postmortem human bladders.

In the venous valve (Fig. 1), the membranous folds within the lumen are inclined in the normal direction of flow toward the heart, and reversal of this direction causes the free edges to come together, preventing reversal of flow. In the muscular sphincter (Fig. 2), contraction of circular muscle squeezes the lumen shut, preventing reversal of flow. The oblique course of the intravesical ureter (Fig. 3) permits the intravesical pressure to compress it against supporting bladder muscle, closing the ureteral lumen and preventing reflux.

Stephens and Tanagho believe that the valvelike action at the ureterovesical junction is active rather than passive, the ureteral lumen being closed by the active contraction of the intrinsic longitudinal muscle fibers of the intravesical ureter and trigone.

Whether the ureterovesical valve is passive or active, the main determinant of reflux is the *length of the submucosal ureteral tunnel.*

1. In animals and humans, the shorter the tunnel, the greater the probability of reflux.

70

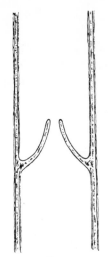

Fig. 1.

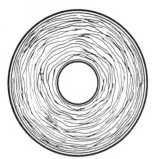

Fig. 2.

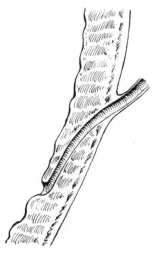

Fig. 3.

2. Clinically, over 90% of patients exhibiting reflux have a short or absent submucosal tunnel.

3. The formation of a submucosal ureteral tunnel of adequate length is the basis of all successful antireflux operations.

4. Paquin emphasized the importance of the ratio of the length of the intravesical ureter to the diameter of the ureteral orifice.

A. Ratio = $\dfrac{\text{intravesical length}}{\text{diameter of ureteral orifice}}$

1) Normal (no reflux) $\dfrac{2.5\text{--}16}{1}$ with average $\dfrac{6\text{--}7}{1}$

2) Refluxing ureters $\dfrac{0.1\text{--}1.4}{1}$ with average $\dfrac{0.75}{1}$

3) All ureters with ratio $< \dfrac{1.4}{1}$ refluxed

$> \dfrac{2.5}{1}$ did not reflux

4) At surgery, he aimed for at least a 5 to 1 ratio.

B. Normal values and ratios per age (Cussen).

Age	$\dfrac{\text{intravesical length (cm)}}{\text{diameter of ureteral orifice (cm)}}$	Ratio
1) 0 to 3 months	$\dfrac{0.5}{0.11}$	$\dfrac{4.5}{1}$
2) 1 to 3 years	$\dfrac{0.7}{0.14}$	$\dfrac{5}{1}$
3) 3 to 6 years	$\dfrac{0.7}{0.17}$	$\dfrac{4.1}{1}$
4) 6 to 9 years	$\dfrac{0.9}{0.2}$	$\dfrac{4.5}{1}$
5) 9 to 12 years	$\dfrac{1.2}{0.19}$	$\dfrac{6.3}{1}$

Note that both the length of the intravesical ureter and the diameter of the ureteral orifice increase with age, but the *ratio is essentially unchanged.*

IS REFLUX HARMFUL?

Patients with unilateral reflux tend to have some dilation of the involved upper urinary tract with varying degrees of caliectasis as contrasted to the normal appearance of the nonrefluxing side. With complete duplication of the ureters, the lower pelvis ureter often permits reflux, whereas the upper pelvis ureter usually does not. Pyelonephritic changes appear only in the lower kidney segment, the one with the refluxing ureter. Reflux is therefore *both abnormal and potentially harmful.*

HOW DOES REFLUX DAMAGE THE UPPER URINARY TRACT?

1. Infection.

A. Bacteria that get into the bladder are transported to the ureter and kidney with resultant ureteritis and pyelonephritis.

1) This causes loss of renal function and impairment of ureteral peristalsis.

2) The refluxed urine usually returns to the bladder within 30 min, but the bacteria may adhere to the renal pelvis and calyces for many hours.

3) Corriere and Lipschultz[4] introduced radioactive colloidal particles the size of bacteria into the bladders of patients with vesicoureteral reflux.

    a) Refluxed fluid returned to the bladder within 30 min, but the particles remained in the kidney for up to 5 hours in many patients.

B. Most patients with reflux have recurrent urinary infections.

C. Reflux appears to be the most common cause of chronic pyelonephritis.

D. Infection may cause reflux, probably by rendering the intravesical ureter rigid and pipelike so that it cannot be closed by the intravesical pressure.

1) When the infection is eradicated, reflux stops.

2) Auer and Seager[2] produced reflux in normal dogs by infiltrating saline around the ureteral orifice.

E. Reflux does not cause infection, but the residual urine present after voiding makes the urinary tract more vulnerable to invading bacteria.

2. Pressure.

A. When free reflux is present, there is an intact fluid column from the bladder to the kidney, and when this fluid is compressed by the contracting detrusor muscle, the intravesical pressure is *transmitted to the renal pelvis*.

1) Gruber,[6] over 40 years ago, produced unilateral reflux in excised animal and human bladders by excising the ventral half of the right intravesical ureter and firmly ligating the urethra.

    a) When he raised the intravesical pressure, he noted an *identical increase* in the intraureteral pressure on the right refluxing side with no change on the left nonrefluxing normal side.

2) Williams and Eckstein[15] studied two patients with reflux and recorded a 41-cm rise of pressure in the renal pelvis during voiding.

B. The intravesical pressure during voiding may be as low as 25 cm of water or as high as 150 cm of water, but it always far exceeds the normal resting pressure in the renal pelvis of less than 10 cm of water.

1) These transmitted high pressure waves pound the kidney against its relatively unyielding capsule, slowly destroying it.

C. When infravesical obstruction accompanies reflux, the resultant abnormally high intravesical pressure may accelerate renal damage.

D. Clinically, the renal damage secondary to reflux is usually due to the combined effects of infection and back pressure.

1) We have seen two patients with terminal renal insufficiency secondary to reflux and *there was no evidence, past or present, of infection or obstruction*.

    a) This indicates that back pressure alone may destroy the kidneys.

3. Intrarenal reflux of urine.

A. Hodson and others have demonstrated *intrarenal* reflux with contrast material escaping into the substance of the kidney with resultant *chemical pyelonephritis*.

B. The significance of this factor in causing reflux-induced pyelonephritis awaits further studies.

C. This mechanism may explain the renal damage sustained by some reflux patients despite a negative history for urinary infection or obstruction.

ETIOLOGY AND CLASSIFICATION OF REFLUX

To maintain competence, the normal ureterovesical valve has:
1. Adequate length submucosal ureteral segment.
2. Firm muscle backing.
3. Compressibility.

When one or more of these three essential anatomical factors is absent, the valve becomes incompetent and reflux results.

CLASSIFICATION

1. Short or absent submucosal ureteral segment.
   A. Congenital.
      1) Lateral ectopia or megatrigone—megacystis.
      2) Complete duplication of ureters.

   a) The ureter to the lower segment of the kidney has the shorter tunnel and is the one most likely to reflux.
   B. Iatrogenic—destruction of roof of submucosal tunnel.
      1) Ureteral meatotomy.
         a) Ureterocele.
         b) Calculus in intravesical ureter.
         c) Transurethral resection (TUR) of bladder tumor.
2. Loss of firm muscle backing.
   A. *Paraureteral diverticulum* or saccule secondary to bladder outlet obstruction or neurogenic bladder.
      1) Hutch[9] first demonstrated this mechanism of reflux.
      2) With infravesical obstruction, the forceful bladder contractions required to empty the bladder raise the pressure inside the bladder and may force the mucosa between the thickened, spread apart muscle fibers producing cellules and diverticula.
      3) These weak blowout pouches often develop near the intravesical ureter since its entry point into bladder is a weak area.
      4) When a saccule or diverticulum is present behind the intravesical ureter, the firm backing is lost, the submucosal ureteral segment is shortened, and reflux occurs.
      5) In the upper motor neuron neurogenic bladder, repeated uncon-

trolled impulses from the isolated stump of the spinal cord cause frequent detrusor contractions.

    a) The external urethral sphincter does not relax when the detrusor contracts, but it is *hypertonic and obstructive.*

  B. Congenital paraureteral diverticulum.

  C. Weakness of bladder muscle behind the intravesical ureter.

    1) Prune-belly syndrome.

    2) Lower motor neuron neurogenic bladder.

3. Loss of compressibility.

  A. Inflammation of the bladder.

    1) The intravesical ureter becomes rigid and it cannot be closed by the intravesical pressure.

4. Mechanism obscure.

  A. Bladder outlet obstruction without any associated loss of muscle backing.

  B. Ectopic ureter opening near the bladder neck or in the midurethra.

CLINICAL FINDINGS

Signs and Symptoms

Patients are *most commonly children* with a history of recurrent urinary infections, often accompanied by fever, sometimes by flank pain. There are two symptoms which specifically suggest reflux.

1. Flank or CVA pain during voiding.

  A. With free, complete reflux, the patient actually voids into the involved kidney, distending the renal pelvis with resultant pain.

    1) When voiding ceases, the refluxed urine returns to the bladder and the pain disappears.

2. After voiding.

  A. Urine that has refluxed to one or both kidneys returns to the bladder within 10 min after voiding as *residual urine.*

  B. This residual urine may be passed or may dribble out only 10 to 15 min after initial voiding, and this is called *after voiding.*

X-RAY STUDIES

Intravenous Urogram

1. Early finding—segmental dilation of the ureter with flabby appearance.

  A. Ureter that is subject to reflux is usually abnormally distensible but normally contractile.

2. Late finding—changes seen in chronic pyelonephritis.

  A. Calyectasis, usually generalized, is commonly first detected and most severe in the upper calyx.

  B. Loss of renal substance may be evident by the decreased distance between calyx and the outer margin of the kidney.

1) This occurs most commonly in the upper pole region.

2) A 1- or 2-min film usually gives a good nephrogram effect facilitating measurement of the thickness of the renal substance.

Cystogram

Although the presence of reflux may be suggested by the intravenous urogram, it is established by properly performed cystograms.

1. Since infection may cause reflux, perform cystograms when the patient is *uninfected* or has been treated with antibacterial agents.

2. To standardize our studies and to roughly quantitate reflux, we perform cystograms at 15-cm pressure and at 40-cm pressure, or during voiding.

A. If reflux is detected at both 15-cm and 40-cm pressure, we call it *low pressure reflux*.

B. If reflux is detected only at 40-cm pressure or during voiding, we call it *high pressure reflux*.

C. If reflux occurs, an additional drainout film is taken 10 min after the high pressure study to rule out obstruction.

CYSTOSCOPY

1. The location and configuration of the ureteral orifices are important indicators of the probability of reflux.

A. The more laterally placed and the larger the lumen, the greater the probability of reflux.

B. Patulous and golf-hole orifices usually permit reflux.

C. With complete duplication of the ureters, the upper ureteral orifice draining the lower kidney segment often permits reflux.

D. Ectopic ureteral orifice near the bladder neck often permits reflux.

2. Fully distend the bladder and look for a saccule or a diverticulum near the ureteral orifice.

3. Check for evidence of prior surgery which might have damaged the roof of the submucosal tunnel.

4. When cystograms are not feasible, the presence of reflux can be established by cystoscopy.

A. Instill Indigo carmine-stained saline into the bladder until the intravesical pressure is 40 cm of water.

B. Remove the catheter and insert a cystoscope without allowing any fluid to escape from the bladder.

C. Gradually exchange clear irrigating fluid for blue bladder fluid, keeping bladder pressure around 40 cm of water.

1) This prevents efflux from the ureters.

D. When the bladder fluid is minimally blue-stained, let the fluid drain out gradually and carefully observe both ureteral orifices.

1) Efflux of blue fluid from either orifice indicates reflux.

MANAGEMENT OF REFLUX

Patients with milder degrees of reflux who are not deemed candidates for antireflux operations are placed on the following regimen.

1. Double voiding.

A. Five minutes after voiding, the patient voids a second time, making every effort to empty the bladder on each occasion.

B. The aim is to reduce the amount of residual urine to the minimum to prevent urinary infection.

2. Voiding by the clock.

A. The patient voids every 2 to 3 hours whether she feels like it or not.

B. The desire to void occurs when a critical level of intravesical pressure is reached.

1) Voiding before this critical level is reached is believed to place less stress on the incompetent ureterovesical junction.

3. Long-term antimicrobial therapy.

A. Reflux creates residual urine in the bladder, and this makes the bladder more vulnerable to invading bacteria.

B. Nitrofurantoin, 50 mg b.i.d., is excellent for this purpose.

Surgery

The formation of a submucosal tunnel of adequate length is the basis of all successful antireflux operations. If the ureter is of normal size, antireflux surgery eliminates reflux over 90% of the time, but if the ureter is grossly dilated and thick walled, the success rate is significantly lower.

Our chief indication for surgery is a history of recurrent episodes of urinary infection plus *evidence of progressive damage to the involved ureter and kidney*. These patients usually have the following.

1. Reflux occurs at both low and high pressure and is complete.

2. Intravenous urogram reveals changes of chronic pyelonephritis with loss of renal substance.

3. On cystoscopy, refluxing orifice is usually more laterally placed than normal and is patulous or golf-hole in appearance.

4. Renal function is decreased in the involved kidney.

REFERENCES AND SUGGESTED READING

1. Ambrose, S. S. and Nicolson, W. P., III. The causes of vesicoureteral reflux in children. J. Urol. 87:688, 1962.
2. Auer, J. and Seager, L. D. Experimental local bladder edema causing urine reflux into ureter and kidney. J. Exp. Med. 66:741, 1937.
3. Castro, J. and Fine, H. Passive antireflux mechanisms in human cadaver bladders. Br. J. Urol. 41:559, 1969.
4. Corriere, J. N., Jr. and Lipschultz, L. I. The clearance of refluxed bacteria sized sulfur colloid particles from the human kidney. Curr. Top. Surg. Res. 3:191, 1971.
5. Cussen, L. J. Dimensions of the normal ureter in infancy and childhood. Invest. Urol. 5:164, 1967.
6. Gruber, C. M. The uretero-vesical valve and experimental production of hydroureter without obstruction. Proc. Soc. Exp. Biol. Med. 25:329, 1927–28.

7. Gruber, C. M. I. A comparative study of the intra-vesical ureters (uretero-vesical valves) in man and in experimental animals. J. Urol. 21:567, 1928.
8. Gruber, C. M. II. The uretero-vesical valve. J. Urol. 22:275, 1929.
9. Hutch, J. A. *The Ureterovesical Junction.* University of California Press, Berkeley 1958.
10. Jones, B. W. and Headstream, J. W. Vesicoureteral reflux in children. J. Urol. 80:114, 1958.
11. King, L. R., Surian, M. A., Wendel, R. M., and Burden, J. J. Vesicoureteral reflux—a classification based on cause and the results of treatment. J.A.M.A. 203:169, 1968.
12. McGovern, J. H., Marshall, V. F., and Paquin, A. J., Jr. Vesicoureteral regurgitation in children. J. Urol. 83:122, 1960.
13. Stephens, F. D. and Lenaghan, D. The anatomical basis and dynamics of vesicoureteric reflux. J. Urol. 87:669, 1962.
14. Tanagho, E. A., Guthrie, T. H., and Lyon, R. P. The intravesical ureter in primary reflux. J. Urol. 101:824, 1969.
15. Williams, D. I. and Eckstein, H. B. Surgical treatment of reflux in children. Br. J. Urol. 37:13, 1965.

6

Urinary Tract Infection

JAY Y. GILLENWATER

INTRODUCTION AND DEFINITIONS

Urinary tract infections are second in frequency only to infections of the upper respiratory tract. The incidence and degree of morbidity and mortality from infections are greater with those in the urinary tract than with those of the upper respiratory tract. About one-third of patients dying of renal failure have infection as the primary kidney disease. To provide a common frame of reference, it is necessary to define the terms.

A. *Bacteriuria* means bacteria in the urine. It can represent colonization of bacteria in the urine both with and without infection and inflammation of the various structures in the urinary tract.

B. The term *urinary tract infection* is believed by many to imply bacteriuria *plus* bacterial invasion of the tissues of the urinary tract. However, since it is difficult to assess clinically how much inflammation and bacterial invasion of the tissues actually exists, the terms *bacteriuria* and *urinary tract infection* are used synonymously in this chapter.

C. Infection of the urinary tract predominately in the urethra is called *urethritis, cystitis* in the bladder, *prostatitis* in the prostate, and *pyelonephritis* in the kidney.

D. *Asymptomatic bacteriuria* refers to colonization of bacteria in the voided urine without any signs or symptoms.

E. *Reinfection* of bacteriuria is the recurrence of bacteriuria with a different microorganism after the successful treatment of the original infection.

F. *Relapse of bacteriuria* is the recurrence of bacteriuria with the same microorganism after therapy.

G. Uncomplicated *acute urinary tract infection* is defined as infection of the upper or lower urinary tract without structural or neurological abnormalities. The organism is usually *Escherichia coli*, and the clinician expects excellent results with appropriate antimicrobial therapy.

H. *Complicated (or surgical) urinary tract infections* are infections associated with structural changes (stones, obstruction, and scarring), neurological changes, or bacterial species resistant to many antimicrobials (such as *Pseudomonas*). The results of therapy are likely to be less successful than with the uncomplicated infection.

PATHOGENESIS

Bacteria may enter and spread within the urinary tract by three mechanisms: 1) ascending, 2) hematogeneous, 3) lymphatic.

Ascending

The ascending pathway is considered to be the most frequent means of introduction of bacteria into the urinary tract. Bacteria from the intestinal tract have been shown to be the reservoir for urinary tract infections. Retrograde or ascending infections historically have been considered important because urinary tract infection occurs much more frequently in females than in males, attributed to the contamination through the short urethra of girls. The high rate of infections after instrumentation (2%) suggested that passage of the catheter through the urethra pushed bacteria into the bladder. Urethral catheters left indwelling invariably result in bacteriuria, again presumably ascending infection. Studies of females by Cox and Hinman and of males by Helmholz showed a few bacteria present in the normal female and male urethra. Recently, studies by Stamey[5] were somewhat conflicting with the above reports, but they graphically showed that the ascending route of infection is probably the most important in the female. Stamey demonstrated that the normal vaginal vestibule and urethral meatus contained only Lactobacilli, Corynebacterium, *Haemophilus vaginalis*, *Staphlococcus albus*, and nonhemolytic Streptococci. That is, few individuals who had never had a urinary tract infection had colonization of the common urinary pathogens. However, when he studied patients having frequent urinary tract infections, he found that the urinary tract infections were preceded by colonization of that bacteria on the vaginal and urethral openings. These studies were interpreted as showing that in most ascending urinary tract infections, the first event may be the breakdown of host resistance to allow colonization of the pathological bacteria on the introitus.

Hematogenous

Hematogenous infection of the kidney has been shown to occur clinically and experimentally and is certainly the route of infection in some patients.

Lymphatic

The importance of the lymphatic route of infection has not been ascertained. It has been shown that particles introduced into the bladder under increased pressure (70 to 100 cm H_2O) can be transmitted by the lymphatics to the kidneys. Possible lymphatic connections between the intestinal tract and the kidney have been postulated, but this has not been clearly proven.

NORMAL HOST RESISTANCE

Lower Urinary Tract

Despite the relatively easy access of bacteria to the urinary tract, normally it is fairly resistant to infection. Cox and Hinman showed that after introduction of 10^5 E. coli into normal male bladders, the urine was sterile after 72 hours. None of these individuals had any clinical signs or symptoms of urinary tract infection. Complete emptying of the bladder is certainly an important factor; however, there will always be a thin film of infected urine left in the bladder. It has been shown experimentally at least that the bacteria close to the mucosal surface of the bladder can be killed. Whether this is due to phagocytosis by leukocytes or secretion of an antibacterial substance by the bladder mucosal cell is not known. The urine normally supports bacterial growth except in conditions of high or low pH and extremes of dilution or concentration.

Upper Urinary Tract

The renal medulla has been found to be much more susceptible to infection than the renal cortex. The postulated reasons for this will be discussed.

1. The medulla has high concentrations of ammonia which have been shown to inhibit the fourth component of complement.

2. Hypertonicity of the medulla decreases the phagocytosis of the leukocytes, and the lower blood supply to the renal medulla would make fewer leukocytes available than in the renal cortex.

3. The high osmolality of the renal medulla would favor persistence of protoplasts (a form of bacteria deficient in cell walls and thus resistant to many antibiotics that kill bacteria through degradation of the cell wall).

CLINICAL MANIFESTATIONS
Upper Urinary Tract

Classical symptoms of upper urinary tract infections (pyelonephritis) are fever, chills, flank pain, and tenderness, as well as the lower urinary tract symptoms of frequency and dysuria. It should be stated that some patients may have few symptoms and yet lose renal function with chronic pyelonephritis. Especially in children, there are frequently the additional gastrointestinal symptoms of anorexia, nausea, vomiting, diarrhea, and abdominal pain.

Lower Urinary Tract

Lower urinary tract symptoms of infection are (in cystitis or prostatitis) vesical irritability (frequency, urgency, dysuria), sometimes hematuria, and vague lower abdominal or perineal discomfort. Many patients describe a pressure feeling over the suprapubic area. Fever is not seen as frequently when the infection is confined to the lower urinary tract.

DIAGNOSIS

Urinary tract infections are diagnosed by quantitatively culturing bacteria from the urine. Normally, urine is sterile and the presence of bacteria (the quantity depends on method and location of collection) in the urine is used to represent tissue involvement, although theoretically one could have colonization of bacteria in the urine without tissue invasion. Presumptive evidence of urinary tract infection is sometimes made by observing bacteria in a centrifuged urine specimen under the microscope. This method is reported to be 20% inaccurate. The finding of five or more white blood cells per high power field in the centrifuged urine specimen is reported to occur in only about 50% of patients with asymptomatic bacteriuria.

Thus, if the diagnosis of urinary tract infections is going to be based on quantitatively culturing bacteria, it is important for the student to understand how and why this is done. In 1941, Marple was the first to measure quantitatively the number of bacteria in the urine, and the concept was popularized by Kass in 1955. Strict control over the methods of urine collection, storage, and transportation of specimens proved necessary because of bacterial contamination of the samples. Although urine normally is sterile, it is an excellent culture medium. Thus, if small numbers of bacteria (with a doubling time of 20 to 45 min) are introduced into the urine from the urethra or labia, counts of 10^8 to 10^9/ml can be achieved in a short time. It was shown by these investigators that if the perineum was cleansed, a midstream or catheterized specimen obtained and immediately cultured or refrigerated at 4°C until culture, most of the bacterial counts in the urine cultures were either greater than 100,000 col/ml or less than 1,000 col/ml. Those specimens less than 1,000 were assumed to represent contamination and those over 100,000 were assumed to represent urinary tract infections. In general, these concepts have withstood the test of time and are accepted by all physicians. Therefore the method of urine collection is important. The most accurate method is suprapubic needle aspiration of the bladder. Stamey[5] reported 2,500 aspirations without complications. When the patient has a full bladder, a $3\frac{1}{2}$-inch sterile, 22-gauge needle attached to a syringe is inserted into the bladder through the skin one finger-breadth above the symphysis pubis, with or without anesthetizing the skin. Similar accuracy can be obtained by having a trained nurse collect a midstream specimen as the patient voids from a cystoscopy table after being carefully prepped. The specimen can be obtained by bladder catheterization, but this method carries about a 3% risk of introducing an infection. Most urine specimens from females are obtained by having the patient sit backwards on the toilet seat, cleanse the labia, spread the labia with one hand, and then collect a midstream specimen. This method has a reported reliability of 80 to 95% with a single collection. Falsely low bacterial counts will occur if urine is collected during a diuresis, contamination of the urine with antibacterial detergents, presence of antibiotics or urinary acidifiers. Falsely high counts may occur with contamination of the specimen or failure to refrigerate promptly the specimen to prevent bacterial multiplication. Quantification of bacteria is performed by obtaining proper dilutions of the urine and counting the number of bacteria on the culture plate. Since normal urine is sterile, the identification of even small numbers of bacteria from direct aspiration or collection from the bladder, ureter, or renal pelvis is considered to represent infection. It should be stated that with most urinary tract infections, the bacteria will number more than 10^8/ml of bladder urine.

Localization of Infection

In general, accurate localization of the exact portions of the urinary tract which are involved in an infection is difficult, and one could argue the importance, since the goal of therapy is to eradicate bacteria from all parts of the urinary tract. The localization of the infection to the upper or lower urinary tract, however, does have some prognostic and therapeutic implications. The presence of renal infection may necessitate a more vigorous course of treatment. In the male, it is important to determine whether or not the infection involves the prostate since eradication of bacteria from the prostate is difficult. In the well hydrated male, the foreskin is retracted, the glans cleansed, and the specimen collected in four parts:

A. *First voided* 10 ml (assumed to represent urethra).

B. *Second voided* (assumed to represent bladder and kidney).

C. *Prostatic secretions* expressed by rectal examination.

D. *A voided specimen after prostatic massage* (representing the prostate).

Localization of the infection to the upper or lower tract can be determined by the urologist obtaining a urine specimen from the bladder and renal pelvis. There has been some correlation with renal involvement of infection causing impairment of urinary concentration and high specific serum antibody titers. Clinically, the kidney usually is assumed to be infected if the patient has fever, flank pain, and tenderness.

EPIDEMIOLOGY

E. coli is cultured from most initial urinary tract infections, principally strains 04, 06, 075, 01, 02, and 07. Serotyping the bacteria allows differentiation between *relapse* (reappearance of the original organism) and *reinfection* (appearance of a different organism, seen in over 80% of recurrent infections). With hospital-acquired infections and those associated with structural abnormalities of the urinary tract, one sees a higher incidence of infections caused by *Proteus*, *Pseudomonas*, and *Klebsiella-Enterobacter*. The prevalence of bacteriuria in young adults is about 1.2% in women and 0.5% in men. As age increases to about 60 years, the prevalence is about 15% in men and women.

The prevalence of bacteriuria among newborns having suprapubic puncture is reported to be 1% with two-thirds of these being males. Autopsy series in children show about 2% incidence of pyelonephritis. Kunin studied children of school age in Charlottesville between 1959 and 1969 and showed that prevalence of bacteriuria (frequency at one point in time) is 1.2% in girls and 0.03% in boys. Each year, 0.3 to 0.4% of the girls who were previously uninfected developed bacteriuria. Thus, during their 12 years of primary and secondary education, 4.5 to 6% of school girls would be expected to have at least one episode of bacteriuria. When these girls were studied, 20% had reflux on cystograms, and 13% had evidence of caliectasis on intravenous urogram. The bacteriuria was treated by appropriate antimicrobial therapy for 2 weeks which eradicated the bacteriuria in 85% (15% single treatment failure). Sixty-five percent developed bacteriuria again within 2 years, and most recurrences (80%) appeared to be caused by infection with new organisms. Thus, each treatment did cause remission in 20% of the girls, and the parents can justifiably be told that with a 10-day to 2-week course of the appropriate antibiotic for each episode of urinary tract infection most children will eventually "outgrow" the tendency to have urinary tract infections during their school years. About one-third of the patients who were found to have "asymptomatic bacteriuria" did reveal symptoms of some urgency, frequency or dysuria on careful questioning.

BACTERIURIA OF PREGNANCY

The prevalence of bacteriuria during pregnancy is reported to be 4 to 6%. Kass (1959) and others have shown that early treatment of bacteriuria prevented the 20% incidence of acute symptomatic pyelonephritis observed in a control bacteriuric group tested by placebo. The incidence of bacteriuria in pregnancy increases with parity and is reported to be higher in the lower socioeconomic groups. Studies by Fairley (1966) showed that about 50% of pregnant bacteriuric patients had bacteria in the upper tracts. Prematurity seems to be increased in mothers with bacteriuria and with symptomatic pyelonephritis. However, treatment of the bacteriuria has not altered statistically the incidence of prematurity. It has been suggested but not conclusively proven that there is a relationship between bacteriuria and toxemia of pregnancy. Radiological studies of the kidney after delivery of patients with bacteriuria showed abnormalities in about one-half. Cystograms showed reflux in 21%. Brumfitt's investigations (1967) showed that those patients cured of bacteriuria by a single course of therapy had 23% upper tract abnormalities on x-ray, while those who remained bacteriuric despite therapy had a 65% incidence of radiological abnormalities.

The lesson seems quite clear that the patient who is refractory to treatment should have urological workup at some time after delivery. With a life-threatening infection during pregnancy, an intravenous urogram should be performed to rule out an infection behind some form of obstruction, *e.g.*, stone. Studies show that if the bacteriuria during pregnancy is untreated, 35 to 80% of patients will continue to have bacteriuria 3 to 12 months after delivery. Antimicrobial therapy in bacteriuria of pregnancy is justified, if for no other reason than to prevent the morbidity of subsequent pyelonephritis. A short course of therapy with the appropriate antibiotics and a close followup are recommended.

MANAGEMENT

Adequate therapy for bacteriuria is justified to manage the morbidity associated with upper and lower urinary tract infections and, in addition, to attempt to prevent deterioration of renal function. Therapy should be determined by the *in vitro* sensitivity studies, and one should strive for eradication, not suppression of the bacteria. Urine cultures should be sterile after 2 or 3 days of therapy. Most investigators have found a 10- to 14-day course of therapy is sufficient with little to be gained by continuing medication for 6 to 12 weeks. Many investigators now believe that in eradicating urinary tract infections, urinary levels of the antimicrobial drugs are more important than the serum levels.

Adequate Follow-up

It is essential that the physician determine sometime after therapy that the drugs have, in fact, sterilized the urine, since this is the goal of therapy.

Treatment in Renal Failure

The dosage of many antimicrobial agents must be modified in patients with renal insufficiency. Therapy in these patients presents several problems.

1. Accumulation of drugs with resultant nephrotoxicity and ototoxicity and providing effective levels of the drugs in the urine to eradicate the bacteriuria.
2. Drugs such as the penicillins, cephalosporins, and aminoglycosides may achieve adequate urinary levels, while nitrofurantoin may not.
3. The tetracyclines (have antianabolic effect), organic acids (cause acidosis), and sulfonamides (may crystallize in the tubules in oliguric patients) should be avoided in severe renal failure.
4. In administering antibiotics to patients in renal failure, it should be remembered that the initial loading dose is the same as normal. The frequency of administration of subsequent doses will depend upon the degree of renal failure and the persistence of the drug in the serum. Reinfections should also be treated with short courses of appropriate antibiotics.

Complicated Infections

1. In some circumstances, it is not possible to eradicate the bacteria and prolonged therapy will only cause the development of a resistant flora, and if the patient has septicemia, the infection will be much more difficult to cure. Some examples are patients with long-term indwelling catheters, conduits, stones, cystoceles, etc.
2. Patients who have frequent episodes of reinfection should be instructed to void after intercourse, to void frequently, and to decrease perineal bacterial flora by cleansing with Phisohex or Betadine, all of which may be helpful.
3. Prophylactic therapy with urinary acidification or small doses of nitrofurantoin sometimes is justified. Nitrofurantoin has the advantage of leaving the fecal flora, which is thought to be the reservoir of bacteria, unaltered. Thus, a subsequent infection should not occur from a resistant organism.
4. Therapy for patients with prostatitis is more difficult because of the blood prostatic barrier which prevents an adequate antibiotic level from being achieved in the prostatic ductal lumens. Trimethoprim, which was recently introduced in the United States, in combination with sulfamethoxazole does achieve adequate levels in the prostate. Chronic bacterial prostatitis is believed to cause relapse of urinary tract infections in the male.

Patients having acute complicated urinary tract infections should be started immediately on one of the more potent bactericidal broad spectrum drugs such as gentamicin.

It is my feeling that, after therapy for the first episode of bacteriuria, every patient should have an intravenous urogram. If an abnormality is noted on the urograms, then cystograms and cystoscopy should be performed. In frequent infections or pyelonephritis, the patient initially should have the cystograms and cystoscopy performed as well as the intravenous urograms.

It is important for the student and physician to remember that when an individual patient has a severe episode of pyelonephritis, with or without associated bacteremia, the underlying problem may be an infection behind an obstruction. Relief of the obstruction is more essential to the survival of this patient than the administration of antibiotics. When an obstruction is present, the infected urine is forced into the renal venous and lymphatic circulation and thus into the systemic circulation. We have seen many patients come immediately out of endotoxemia and shock after release of the obstruction by passing a catheter or surgical removal of a stone. Thus, in these patients it is necessary to perform the intravenous urogram during the infection and not postpone it until later—since the patient would not be around later.

REFERENCES AND SUGGESTED FURTHER READING

1. Brumfitt, W., Grünberg, R. N., and Leigh, D. A. Bacteriuria of pregnancy with reference to prematurity and long-term effects on the mother, in *Symposium on Pyelonephritis*, Edinburgh, 1966, p. 20.
2. Cox, C. E. and Hinman, F., Jr. Experiments with induced bacteriuria, vesicle emptying, and bacterial growth on the mechanism of bladder defense to infection. J. Urol. 86:739, 1961.
3. Helmholz, H. F., Sr. Determination of the bacterial content of the urethra: a new method with results of a study of 82 men. J. Urol. 64:158, 1950.
4. Kaye, D. *Urinary Tract Infection and Its Management*. C. V. Mosby Company, St. Louis, 1972.
5. Kunin, C. M. *Detection, Prevention and Management of Urinary Tract Infections*. Lea and Febiger, Philadelphia, 1972.
6. O'Grady, F. and Brumfitt, W. *Urinary Tract Infection*. Oxford University Press, London, 1968.
7. Smallpiece, V. *Urinary Tract Infection in Childhood and Its Relevance to Disease in Adult Life*. C. V. Mosby Company, St. Louis, 1969.
8. Stamey, T. A. *Urinary Infections*. Williams and Wilkins Company, Baltimore, 1972.

7

Embryology and Congenital Anomalies of the Genitourinary System

E. DARRACOTT VAUGHAN, JR.
GEORGE W. MIDDLETON

INTRODUCTION

The recognition, classification, interpretation, and management of congenital abnormalities of the genitourinary system are dependent on a clear understanding of normal genitourinary embryology. Hence the present chapter is primarily concerned with the embryological development of the normal genitourinary tract.

This information would appear to be pertinent in view of the fact that about 10% of all infants are born with some anomaly, and about 30 to 40% of these anomalies involve the genitourinary system.

KIDNEY

1. The nephrogenic cord arises by longitudinal fusion of the intermediate mesoderm which arises between the medial paraxial mass and the lateral plate.

A. Pronephros. Seven paired segments can be identified by the 28th day with complete regression by the 5th week.

B. Mesonephros. Thirty units arise from the nephrogenic cord and divide into mesonephric vesicles at the cephalic end while growing in a caudal direction. The prime role of the mesonephros is in the later development of the ureter and genital systems, which will be discussed subsequently.

C. Metanephros. This structure arises (1) from the caudal portion of the nephrogenic cord (S-2 to S-3), *i.e.*, the metanephric blastema, and (2) from the ureteric outgrowth from the caudal part of the mesonephric duct, *i.e.*, the ureteral bud. Both of these components are mesodermal in origin.

1) Metanephric blastema. Further development of this blastema into the definitive metanephros appears to be dependent on contact with the ureteral bud. Therefore, development of this component can be discussed in conjunction with discussion of the development of the ureteral bud.

2) Ureteral bud. The development of the ureteral bud has been extensively studied by Potter, who divides its maturation into 4 periods (Fig. 1).

a. Period I (5th to 14th week). The ureteric bud arises from the posteromedial wall of the mesonephric duct near the cloaca. Caudal to the

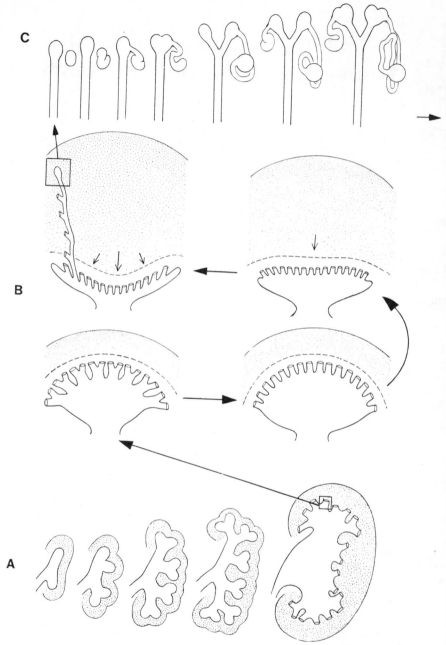

Fig. 1. Schematic representation of the development of the ureteric bud, calyces, papillae, and ampullae in the metanephros. *A*, the early formation of the pelvis and major and minor calyces by division of the ureteric bud; *B*, the development of the calyces and papillae; *C*, the division of ampullae and the induction of nephrogenic vesicles by the ampullae during the first period of metanephric development; *D*, further induction by an ampulla of arcades of nephrons, during the second period of metanephric development; *E*, the migration of the ampulla into the

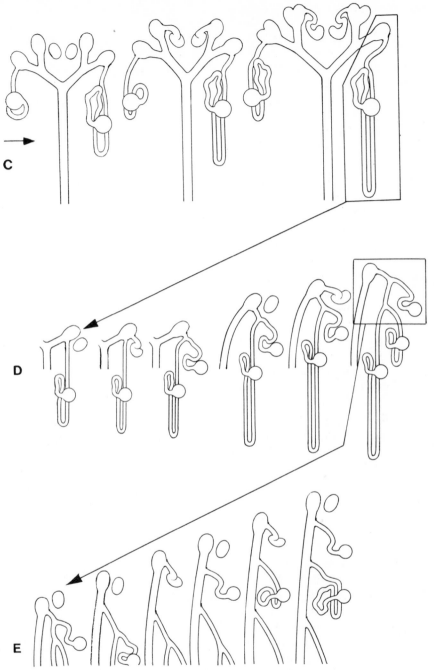

Fig. 1.

peripheral part of the cortex with the formation of more nephrons, during the third period of metanephric development. (Redrawn after Osathanondh and Potter.) (Reproduced with permission from Hamilton, W. J., Boyd, J. D., and Mossman, H. W.: The urogenital system, in *Human Embryology*, Ed. 4, Chap. 12, edited by Hamilton, W. J. and Mossman, H. W., The Williams and Wilkins Company, Baltimore, 1972.)

bud, the mesonephric duct is called the common duct. The ureteral bud grows dorsally and its origin migrates to the posterolateral wall of the mesonephric duct. The cranial end swells forming an ampulla with further growth taking place at the ampulla as it contacts and pushes the metanephric blastema cranially. There is evidence that there is a reciprocal induction at this point. The ampulla branches in a dichotomous fashion, each branch having an ampulla at its tip. Branching is symmetrical toward the poles but shorter toward the interpolar area giving rise to the characteristic kidney shape. Three to five generations of branches contribute to the renal pelvis and major calyces. One generation forms minor calyces, and generations 7 through 11 form medullary collecting tubules. These changes occur by the 14th week.

At the 7th week, early nephrogenic vesicles derived from the metanephric blastema are induced by the sixth division ampullae from which the glomerular complex forms. At the next branching, one ampulla differentiates into a nephron while the other continues to divide and advance.

b. Period II (14th to 22nd week). This period is characterized by the formation of nephron arcades with an ampulla carrying the nephron being able to induce another. This is possible because the collecting tubule of the older nephron shifts away from the ampulla to attach as a collecting tubule for the younger nephron also.

c. Period III (20th to 36th week). Ampullary cortical advancement with formation of a series of nephrons occurs at this period. These nephrons are peripheral to the arcades.

d. Period IV (36th week to term). During this period, formation of nephrons ends and this is primarily a period of interstitial growth.

2. Position of the metanephros. Initially the metanephros is at the level of the upper sacral segments. Early blood supply is from the lateral sacral branches of the aorta. "Ascent" occurs from the 5th to 8th week and is primarily due to "unfolding" of the embryo with rapid longitudinal lumbar and sacral growth. The ventral hilum rotates to a medial position. The blood supply arises at progressively higher origins on the aorta.

3. Anomalies.

A. Failure of development.

1) Agenesis. Agenesis or absence of the kidney can occur alone or with associated anomalies of the ureter and genital system.

a. Absence of the metanephros, mesonephric derivatives, i.e., ureter, vas deferens, superficial trigone.

b. Presence of the ureter with absence of the definitive metanephros.

c. Abnormal ureter with absent kidney.

2) Hypoplasia. Failure of the kidney to reach normal size should be contrasted with aplasia, where there is only embryological renal tissue which is nonsecretory. Hypoplasia is almost always unilateral. The term dysplasia is used only if primitive elements or elements foreign to the kidney persist. Potter has suggested that this defect is one of normal

branching of the ureteral bud (group II defect) with decreased number of generations of branching.

B. Disturbances of position.

1) Simple ectopy. Malascent without crossing the midline.

2) Crossed renal ectopia. Both renal masses present on one side of the abdomen and are usually associated with fusion. Rarely, there is a single fused kidney in the pelvis. Especially rare is drainage of the entire metanephric mass by only one ureter with arrest of the other ureteral bud.

3) Malrotation. The kidney fails to rotate so that there is ventral positioning of the pelvis with a typical position of the renal hilum.

C. Vascular abnormalities.

1) Accessory vessels. The presence of multiple arteries and veins has been studied in detail with the finding that multiple veins are rare on the left. However, only 39% of autopsies show two vessels (one artery, one vein) to both sides. Additional renal veins are less common than arteries. Venous hiatuses occur most commonly on the right. These vessels may cause ureteropelvic junction obstruction or malascent.

D. Fusion anomalies.

1) Horseshoe kidney. Fusion of the upper or lower poles of the kidney, probably occurring in the 4th to 7th week of embryological development, can occur with the usual fusion being in the lower poles. There is subsequent failure of lateral motion of the lower poles and failure of normal ascent.

2) Unilaterally fused kidney. See crossed renal ectopia.

E. Cystic abnormalities.

1) Congenital infantile polycystic disease is an uncommon defect usually resulting in death within the first days or months after birth. Potter has classified this as a group I defect where there is differentiation of the kidney into collecting tubules and nephrons but hyperplasia of the collecting tubules. There is sacular dilation of the earlier collecting tubules and diffuse dilation of the later tubules. Defects are always bilateral and the nephrons are normal.

2) Multilocular cystic disease. When unilateral, this is called unilateral multicystic kidney. These kidneys are nonfunctional by conventional studies and often present as abdominal masses in children. Alternatively, a portion of the kidney may contain a multilocular cystic segment with distortion of the remainder of the collecting system and present as a renal mass in the adult. Potter has suggested that this is a type II defect (see Hypoplasia) with failure of branching of the ureteral bud.

3) Adult polycystic disease. Both kidneys show displacement of small islands of normal nephrons by multiple cysts arising in both glomerular and tubular elements. This disease is an autosomal dominant and is characterized by slowly progressive deterioration of renal function. Potter feels that this is a group III defect with variable patterns of abnormalities, with generations of nephrons being normal or reduced. However, there is also

irregular ureteral bud division, tubules show dilation, and nephrons may be normal or abnormal.

URETER

1. Cranial development. A considerable portion of ureteral embryology has already been discussed, as we have reviewed the integral part that ureteral bud development plays in the formation of the metanephros or definitive kidney.

2. Caudal development. At the time of cephalic extension of the ureteral bud, transformations occur at the caudal portion of the mesonephric duct that will subsequently determine the mesodermal components to the ureterovesical junction and trigone. At 3½ to 4 weeks, the ureteral bud appears along the dorsal medial wall of the mesonephric bud at the point of its caudal sagittal bend or "knee" (Fig. 2). The mesonephric duct distal to the ureteral bud is a common duct which becomes absorbed into the dorsal wall of the vesicourethral canal. With rapid growth of the bladder (after the cloaca is divided by the urorectal septum), there is increasing separation of the orifices of the ureter from the mesonephric ducts (see Fig. 2). The ureteral orifices move cranially and laterally while the mesonephric openings remain closed and move caudally. Thus the final opening of the orifice of the ureteral bud is lateral, and that of the mesonephric duct is medial. The tissue between the ureteral orifices and the future ejaculatory ducts (metanephric openings) is mesodermal in origin (the future trigone). Also the most distal (caudal) extension of this mesonephric component is the ejaculatory duct (male) or most of the definitive urethra (female). Thus the inner longitudinal muscular layer of the ureter persists downward past the ureteral orifice to the bladder neck as Bell's muscle and the superficial trigone. It then passes on to the verumontanum along the dorsal wall of the urethra. The connection between the bladder and ureter is derived from Waldeyer's sheath of connective tissue and muscle which surrounds the lower 2 to 3 cm of the extravesical ureter. The origin of Waldeyer's sheath appears to be derived from both ureteral and bladder components. Its medial components form the superior border of the deep trigone, while the lateral components form the lateral border of the deep trigone.

3. Anomalies.

A. Anomalies in number.

1) Partial duplication. This defect is the most common anomaly of the upper urinary tract. It is probably due to early initial branching of the ureteral ampulla prior to ascent to the level of the metanephric blastema.

2) Total duplication. In this situation, the ureters will cross before entering the bladder. The ureter whose orifice is lower and more medially placed drains the smaller, upper segment of the metanephric tissue. Being lower and more medial, its intravesical tunnel is longer, and so it is less likely to reflux than the ureter draining the lower segment. The second ureteral bud forms the duplicated ureter and arises from the mesonephric

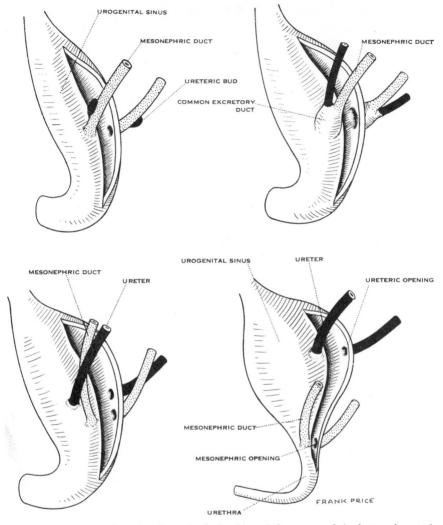

Fig. 2. Schemes to show the changed relationships of the mesonephric duct and ureteric openings into the bladder and the primitive urethra. (Reproduced with permission from Hamilton, W. J., Boyd, J. D., and Mossman, H. W.: The urogenital system, in *Human Embryology*, Ed. 4, Chap. 12, edited by Hamilton, W. J. and Mossman, H. W., The Williams & Wilkins Company, Baltimore, 1972.)

duct cranial to the initial bud. This cranial bud enters the cranial portion of the metanephric blastema, while the caudally located bud enters the lower portion. At the point of entrance into the bladder, the caudal orifice (orthotopic) is established first, but then with rapid bladder growth and incorporation of the common duct into the dorsal bladder wall, the orthotopic (normally placed) ureteral orifice rises cranially and laterally, so that as a second orifice separates from the mesonephric opening, it is located lower and more medial. Thus the orifice that drains the superior renal pelvis emerges at a point lower and medial to that draining the lower segment (Weigert-Meyer law). This caudal movement also explains why the duplicated ureters always cross in the lower one-third as they ascend to the metanephric blastema.

B. Anomalies of the ureteral orifice.

1) Duplication. Position of multiple ureteral orifices within the bladder occurring with complete duplication has been discussed.

2) Ectopia. There are two definitions of ureteral ectopia. Any orifice which is not in the orthotopic position may be considered ectopic. However, more commonly, the term has been used when the ureteral orifice is outside of the bladder. Approximately 70 to 80% of ectopic ureteral orifices are associated with duplicated ureters. In the male, the most common site of opening outside of the bladder is into the prostatic urethra (58%) and the ectopic orifice will always be proximal to the external sphincter. In the female, the most common site is in the vestibule (34%), and the presenting complaint is constant leakage of urine despite a concurrent normal voiding pattern.

3) Ureterocele. A ureterocele is a congenital or acquired cystic dilation of the distal end of the ureter. The embryological defect here is unclear, but it is generally thought to be incomplete perforation of a membrane or spur that exists between the ureteral orifice and the mesonephric opening (Chwalla).

a. Simple. A simple ureterocele arises in a ureter in which the orifice opens into the bladder.

b. Ectopic. As implied, these cystic dilations occur in a ureter whose orifice is outside of the bladder, or the ureterocele appears outside of the bladder because it is prolapsed from the interior of the bladder.

C. Agenesis. Absence of the ureter and its consequence has been discussed under Kidney above, concerning definitive formation of the metanephros.

D. Anomalies of position. Generally these are actually anomalies of the vasculature of the lower abdominal venous inferior vena caval system with the ureter following its normal course. The most common anomaly is the retrocaval ureter where the ureter passes dorsally to the inferior vena cava.

BLADDER

1. The caudal portion of the hindgut which receives the allantois ventrally is a blind pouch: the cloaca. It is separated from the exterior by the cloacal membrane. This membrane is composed of tightly adherent endodermal and ectodermal layers and is bordered by mesoderm which subsequently migrates between ectoderm and endoderm to form the lateral genital folds and the midline genital tubercle.

At 4 weeks, a transverse ridge, the urorectal septum (with its free edge in a coronal plane), grows down to the cloacal membrane dividing the cloaca into the dorsal rectum and the larger primitive ventral urogenital sinus (Fig. 3).

The ventral urogenital sinus can be subdivided into the portion cranial to the mesonephric opening from which will derive the bladder and primary urethra (essentially the entire female urethra and the cranial portion of the pars prostatica in the male) and that caudal to the mesonephric openings, the definitive urogenital sinus.

The mucosa of the bladder arises from the endodermal lining of the vesicourethral canal. The vesical musculature arises from splanchnopleuric mesoderm and the trigone primarily from mesonephric components as previously described.

The fate of the urogenital sinus is intimately related to gonadal

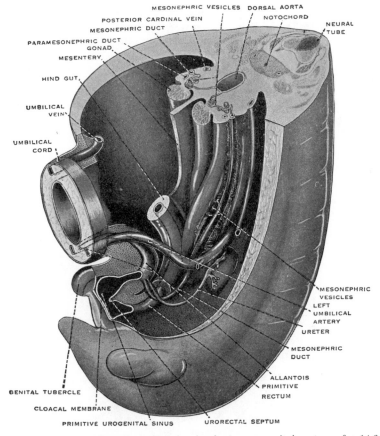

Fig. 3. Schematic ventrolateral view of the developing urogenital system of a 14 6 mm human embryo. (Based on Kelly and Burnam, and Shikinami.) (Reproduced with permission from Hamilton, W. J., Boyd, J. D., and Mossman, H. W.: The urogenital system, in *Human Embryology*, Ed. 4, Chap. 12, edited by Hamilton, W. J. and Mossman, H. W., The Williams & Wilkins Company, Baltimore, 1972.)

development and thus discussion will be deferred to that section.

2. Anomalies.

A. Agenesis. Agenesis is rare but compatable with life if the ureters are unobstructed.

B. Duplication. Again, rare presence of complete or incomplete saggital septae dividing the bladder has been reported. In complete form, there are two bladders each receiving one ureter and emptying through its own urethra.

C. Exstrophy-epispadias complex. Deformities which vary in severity from total ectopic viscera abdominalis to only mild musculoskeletal defect can occur, which in essence represent derangements of the organs and musculoskeletal elements of the lower abdominal wall. The gradations of this complex have been elegantly characterized by Marshall and Muecke.

The most common form is classical exstrophy (see Fig. 4). It is not familial and occurs more commonly in males. The classical exstrophy is characterized by eversion of the bladder onto the lower abdominal wall, epispadiac urethra on the spade penis in the male, separation of the pubic bones, divergent recti, bilateral hernia, and often cryptorchism. For variations of the whole complex, one is referred to Marshall and Muecke. The defect here is an overdevelopment of all or a portion of the cloacal membrane without normal regression, thus retarding the midline migration of mesenchymal mesoderm, creating what has been termed a "wedge

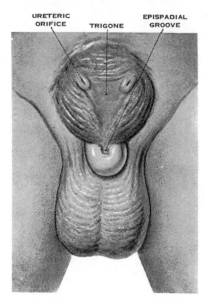

Fig. 4. A semi-schematic drawing to show ectopia vesicae and epispadias. (Reproduced with perimssion from Hamilton, W. J., Boyd, J. D., and Mossman, H. W.: The urogenital system, in *Human Embryology*, Ed. 4, Chap. 12, edited by Hamilton, W. J. and Mossman, H. W., The Williams & Wilkins Company, Baltimore, 1972.)

effect." This defect has been experimentally produced in the laboratory using chick embryos.

GENITAL SYSTEM

The genital system consists of the gonads, internal ductal system, and the external genitalia. In sexual differentiation, the testes or ovaries develop from a common indifferent gonad, and the external genitalia are derived from the urogenital sinus. However, the internal ductal system arises from two different origins: the male, mesonephric (wolffian) ducts and the female, paramesonephric (müllerian) ducts. Moreover, the direction of differentiation of the gonad (male or female) is responsible for future development of the internal ductal system and the external genitalia.

Thus in early embryological development (up to 17 mm), no indication of future sex can be obtained by examination of the gonad, or the paired mesonephric or paramesonephric ducts.

1. Gonad.

A. Indifferent stage. The primordia of the gonad appear (4- to 5-mm stage) as paired thickenings medial to the mesonephros and lateral to the dorsal mesentary. The early gonad consists of mesodermal cells of coelomic epithelial origin and becomes interspersed with primordial germ cells (gonocytes) which probably migrate from the yolk sac. For further development, both elements appear to be necessary. There is arrest of genital ridge formation if either is absent.

The newly formed genital blastema are supported by the urogenital mesentary, and with the mesonephros compose the urogenital ridge. Grooves then separate the regressing mesonephros forming the gonadal mesentary (mesovarium of mesorchium). The caudal portion of the urogenital ridge fuses in a coronal plane forming the urogenital septum between the bladder and the hindgut.

B. Gonadal differentiation.

1) Testis. By the 17-mm stage (7th week) the gonadal blastema becomes divided into sex cords which later include the primordial germ cells and form the rete testis near the mesorchium. These cords canalize to become the seminiferous tubules, the walls of which are supported by Sertoli cells. The interstitial cells (Leydig) are probably derived from mesenchymal cells of the stroma. The rete testis canalizes later and connects with the mesonephric tubules (efferent ductules), thus establishing contact with the mesonephric ductal system. Influence of the developing testis on the mesonephric and paramesonephric ductal systems will be discussed.

2) Ovary. Here the developing sex cords become fragmented and group to form the primordial ovarian follicles which incorporate the primordial ova (germ cells). Structures analogous to the rete testis do not differentiate and thus connection to the mesonephric ductal system does not occur, nor does a definitive tunica albuginea form.

C. Gonadal descent.

1) Testis. With formation of the urogenital septum, the urogenital ridge, as it passes the brim of the embryonic pelvis, is joined by a mesenchymatous band, the inguinal fold or plica inguinalis, in which the plica gubernaculi form. In the cranial portion, the mesonephric fold has regressed with the mesonephros, and by the 13th week the residual diaphragmatic ligament (suspensory ligament) of the mesonephros disappears. Thus the testicle is attached by the dorsal mesorchium and by the postgonadal inguinal ligament of the mesonephros in which lies the inguinal fold. With the development of the pelvis, the testis remains at the apex of the plica gubernaculi lying in close proximity to the inguinal region. Therefore "descent" occurs. At the 6th month, the processus vaginalis, which arose as a dimple on the ventral aspect of the inguinal ligament, grows to form a ventral crescentric sac. The region around the processus vaginalis and the inguinal ligament of the mesonephros contain the gubernaculum. During the 7th month, the testis passes through the inguinal canal. The gubernaculum, with components from both the inguinal ligament of the mesonephros and the scrotal ligament, does not shorten during final descent and thus acts as a guide but does not "pull" the testis down.

2) Ovary. In the female, the plica gubernaculum becomes attached to the enlarging uterovaginal canal, that part passing between the ovary and uterus persists as the round ligament of the ovary, and that between the uterus and the labia majora as the round ligament of the uterus. Attachment to the uterus may prevent extra-abdominal descent.

D. Anomalies.

1) Anomalies in number. These anomalies are rare, but cases of synorchism and polyorchism have been reported.

2) Anomalies of descent. The primary anomalies of concern in the testicle are of position with absence (unilateral or bilateral) of the testis in the scrotum. The possibility of intersexuality should be considered in the bilaterally cryptorchid child.

a. Retractile testis. Absence of the testis in the scrotum which is intermittent and due to hyperactivity of the cremasteric muscle can occur, should be considered a normal situation, and is only mentioned as part of the differential diagnosis.

b. Ectopic testis. The ectopic testis is a normal gonad which during descent has deviated from the normal path. The testis may be abdominal, femoral, suprapubic, penile, perineal, or in the opposite side of the scrotal sac.

c. Cryptorchism. Here there is an arrest of normal testicular descent somewhere along the path between the renal and scrotal areas (see Chapter 18).

3) Anomalies of the testicular tunics.

a. Inguinal hernia. An indirect inguinal hernia may occur alone or in conjunction with the presence of cryptorchid testis. This defect is due to incomplete obliteration of the processus vaginalis.

b. Hydrocele of the tunica vaginalis or of the cord is a collection of fluid within the layers of the tunica vaginalis or portions which are normally obliterated.

c. Torsion of the testis. Rotation of the spermatic cord causing strangulation of blood supply to the testis and testicular infarction is usually seen in postpubertal males but has been reported as early as the neonatal period. In this disease, there is either persistence of a voluminous tunica albuginea or defective scrotal ligamentous attachments to the gubernaculum.

2. Genital internal ductal system. During the indifferent stage, there are paired mesonephric and paramesonephric structures with subsequent development of gonadal and mesonephric relationships in the male and gonadal and paramesonephric relationships in the female. Although gonadal sexual differentiation is due to chromosomal influence, the differentiation of the internal ductal system appears to depend on elaboration of gonadal substances. Testicular formation appears to be dominant, since the castrated male fetus will develop female (müllerian, paramesonephric) structures with regression of male (wolffian) mesonephric ducts. Thus the testis elaborates substances that induce regression of the müllerian ducts (müllerian inhibitory substance) and stimulation of wolffian structures (testosterone). In the castrated female fetus, normal female development occurs.

A. Mesonephric duct.

1) In the male, the ductuli efferentes (from persistent mesonephric tubules) becomes connected with the rete testis. The portion of the mesonephric duct caudal to this junction elongates to form the epididymis, while the remainder of the duct forms the ductus deferens. Each ductus deferens close to the mesonephric opening becomes dilated to form a glandular diverticulum from which the seminal vesicle forms. The part of the duct between the seminal vesicle and the urethra becomes the ejaculatory duct.

2) In the female, remnants of the mesonephric duct persist to form the paraoophoron and epoophoron cranially and Gartner's duct caudally.

B. Paramesonephric duct.

1) Female. At the 6th week of development, a cleft appears between the pronephric and gonadal portions of the urogenital ridge. It is open to the coelom cranially and the solid mesonephric cord caudally, and it is termed the müllerian cleft. At the caudal end, it grows caudomedially, crosses the mesonephric duct, upon the presence of which it is dependent for normal development. It meets and fuses with the opposite duct on the urogenital septum (8th to 12th week). The caudal tip reaches the urogenital sinus and forms an elevation called the müllerian tubercle. Fusion (12th to 16th week) progresses cranially resulting in a vertical single tube (uterus) and laterally coursing separate tubes (fallopian tubes) in the mesovarium which opens

into the coelom. The cranial portion and intermediate transverse part become the uterine tube, while the caudal ligamentus part forms the uterovaginal canal. Proliferation of the tip of the canal forms a solid vaginal cord, increasing the distance between the uterovaginal junction and the urogenital sinus. Later evaginations (sinovaginal bulbs) in this region probably form one-fifth of the vagina, although some investigators feel that the entire vagina arises from the endoderm of the urogenital sinus. That portion of the urogenital sinus (vesicourethral canal) immediately cranial to the sinovaginal bulbs becomes narrowed and elongated to form the female urethra.

2) Male. The paramesonephric ductal system almost totally degenerates. The caudal portion of the paramesonephric duct may disappear entirely or persist as the prostatic utricle or uterus masculinis. The most cranial portion of the paramesonephric duct persists only as the appendix testis, a structure homologous to the fimbriated end of the fallopian tube. It is the most common testicular appendage.

C. Anomalies.

1) Male.

a. Absence. See the section on the kidney with defects in initial mesonephric duct development.

b. Nonunion with the testis. This is a rare occurrence with nonunion of the epididymis to the testis.

c. Müllerian remnants. Persistence of a diverticulum or cyst from the prostatic utricle can occur.

d. Ureteral ectopia. Ureteral ectopia into the male ductal system has been considered in the section on ureteral abnormalities.

2) Female ductal system anomalies.

a. Agenesis. Total absence of the fallopian tubes, uterus, and cervix has rarely been reported.

b. Septal deformities. Deformities exist either in cannulization of the uterus or persistence of a septa forming duplicated or bicornate uteri.

c. Ureteral ectopia. This has been discussed in the section on ureteral abnormalities.

3. External genitalia. The point of entrance of the mesonephric ducts into the primitive urogenital sinus divides the latter into a cranial (vesicourethral) canal which forms the bladder and prostatic urethra (male) or the entire urethra (female) and a caudal definitive urogenital sinus. The definitive urogenital sinus will develop into the external genitalia.

A. Male. The upper portion of the urogenital sinus (pars pelvina) forms the lower part of the prostatic urethra and the membranous urethra. A series of endodermal buds arise from the prostatic urethra and grow into dense mesenchyme to form the prostate. The prostatic utricle arises from the region of the müllerian tubercle on the dorsal wall of the prostate at the junction of the vesicourethral canal and urogenital sinus.

The lower portion (pars phallica) forms the male external genitalia in the presence of testes. Otherwise female genitalia will develop. In the indifferent state, anterior to the cloacal membrane is the genital tubercle and on either side are the genital swellings derived from mesodermal ingrowth (Fig. 5). At the 10-mm stage, an endodermal urethral plate forms along the ventral surface of the genital tubercle with its axis parallel to the long axis of the growing phallus. Lateral mesenchymal ingrowths with their endodermal covering form the urethral folds with the primitive urethral groove in between. At this time, the urorectal septum has grown caudally, separating the cloacal membrane into the urogenital membrane (floor of the urogenital sinus) and the anal membrane. With disintegration of the urogenital membrane, the endodermal urethral plate becomes continuous with the urogenital orifice. Further ectodermal degeneration overlying the urethral plate results in the deepening of the urethral groove.

Further development is under testicular control. The genital tubercle becomes elongated and the urethral folds grow together or fuse, so that the lining of the penile urethra is only endodermal. The fusion also results in the formation of the penile raphe, and the genital swellings fuse to form the scrotum. Only the lining of the glandular urethra is derived from ectoderm (see Fig. 5).

B. Female. In development, the urethral groove is short, and the genital tubercle becomes bent caudally and forms the clitoris. It is not encroached upon by the urethral plate; hence there is no counterpart of the male penile urethra in the female. The lateral portion of the labial swellings form the labia majora and the urethral folds, the labia minora.

C. Anomalies.

1) Hypospadias. Incomplete development of the urethra in which the canal terminates ventral or proximal to the normal opening is termed hypospadias (see Fig. 5). It occurs in both sexes but predominantly in the male. It occurs with a hooded prepuce, absent frenulum, and chordee, (a downward curve to the penile shaft) and often with scrotal and testicular abnormalities. The most common locations of the urethral orifice are glandular (40 to 50%), penile (25 to 30%), and penoscrotal or perineal (10 to 15%). In this situation, there is failure of the margin of the urethral folds to grow together and fuse; therefore, the urethral groove does not form into a tube. Some controversy exists as to whether this is a purely developmental arrest or a hermaphroditic manifestation due to testicular hypogonadism and deficiency of an evocator substance (see Chapter 20). The chordee present is due to the insertion of abortive corpus spongiosum into the corporal bodies.

2) Anomalies in number. Rare complete or incomplete duplication of the urethra occurs in the penile portion of the urethra. The accessory urethra may be dorsal or ventral to the normal urethra.

3) Anterior urethral valves. These valvular folds are rare yet can

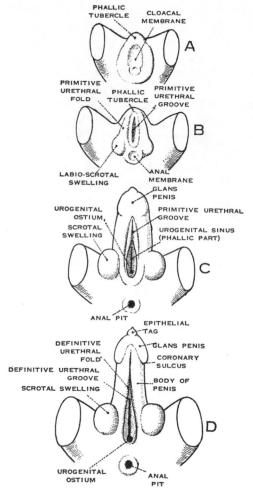

Fig. 5. Schemes to show the development of the phallus and urethral grooves (seen from below). (Reproduced with permission from Hamilton, W. J., Boyd, J. D., and Mossman, H. W.: The urogenital system, in *Human Embryology*, Ed. 4, Chap. 12, edited by Hamilton, W. J. and Mossman, H. W., The Williams & Wilkins Company, Baltimore, 1972.)

obstruct urinary flow and lead to severe upper tract decompensation.

4) Posterior urethral valves. These are mucosal folds located in the posterior urethra attaching to the veru montanum which are obstructive to urinary flow. This anomaly should be considered in any newborn male with azotemia, urinary tract infection, or signs and symptoms of obstructive uropathy. It is the most common cause of hyperkalemia in the newborn male. The valves have been classified into three types by Young in respect to their configuration. The embryological defect involved in this situation is controversial.

5) Abnormalities of the external genitalia in both male and female

which are associated with intersex problems are discussed in Chapter 20.

REFERENCES AND SUGGESTED FURTHER READING

1. Alken, C. E., Dix, V. W., Goodwin, W. E., Weyrach, H. M., and Wildbolz, E. W. (Editors). *Encyclopedia of Urology, VII/I Malformations.* Springer-Verlag, Berlin, Heidelberg, New York, 1968.
2. Hamilton, W. J. and Mossman, H. W. *Human Embryology.* Williams & Wilkins, Baltimore, 1972.
3. Marshall, V. F. and Muecke, E. C. Variations in exstrophy of the bladder. J. Urol. 88:766, 1962.
4. McCrory, W. W. *Developmental Nephrology.* Harvard University Press, Cambridge, Mass., 1972.
5. Potter, E. L. *Normal and Abnormal Development of the Kidney.* Year Book Medical Publishers, Chicago, 1972.
6. Vaughan, E. D., Jr. and Middleton, G. W. A review of pertinent genitourinary embryology for the practicing urologist. Urology (in press).

8

Trauma

ARTHUR W. WYKER, JR.

The urinary tract's chief defense against trauma is its *ability to move.* This mobility prolongs the period of deceleration, thereby decreasing the *rate* of energy release and blunting the effect of the impact on the urinary tract. This is similar to the football player who, in diving for a loose ball, ducks his head and shoulder and rolls, prolonging the period of deceleration and minimizing the impact to his shoulder.

The only portion of the urinary tract that lacks this protection is the membranous urethra, for it is immobilized in the muscular grasp of the urogenital diaphragm.

KIDNEY

1. The kidneys are located behind the posterior peritoneum in shallow depressions adjacent to the vertebral column.

A. Supine, T12 to L3; upright, L1 to L4.

B. They are much closer to the posterior abdominal wall than to the anterior abdominal wall.

2. The lower ribs and lumbar vertebrae partially shield the kidney and when they are fractured, the likelihood of renal injury is increased.

ANATOMY OF THE KIDNEY
(lateral view)

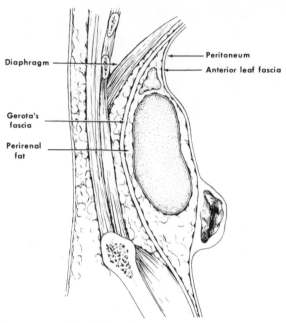

Fig. 1. Lateral view of the kidney.

3. The kidney is a mobile organ, surrounded by fat and fixed *only* at its vascular attachments to the aorta and vena cava.

A. The kidney descends about one vertebral length on deep inspiration or in going from supine to the standing position.

B. The normal mobility of the kidney permits it to slide away from the full force of most injuries, but if it is immobilized by perirenal inflammation, it is more vulnerable to trauma.

C. Children have a relatively thin perirenal fatty envelope and, in addition, their kidneys are less protected by the skeletal framework—both factors making them more at risk.

4. The renal capsule is a *strong membrane which resists rupture*, so when it is torn, there is usually significant damage to the underlying parenchyma.

5. The retroperitoneal space contains many nerves and has a *tremendous potential capacity.*

A. Large quantities of blood and urine must be present before swelling in the flank is detectable.

B. Retroperitoneal bleeding causes *severe ileus* owing to irritation of sympathetic nerves, and the ileus persists until the bleeding stops or the hematoma is evacuated.

6. Gerota's fascia, surrounding the kidney and its fatty envelope, *tends to stop renal bleeding* as accumulating blood within its layers exerts pressure on the bleeding site (tamponade).

A. In contrast, intraperitoneal conditions favor a continuation of bleeding owing to the lack of resistance to the flow of blood into the peritoneal cavity, and a fatal hemorrhage may follow a relatively small laceration of an intraperitoneal organ.

7. Because of its anatomical location, penetrating injuries involving the kidney usually damage other organs as well.

Etiology of Renal Injuries

The majority of renal injuries follow blunt, nonpenetrating trauma.

Causes of Renal Injury

1. Traffic accidents, usually automobile—50 to 60% of all renal injuries.
2. Football—30% of all renal injuries.
3. Fall against the flank.
4. Gunshot or stabbing (penetrating)—incidence higher in areas of violence or in wartime.
5. Indirect injuries—rare.
   A. Fall on the feet, buttocks, or shoulder may cause the renal counterpart of the familiar whiplash injury.
      1. The freely moving kidney, *fixed only at its pedicle*, may continue its downward course, being torn free from its pedicle.

Classification and Pathology

The kidney is enclosed by a *tough, fibrous capsule*, and its integrity, in large part, determines the severity of the renal injury. For this reason, it is the basis of this classification.

1. Intracapsular injuries—usually minor.
   A. Account for 60 to 70% of all renal injuries.
   B. Integrity of the renal capsule is established by seeing contrast medium *confined to the renal outline* on infusion intravenous urogram or on renal angiography.
   C. Most of the injuries may be treated conservatively without surgery, and the large majority heal up without any sequelae.
2. Extracapsular injuries—usually major.
   A. Account for 30 to 40% of all renal injuries.
   B. With damage to the renal capsule, blood and urine may accumulate around the kidney with resultant enlarging mass.
   C. Fifty percent of these patients require surgery.
3. Renal pedicle injuries—always major and often fatal.
   A. Account for 2 to 3% of all renal injuries.
   B. If the patient survives, nephrectomy is usually performed.

KIDNEY INJURIES

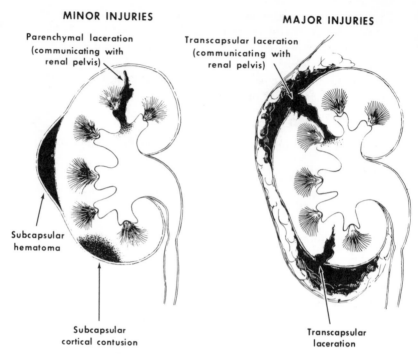

MINOR INJURIES

MAJOR INJURIES

Parenchymal laceration
(communicating with
renal pelvis)

Transcapsular laceration
(communicating with
renal pelvis)

Subcapsular
hematoma

Subcapsular
cortical contusion

Transcapsular
laceration

Fig. 2. Schematic drawing of renal injuries.

Mechanism and Pathology of Renal Injuries

In blunt injuries, the impact is usually *directly over the kidney* either posteriorly or laterally. The kidney may be injured in two ways.

1. Displacement.

A. The moving kidney may strike ribs or vertebrae, producing a contusion.

B. Since the kidney is fixed only at the renal pedicle, unusual sudden movement may *avulse the renal pedicle*; or with undue elongation of the renal artery, an *intimal tear* may be produced with resultant thrombosis.

2. Explosive hydraulic effect.

A. Because of its high fluid content of urine and blood, the kidney reacts to external force like an *enclosed fluid mass*.

1) Küster found that a kidney devoid of blood and urine will withstand great violence without damage, but that if the pelvis and vessels are filled with fluid and tied, the organ is readily ruptured by impact.

a. The experimental renal lacerations so produced are similar in location and character to those which occur in life.

B. Fluid laws are therefore applicable to renal injury.

1) Any additional pressure exerted upon an enclosed fluid mass is

transmitted equally in all directions.

2) Fluids are *almost totally incompressible* and are *incapable of resisting forces,* following pathways of least resistance.

C. The incompressibility of fluid accounts for the increased vulnerability to rupture of the hydronephrotic kidney.

1) Ten to 15% of all renal injuries and 20 to 25% of renal injuries in children occur in *abnormal kidneys,* usually hydronephrotic kidneys.

D. Pathology due to hydraulic effect.

1) The kidney in effect *explodes,* and this bursting produces ragged lacerations of the renal parenchyma.

The extent of renal damage depends upon:

1. The severity of the blunt force.
2. The direction and degree of kidney displacement.
3. The status of the kidney prior to trauma.

Clinical Findings

The most important sign of renal injury is the *presence of blood in the urine,* and this occurs in 85 to 90% of all renal injuries. Hematuria may be absent if the area of renal damage does not communicate with the collecting system or if the urinary drainage system is either interrupted or obstructed by blood clots.

Pain and tenderness in the kidney region are usually present, but this is a nonspecific finding, being normally present with abdominal wall trauma alone. Colicky pain along the course of the ureter may occur if blood clots produce partial ureteral obstruction.

Diagnostic Studies

Urinalysis

1. This should be obtained as *soon as possible* on all patients with significant trauma to the thoracoabdominal area.

MECHANISM OF RENAL INJURIES

A. Displacement   B. Hydraulic bursting

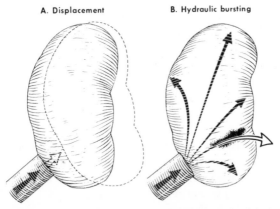

Fig. 3. Schematic drawing illustrating displacement and bursting injuries of the kidney.

2. Catheterize if necessary, using gentle aseptic technique.

A. Traumatic catheterization may cause hematuria.

3. A normal urinalysis *does not rule out renal injury*, being found in 10 to 15% of all patients with documented renal damage.

4. There is no good correlation between the degree of hematuria and the degree of renal injury, and so the emphasis should be placed on the presence or absence of hematuria—not the degree.

Infusion Intravenous Urogram.

1. This should be performed on all patients with *any degree of hematuria* and on those patients without hematuria who are *still suspect for renal injuries*, e.g., fractured ribs or lumbar vertebrae.

2. Infusion intravenous urogram is better than the regular intravenous urogram, giving an adequate study 80 to 90% of the time as compared to 40 to 50%.

A. Since it is a hypertonic solution, it draws fluid from the intracellular compartment into the vascular compartment, and therefore it must be used cautiously in children or in markedly dehydrated patients.

3. Information obtained by infusion urography.

A. Detects presence of renal injury and sometimes the nature and degree of damage.

B. Detects pre-existing pathology such as hydronephrosis or tumor present in 10 to 15% of all renal injuries.

C. Presence and gross functional capacity of the contralateral kidney. *This is extremely important* for it may significantly affect surgical decisions.

4. Findings suggesting a renal injury.

A. Plain film.

1) Evidence of bleeding around kidney—loss of renal outline, obliteration of psoas muscle margin.

2) Damage to protective skeletal framework—fractured ribs or lumbar vetebrae.

B. Urogram phase.

1) Diminished or absent renal function in presence of normal renal function of contralateral kidney.

2) Distortion of collecting system.

3) *Urinary extravasation.*

4) Filling defects in collecting system due to blood clots.

Renal Angiography

1. This should be performed on all patients with significant renal damage on infusion urography, particularly if surgery is anticipated.

2. It gives the most precise assessment of the nature and degree of renal injury, thereby increasing the renal salvage rate.

A. It is the only way to determine the status of renal vasculature.

B. Relatively small areas of damage may be detected by the presence of displacement of segmental branches of the renal arteries.

C. Fractures of the kidney are easily recognized.

D. Subcapsular hematomas may be detected by observing displacement of the capsular artery.

Cystoendoscopy with Retrograde Pyelograms

1. This is *infrequently* indicated. If the infusion intravenous urogram reveals a poorly functioning or nonfunctioning kidney and renal angiography is not feasible, retrograde studies may be performed. If bleeding is not excessive, the collecting system will be defined and the presence or absence of urinary extravasation established.

2. Drawbacks.

A. The procedure itself is somewhat traumatic.

B. Infection may be introduced into the damaged kidney.

C. Pressure of injected contrast medium or of ureteral catheter may aggravate renal bleeding.

Scheme of Workup for Suspected Renal Injury
(Modification of one proposed by Banowsky)

Trauma
↓
Urinalysis

no hematuria but injury suspected

no hematuria, injury not suspected

Hematuria
↓
Infusion Intravenous Urogram

intracapsular injury (mild)

normal

nonfunction or major injury with extracapsular extravasation

repeat infusion intravenous urogram in 2–3 days

renal angiogram

Management of Renal Injuries

Two-thirds of all renal injuries are *intracapsular* and these minor injuries usually heal up without any complication or sequelae. Complete bed rest is advisable until hematuria ceases.

One-half of the *extracapsular* injuries require surgery, and the two major indications are *continuing hemorrhage* and *continuing significant urinary extravasation*. Renal angiography, by accurately pinpointing the pathology, has resulted in more surgical repairs of renal lacerations and few nephrectomies. If feasible, surgery is performed 1 to 2 days after major trauma so that the patient's overall condition is optimal.

One-half of the extracapsular injuries may be managed conservatively but require close follow-up. Extravasation of blood and urine outside the capsule increases the chance of a late complication—loss of renal function, hypertension, obstructive hydronephrosis, persistent flank pain.

URETER

The cause of most ureteral injuries is pelvic surgery. Because of its deep location, small size, and mobility, the ureter is rarely injured by external trauma. Ureteral damage occurs in 2 to 3% of all pelvic operations and in 10 to 15% of all radical pelvic operations with a unilateral-to-bilateral ratio of 6 to 1.

Why is the ureter so vulnerable to surgical injury?

1. It is dangerously close to the surgical field in many pelvic operations.

A. The ureter passes 1 to 2 cm below the uterine artery at the site of its ligation in a total abdominal hysterectomy, and this is the *most common site* of ureteral injury.

B. Another danger point is its entry into the pelvis where it is crossed by the ovariopelvic fold of peritoneum.

C. When troublesome bleeding occurs anywhere in the pelvis, the ureter may be clamped or included in a suture ligature.

2. It is *mobile* so it may be displaced to abnormal locations by pelvic tumors.

3. Ureteral blood vessels are located in the adventitia.

A. T-shaped long arteries reach the ureter from the aorta or its branches and then send long branches up and down.

B. Adventitia and loose periureteral tissue should *not be disturbed* because of the risk of producing ischemic necrosis.

1) This mechanism may account for the late appearing ureterovaginal fistulae following radical hysterectomy.

4. Congenital anomalies of the ureter are relatively common.

A. Significant anomalies such as partial or complete duplication and megaloureter occur in 3 to 5% of people.

5. The ureter is partially adherent to the overlying peritoneum. During reapproximation of the posterior peritoneum, the ureter may be included in a suture.

6. The pressure inside the ureter is relatively low.

A. Retroperitoneal hematomas or other pelvic masses may compress and obstruct the ureter.

Pathology

The majority of traumatic nonsurgical injuries involve the abdominal ureter, whereas the majority of surgical injuries involve the pelvic ureter, usually within 4 to 6 cm of the bladder (Fig. 4). Both injuries occur directly to the ureter, eventually producing a ureteral fistula or a ureteral obstruction, or both.

The most common forms of surgical injury are partial or complete division of the ureter and inclusion or angulation by a mass ligature of blood vessels. Necrosis of a portion of the ureter may follow aggressive removal of its periureteral tissue. Pelvic edema and retroperitoneal bleeding may cause partial obstruction of the ureter.

Clinical Findings

The signs and symptoms of a ureteral injury depend upon whether the damage produced results in ureteral obstruction or ureteral necrosis with formation of a ureteral fistula. A ureteral injury should be suspected in the early postoperative period if the patient has *fever, abnormal pain, or urinary incontinence*. Pelvic pain results from inflammation secondary to

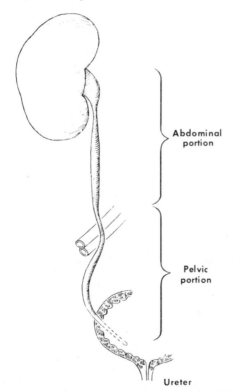

Abdominal portion

Pelvic portion

Ureter

Fig. 4. Drawing of the ureter illustrating the abdominal portion which extends from the renal pelvis to the iliac vessels and the pelvic segment which runs from the iliac vessels to the bladder.

extravasated urine and pelvic infection. Lateral abdominal or costovertebral angle (CVA) pain results from partial ureteral obstruction.

Ureteral Fistula

1. Seventy-five percent of surgical ureteral injuries result in a ureteral fistula, most commonly a ureterovaginal fistula.

A. Prior to the escape of urine into the vagina or the wound, a fistula may be suspected if the patient has an unusual amount of pelvic pain or if a tender mass can be palpated adjacent to the vaginal apex.

2. The ureteral fistula may be detected at any time in the postoperative period, but the *majority appear 1 to 2 weeks after surgery.*

A. First week after surgery—25%.

1) Usually due to partial or complete division of the ureter.

B. Second week after surgery—50%.

1) Usually due to inclusion or angulation by mass ligature of vessels with eventual sloughing of the involved ureteral segment.

C. Third week or later after surgery—25%.

1) Usually due to ischemic necrosis from denudation of ureter during radical pelvic surgery.

3. Some degree of ureteral obstruction often occurs above the site of the ureteral fistula.

Ureteral Obstruction

1. Twenty-five percent of surgical ureteral injuries result in ureteral obstruction.

2. Pain in the lateral abdomen or CVA region is *usually present.*

A. Painless atrophy of a kidney may follow complete obstruction of one ureter.

3. Anuria results if a solitary ureter is completely obstructed or if both ureters are completely obstructed.

4. Fever is commonly present because of associated urinary infection. Transient, reversible mild ureteral obstruction occurs in about 25% of patients after a radical hysterectomy owing to edema from the extensive dissection of the lower ureters.

Urological Workup for Possible Ureterovaginal Fistula

1. Establish the presence of a urinary-vaginal fistula.

A. Inject a dye such as Indigo carmine intravenously, and if a urinary fistula is present, the fluid reaching the vagina will be blue-stained.

B. If the quantity of escaping fluid is small and the above dye test equivocal, determine the urea or creatinine concentration in the *suspect fluid* and the patient's serum.

1) If the fluid is urine, its urea and creatinine concentration will be 25 to 75 times that of serum.

2) Nonurinous fluids will have approximately the same concentrations as serum.

2. Intravenous urogram.

A. Urinary extravasation may be evident, and in most cases there is some hydroureter and hydronephrosis above the site of injury.

3. Cystogram.

A. This is done to rule out a vesicovaginal fistula.

B. Contrast medium with blue dye added is instilled into the bladder and a lateral film is taken.

1) If there is a vesicovaginal fistula, the fistula may be seen on x-ray and the vaginal pack should be stained blue.

4. Cystoendoscopy with *occlusive ureterogram*.

A. Urethrovaginal or vesicovaginal fistulas may be seen if present.

B. With a vaginal pack in place, blue-stained contrast medium is injected into the right ureteral orifice using an occlusive cone catheter.

1) The ureterovaginal fistula, most commonly 2 to 6 cm above the bladder, may be demonstrated on x-ray as well as by blue staining of the vaginal pack.

C. A similar procedure is performed on the left side using red stain (PSP) contrast medium.

D. The ureter is usually *not outlined* above the site of the ureteral fistula on this retrograde study.

Management of Ureteral Injuries

There are a few general principles which are applicable to all ureteral injuries.

1. The area of ureteral repair should *always* be drained to the outside via an *extraperitoneal* Penrose drain.

A. This prevents accumulation of extravasated urine, a source of local inflammation.

2. In most cases, the *entire* ureter should be splinted.

A. A splinting catheter, preferably no. 8 French size Silastic, extends from the renal pelvis to the bladder and exits alongside a cystostomy tube or a urethral catheter.

B. The splint drains the urine from the involved kidney decreasing urinary extravasation and putting the ureter at rest.

3. All suturing is done with fine absorbable suture material.

A. Nonabsorbable sutures (silk) which extend into the ureteral lumen act as a foreign body nidus for calculus formation.

4. The area of repair is surrounded with live fat.

A. This prevents fixation of the ureter to the adjacent fascia or muscle and facilitates return of normal ureteral peristalsis.

Lower Ureter

1. Reimplant the ureter into the bladder.

A. If there is a gap between the ureter and the bladder, mobilize the bladder upwards and suture it to the psoas fascia, or create a bladder flap.

Upper and Midureter

1. Spatulate ends of ureter on opposite sides and perform a watertight, end-to-end anastomosis using interrupted fine, chromic catgut sutures.

2. Avulsion injuries at the ureteropelvic junction require anastomosis of the spatulated end of the ureter to the dependent portion of the renal pelvis.

Massive Ureteral Injuries

1. Defer definitive repair.

2. Divert urine via a nephrostomy and drain the injured area adequately.
   A. This protects the kidney and minimizes urinary extravasation.

3. At a later date, consider the following surgical options.
   A. Replace injured ureter with a segment of small intestine.
   B. Connect proximal viable ureter to opposite normal ureter (ureteroureterostomy).
   C. Transplant the kidney to the pelvis.
   D. Remove the kidney.

Prevention of Surgical Ureteral Injury

1. The best safeguard is to identify the ureter wherever it approaches the surgical field.

2. An intravenous urogram should be performed prior to all major pelvic surgery.
   A. This will detect the 3 to 5% ureteral anomalies and will also show if the pelvic pathology has obstructed or displaced the ureter.

3. Ureteral catheters may be passed prior to surgery in *selected* cases.
   A. This is feasible when difficult surgery is anticipated—extensive endometriosis, large pelvic tumors, pelvic inflammation.
   B. The presence of ureteral catheters decreases, but *does not eliminate*, the chance of ureteral injury. It does permit *easy recognition*.

4. Preserve periureteral tissue if at all possible.
   A. Nerves and blood vessels reside in this adventitial layer and removal or damage to these vessels may cause eventual ischemic necrosis or stricture.

BLADDER

The empty bladder is *relatively invulnerable* to injury, but the distended bladder may be ruptured by a violent blow to the lower abdomen or by direct injury from a bone fragment, knife, bullet, or surgical instrument. A fracture of the pelvis is the most common cause of bladder injury.

There are two physiological factors that play an important role in bladder injuries—degree of bladder distention and state of recti muscles in the lower abdomen.

Degree of Bladder Distention

1. The bladder becomes increasingly vulnerable as it fills with urine.
   A. The empty bladder retreats to a deep position in the pelvis behind a formidable bony shield.

1) Its volume and intraluminal pressure are *minimal*; its wall thickness is *maximal*.

B. The distended bladder rises out of its protected pelvic position, its volume and intraluminal pressure increase, and its walls become progressively thinner.

1) Like a balloon, the more distended it is, the less force is required to rupture it.

2. Older men are particularly vulnerable because many of them have a moderate amount of urine in their bladders at all times owing to bladder outlet obstruction from benign prostatic hypertrophy or carcinoma of the prostate.

3. Infants and children are also more vulnerable because their bladders are more an abdominal organ and thus less well protected.

State of Recti Muscles in the Lower Abdomen

1. *Coordinated* contraction of *sturdy* recti muscles offers great protection against injury by impact.

2. This protective muscular shield fails if the recti muscles are lax or if they are not contracted prior to the impact.

A. Women who have had multiple pregnancies often have lax recti muscles.

B. Intoxicated individuals are unable to contract their recti muscles prior to impact.

1) They are additionally vulnerable to bladder injury because of their combative nature and tendency to have a distended bladder.

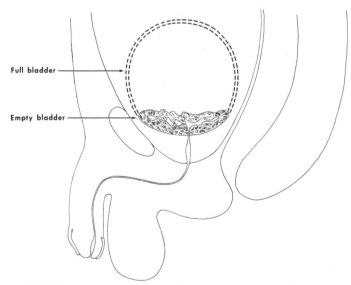

Full bladder

Empty bladder

Fig. 5. Schematic drawing illustrating that the empty bladder is a pelvic organ protected by the pelvis, whereas the full bladder extends into the abdominal cavity where it is vulnerable to trauma.

Pathology of Bladder Injuries

Blow to the Lower Abdomen

1. Damage results from the explosive hydraulic effect on the distended bladder.

A. Since any additional pressure exerted upon an enclosed fluid mass is *transmitted equally in all directions*, bladder rupture occurs at the site of least resistance.

1) If there is no pathology in the bladder wall, a longitudinal tear occurs in the peritonealized portion of the bladder—*intraperitoneal rupture.*

2) When the bladder is distended, the peritoneum over the dome becomes taut, and since it is the least elastic component of the bladder wall, it is the first to tear (Moritz).

Fractured Pelvis

The bladder may be injured in two ways—explosive hydraulic effect or direct injury from broken ends of bone.

1. Ten percent of patients with a fractured pelvis will have an associated rupture of the bladder.

A. Eighty percent of these are extraperitoneal on the anterolateral bladder wall close to the bladder neck.

1) Injury is produced by inward displacement of the broken end of one of the pubic arch bones.

B. Twenty percent of these are intraperitoneal due to hydraulic effect.

2. Fractures of the pubic arch are most likely to cause injury to the bladder.

A. Fracture of one pubic ramus → 5% bladder injury.

B. Bilateral fractures of the pubic rami → 20% bladder injury.

Penetrating Injuries

Bullet, knife, and instrumental injuries can be either intraperitoneal or extraperitoneal depending on the area of the bladder involved.

Extravasation of Urine

With urine extravasation, there is gradually increasing inflammation of *all tissues in contact with the urine.* This urine soon becomes infected because of migration of bacteria from the intestinal tract, and this causes severe sepsis.

Friend produced intraperitoneal and extraperitoneal extravasation of urine in dogs by surgically removing an appropriate segment of the bladder wall. The dogs with intraperitoneal extravasation lived an average of 2 ½ days; those with extraperitoneal extravasation an average of 4 ½ days.

Intraperitoneal Extravasation (Friend)

1. Early—dogs developed anorexia, weakness, gradual distention of the abdomen, and progressive dyspnea.

2. Late—dogs developed markedly distended abdomens and severe respiratory insufficiency.

3. Serum levels of urea, creatinine, and potassium progressively increased up to death.

4. At autopsy, the abdomen was distended with urine and there was marked peritonitis.

Extraperitoneal Extravasation (Friend)

1. Dogs did not appear ill until the 3rd day when weakness and anorexia first appeared.

2. The abdomen did *not* become distended and dogs did *not* become dyspneic.

3. Weakness progressed up to death.

4. Serum levels of urea, creatinine, and potassium were normal for 2 days, then gradually rose; but levels at death were substantially less than in those dogs with intraperitoneal extravasation.

5. At autopsy, there were large amounts of urine in the retroperitoneal space from the pelvis to the diaphragm with inflammation, edema, and some necrosis of tissues lining the retroperitoneal space.

    A. The peritoneal cavity was free of urine.

Clinical Findings

The possibility of bladder injury must be considered whenever suprapubic pain follows a blow to the lower abdomen or a bony injury of the pelvis. If a patient with abdominal pelvic injuries is unconscious because of severe injuries or intoxication, appropriate studies should be performed to rule out bladder injury. Always ask the patient or his family if he had any known urinary tract pathology prior to his injury.

Signs and Symptoms of Bladder Rupture

1. Pain in lower abdomen and pelvic region is *always present.*

    A. The chief cause of pain is chemical inflammation from the extravasated urine.

        1) Sterile urine is nonirritating for a short period of time, but infected urine produces an *immediate and severe tissue reaction.*

    B. A fractured pelvis may produce similar pain whether or not there is an associated bladder injury.

2. Hematuria is almost invariably present.

    A. The initial urine specimen obtained following the injury usually is bloodstained.

3. The patient usually is *unable to void.*

    A. Attempts to void often cause considerable pain.

    B. The ability to void following an injury *does not* rule out a ruptured bladder.

4. Abdominal findings.

A. With intraperitoneal rupture, there may be no swelling present, but within a few hours after injury the signs of peritoneal irritation become evident—tenderness, involuntary muscular rigidity, and ileus.

B. With extraperitoneal rupture, there is marked tenderness and swelling in the suprapubic region, and a fracture of the pubis may be detected on palpation.

5. Rectal findings.

A. The prostate is in its normal position ruling out a complete rupture of the membranous urethra.

B. Above the prostate a doughy mass may be felt because of perivesical bleeding.

6. Evidence of shock is often present.

A. In a previously healthy person, signs of shock after injury indicate a blood loss of 1,000 to 1,500 cc.

B. A fractured pelvis often results in blood loss of this magnitude.

Workup for Possible Bladder Injury

Whenever there is a chance of bladder injury, the integrity of the bladder should be promptly determined by *properly performed cystograms.*

1. If a urethral catheter is not already in place, perform a gentle *retrograde urethrogram* injecting 10 to 15 ml of *undiluted* intravenous contrast medium.

A. A pelvic fracture may damage the prostatomembranous urethra as well as the bladder, and so it is important to establish the integrity of the urethra.

B. Any preinjury urethral abnormality such as stricture will be detected facilitating passing of a urethral catheter into the bladder.

2. A well lubricated no. 20 Foley catheter is then passed into the bladder, and a three-phase cystogram is obtained using a *diluted* solution of intravenous contrast medium.

A. 1st study—instill 50 to 60 ml; 2nd study—instill 250 to 300 ml, fully distending the bladder; 3rd study—empty bladder, lavage with saline, and take third film.

B. The first study is made with a small volume, for if there is a large bladder rupture, the diagnosis may be established and the harmful effects of the escaping contrast medium minimized.

C. The third study is necessary to rule out a perforation of the posterior bladder wall that might be obscured by the contrast medium within the bladder.

1) Lateral or oblique films are often not feasible owing to the danger of aggravating pelvic bleeding by moving the patient.

D. Cystograms, in addition to detecting bladder perforations, also give a fairly reliable estimate of the degree of intrapelvic hemorrhage.

1) Pelvic bleeding due to a fractured pelvis produces a *teardrop bladder*

(Fig. 6) because the blood compresses the bladder *from all sides* and lifts it out of the pelvis.

Intraperitoneal Rupture (Fig. 7)

1. Escaping contrast medium must exit from the *peritonealized superior* portion of the bladder and must be totally confined within the peritoneal cavity.

   A. In the supine position, contrast medium tends to pool in the dependent portion of the peritoneal cavity.

     1) A line extending across the roofs of the acetabular cavities outlines

TEAR DROP BLADDER

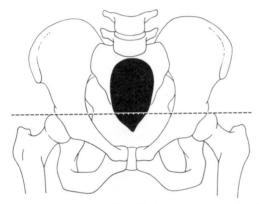

Fig. 6. Pelvic bleeding produces a teardrop bladder by compressing the bladder from all sides and lifting it out of the pelvis.

INTRAPERITONEAL EXTRAVASATION

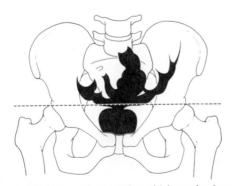

Fig. 7. Drawing showing hourglass configuration which results from the escape of contrast medium from the round, well defined bladder base through a tear in the peritonealized superior portion of the bladder. Within the peritoneal cavity, contrast medium tends to go along paracolic gutters.

the lower limits of the peritoneal cavity so that extravasated contrast medium *must reside above this line*.

2. An *hourglass configuration* often results as contrast medium escapes from round, well defined bladder base through small vertical rent in the superior portion into the general peritoneal cavity.

3. Within the peritoneal cavity, contrast medium tends to go along the paracolic gutters, and these narrow bands of contrast medium are often indented by the adjacent colon, producing scalloped filling defects.

4. If the perforation is large or if a large volume of contrast medium has been instilled, it may coat the pelvic loops of small intestine and may even be seen beneath the diaphragm.

Extraperitoneal Rupture (Fig. 8)

1. The escaping contrast medium penetrates into the prevesical space and the pelvic tissues.

   A. Extravasation occurs *below* the line across the roof of the acetabular cavities.

2. The bladder outline, particularly the base, is often *indistinct and fuzzy* because of the presence of contrast medium in different layers (within and outside the bladder).

3. There is no collection of contrast medium in the dependent portion of the peritoneal cavity, and the intestinal loops are not outlined.

4. Intravenous urogram.

   A. This should be initiated after the second cystogram study, injecting a double dose of intravenous contrast medium.

   B. An adequate study can usually be obtained despite the presence of hypotension.

   C. This rules out any upper urinary tract pathology.

5. *Do not* perform cystoendoscopy.

EXTRAPERITONEAL EXTRAVASATION

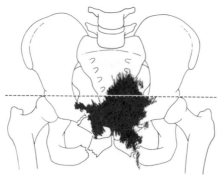

Fig. 8. Urinary extravasation occurs below the line across the roof of the acetabular cavities into the prevesical space and pelvic tissues.

A. The procedure itself is traumatic and visualization is often unsatisfactory.

6. *Do not* instill a measured amount of sterile saline into the bladder and measure the return from the catheter.

A. This is an *unreliable* test for bladder perforation.

Management

If the cystograms and urethrogram show no break in the continuity of the lower urinary tract, the injury is classified as a *bladder contusion* and it is managed by a short period of urethral catheter drainage.

If a bladder rupture is detected, immediate surgery should be performed primarily to eliminate the *continuing damage from extravasated urine.*

Surgery for Ruptured Bladder

1. A vertical subumbilical incision is preferred.

A. If other intra-abdominal injuries are found, the incision can easily be extended upwards.

2. *Always* open the peritoneal cavity even if you are sure that bladder rupture is extraperitoneal.

A. If there is an opening in the peritoneal portion of the bladder, close it with absorbable sutures, aspirate blood and urine from the peritoneal cavity, and close the peritoneum without drainage.

B. Look for signs of other organ damage.

3. Open the bladder, verify the integrity of both ureters, and then close the bladder laceration with absorbable suture.

A. Divert urine via a suprapubic cystostomy tube, not a urethral catheter.

4. Drain both perivesical areas with Penrose drains.

URETHRA

The relatively fixed portions of the urethra are most vulnerable to injury—the *membranous urethra* via a fracture of the pelvis, the *bulbous urethra* via a straddle-type fall. When the urethra is ruptured, the escaping urine proceeds along *well defined fascial planes.*

Anatomical Considerations

1. The urogenital diaphragm, separating the pelvis from the perineum, plays a very important role in urinary extravasation.

A. If the urethra is ruptured above or within the U-G diaphragm—prostatic or membranous urethra—urine escapes *into the pelvis;* if below the U-G diaphragm—bulbous urethra—urine escapes *into the perineum.*

B. Both the superficial (Colles') and deep (Buck's) fascia of the genitalia and perineum attach to the inferior layer of the U-G diaphragm.

2. In urethral injuries below the U-G diaphragm, extravasated urine is *anatomically directed between Buck's and Colles' fascia.*

NORMAL MALE ANATOMY

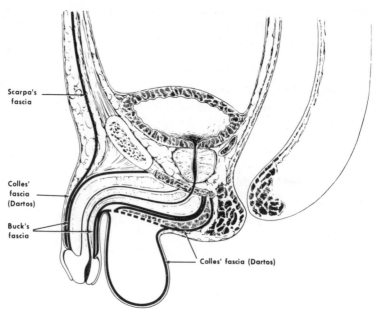

Fig. 9. Lateral drawing of the male pelvis showing the critical role that the fascial attachments play in determining the pathology of urinary extravasation.

A. Nontraumatic urinary extravasation due to infected urine escaping from a necrotic portion of the urethra proximal to a urethral stricture *may not follow this fascial pathway.*

3. Colles' fascia.

A. The superficial fascia of the abdominal wall continues downward over the penis, scrotum, and perineum and fuses with the posterior, inferior margin of the U-G diaphragm.

1) It is called Scarpa's fascia over the abdomen, Colles' or dartos fascia over the penis and scrotum, and Colles' fascia in the perineum.

B. It divides the scrotum into two compartments and forms a roof across the top.

C. *Its attachments define the limits of urinary extravasation.*

1) In the perineum, it is attached to the U-G diaphragm, the inferior pubic rami, and the superior rami of the ischium.

a. Urine is thus prevented from reaching the anus or the ischiorectal fossae.

2) The abdominal continuation of Colles' fascia (Scarpa's) is attached to the fascia lata of the thigh just below the inguinal ligaments.

a. Urine is thus prevented from reaching the legs.

3) Scarpa's fascia is not attached superiorly so that urine may extend *all the way to the clavicles or neck.*

4. Buck's fascia.

A. This tough, *deep fascia of the penis* extends from the U-G diaphragm to the corona, enveloping the copora cavernosa and the corpus spongiosum throughout their entire course.

1) The bulbocavernosus and ischiocavernosus muscles *are not* contained within Buck's fascia.

B. A transverse septum of Buck's fascia encloses the corpus spongiosum and urethra in a *separate compartment*.

C. It is continuous above with the suspensory ligament of the penis.

D. In all significant infradiaphragmatic urethral injuries, Buck's fascia is disrupted, permitting blood and urine to escape into the perineum beneath Colles' fascia.

Pathology

Injuries to the Membranous Urethra

The membranous urethra is about 2 cm in length and extends from the apex of the prostate to the inferior margin of the U-G diaphragm. The first portion above the U-G diaphragm is *fragile and unprotected*, and when the pubic rami are fractured and the puboprostatic ligaments torn, this segment is *avulsed from the U-G diaphragm*. The diaphragm usually remains partly or completely intact so that extravasated urine and blood escape into the pelvis, but if the diaphragm is lacerated, they may gain access to the perineum and scrotum.

URETHRAL TRAUMA
(Rupture of the membranous urethra)

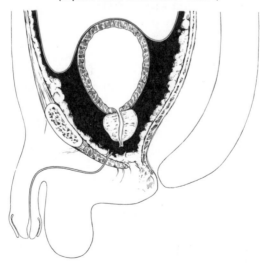

Fig. 10. With a complete rupture, the puboprostatic ligaments are usually torn so that the prostate retracts into the pelvis creating a 3- to 4-cm gap between the prostatic urethra and the distal remnant of the membranous urethra.

Less commonly, the membranous urethra may be damaged by the sharp ends of bone fragments.

Contusion and incomplete division of the membranous urethra may occur, but the most common injury is *complete rupture*.

Injuries to the Bulbous Urethra

The bulbous urethra is a relatively fixed segment just below the U-G diaphragm. Straddle-type falls on the perineum compress the bulbous urethra against the overlying symphysis pubis, causing either a contusion or a laceration of the urethra. If there is a break in the continuity of the urethra, blood and urine may be evident in the perineum.

Injuries to the Penile Urethra

This portion of the urethra is a common site for urethral strictures, and urethral dilation with metal sounds may occasionally produce lacerations and false passages.

Clinical Findings

Injuries of the Membranous Urethra

1. The combination of a *fractured pelvis and blood at the urethral meatus* points to an injury of the membranous urethra.
2. With a complete rupture, the puboprostatic ligaments are usually torn so that the prostate *retracts into the pelvis* creating a 3- to 4-cm gap between the prostatic urethra and the distal remnant of the membranous urethra.
   A. On rectal examination, the prostate is displaced *upward and posteriorly* and in its customary place there is a soft, boggy mass.
      1) This finding is *pathognomonic of a complete rupture.*
   B. The urethral gap and the change in alignment of the urethral ends account for the usual inability to pass a catheter into the bladder.
3. The bladder is usually distended and may be palpable in the suprapubic region.
   A. Spasm of the internal sphincter usually prevents any urine from escaping from the bladder.
      1) This accounts for a full bladder and lack of extravasated urine in the pelvis.
      2) The patient is usually *unable to void* but he should still be advised not to make the attempt.
4. The perineum and genitalia usually show no sign of bleeding.
   A. Blood collects above the U-G diaphragm in the pelvis.
   B. With extensive retroperitoneal hemorrhage, flank, inguinal, or scrotal ecchymosis may be present.
5. A gentle retrograde urethrogram should be performed to establish the diagnosis, injecting 10 to 15 ml of undiluted intravenous contrast medium.

Injuries of the Bulbous Urethra

1. There is usually a history of a fall astride a fixed object with resultant *immediate* pain, swelling, and ecchymosis in the perineum.

2. Escaping blood is confined within the boundaries of Colles' fascia.

A. With significant hemorrhage, the penis, scrotum, and the anterior perineum may be ecchymotic.

3. There is usually no urinary extravasation initially but later, if not warned, the patient may in effect void into his perineum.

A. As with blood, escaping urine is confined within the boundaries of Colles' fascia.

4. On rectal examination, the prostate is in normal position.

5. Diagnosis is established by a *retrograde urethrogram* and this should always be performed *before* passing a urethral catheter.

A. The passage of a urethral catheter may convert a partial rupture into a complete rupture.

B. The successful passage of a catheter into the bladder may obscure the presence of a complete rupture.

1) A catheter may be passed into the bladder in about 50% of complete bulbous urethral ruptures as compared with less than 10% in complete ruptures of the membranous urethra.

Management of Urethral Injuries

Minor Injuries

With contusions or small lacerations of the urethra, insert a no. 20 Silastic Foley catheter into the bladder and tape it to the lower abdomen to

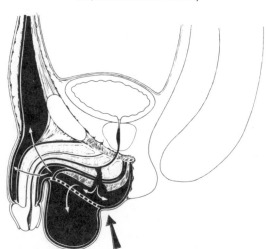

SADDLE INJURY
(Rupture of bulbous urethra)

Fig. 11. Lateral drawing showing extravasation of urine into the scrotum, perineum, and lower abdominal wall secondary to a rupture of the bulbous urethra.

prevent injury at the penoscrotal angle. After 10 days the catheter may be removed. Healing is usually satisfactory without any stricture but a stricture may result if there is a periurethral hematoma or infection.

Complete Rupture of the Membranous Urethra

This is the *most serious* injury of the lower urinary tract because of the frequency of major complications—stricture 50%, impotence 30%, and incontinence 5%.

Surgery

1. *All* patients require urinary diversion via suprapubic cystostomy.
2. If the patient's condition is precarious, primary urethral reconstruction is not done.

   A. Secondary repair may be performed 3 to 6 weeks later using the one-stage transpubic repair advocated by Waterhouse or the two-stage Turner-Warwick scrotal flap urethroplasty.

3. Primary repair is best accomplished with a combined suprapubic-perineal approach.

   A. Suprapubic.

     1) Explore the peritoneal cavity to rule out any associated injuries.

     2) Open the bladder, insert a cystostomy tube, and repair any bladder perforations.

     3) Evacuate any blood and urine, control bleeding, and remove or retract bone fragments away from the urethra.

     4) If the patient is doing poorly or if the lithotomy position is not feasible because of a fracture of the hip joint, the perineal approach is omitted and a Foley catheter is negotiated per urethra into the bladder.

       a. To eliminate or minimize the gap between the injured urethral ends, the prostate should be pulled down to the U-G diaphragm by traction sutures placed on either side of the prostatic urethra and brought out through the U-G diaphragm and tied over rubber tubing in the perineum.

   B. Traction on the prostate is preferred to traction on the bladder neck via Foley catheter balloon. Prolonged bladder neck traction sometimes causes damage to the internal sphincter mechanism with resultant urinary incontinence.

   C. Perineal.

     1) This approach permits *direct visualization* of the injured area.

     2) The urogenital diaphragm and displaced bone fragments may be properly positioned.

     3) The urethral ends may be approximated with interrupted fine chromic catgut sutures. Eliminating the gap between the urethral ends is the *best way to avoid urethral stricture.*

     4) A no. 16 Silastic catheter is left in the urethra as a splint for 2 weeks but is not placed on traction.

     5) A rubber tissue drain is left in place for dependent drainage.

Complete Rupture of the Bulbous Urethra

1. A vertical perineal incision is made over the area of injury, and all blood and urine are evacuated.

2. The urethral ends are identified, debrided, and spatulated in reverse directions to minimize chances of stricture.

A. To prevent tension on the anastomosis, the urethra is *extensively mobilized, both proximally and distally.*

B. The anastomosis is made with fine chromic catgut suture.

3. The area is drained and a Silastic no. 16 Foley catheter is left in place only 2 days.

4. Urinary diversion is always via a suprapubic cystostomy.

5. After 2 weeks, a voiding cystourethrogram is obtained, and if the urethra is well healed, the cystostomy tube is removed.

REFERENCES AND SUGGESTED FURTHER READING

General

1. Charron, J. W. and Brault, J. P. Recognition and early management of injuries to the urinary tract. J. Trauma 4:702, 1964.
2. Guerrier, K. R., Albert, D., and Persky, L. Urinary extravasation and urosepsis. Surg. Forum 19:529, 1968.
3. Moritz, A. R. Mechanical injuries of the urogenital tract. In *The Pathology of Trauma,* Chap 8. Lee and Febiger, 1954.

Kidney

1. Banowsky, L. H., Wolfel, D. A., and Lackner, L. H. Considerations in diagnosis and management of renal trauma. J. Trauma 10:587, 1970.
2. Halpern, M. Angiography in renal trauma. Surg. Clin. N. Am. 48:1221, 1968.
3. Marshall, V. F., Witsell, J., McGovern, J. H., and Miscall, B. G. The practicality of renal autotransplantation in humans. J.A.M.A. 196:1154, 1966.
4. Scott, R., Jr., Carlton, C. E., Jr., and Goldman, M. Penetrating injuries of the kidney: an analysis of 181 patients. J. Urol. 101:247, 1969.

Ureter

1. Badenoch, A. W. Injuries of the ureter. Proc. R. Soc. Med. 52:101, 1959.
2. Carlton, C. E., Jr., Scott, R., Jr., and Guthrie, A. G. The initial management of ureteral injuries: a report of 78 cases. J. Urol. 105:335, 1971.
3. Green, T. H., Jr., Meigs, J. V., Ulfelder, H., and Curtin, R. R. Urologic complications of radical Wertheim hysterectomy: incidence, etiology management and prevention. Obstet. Gynecol. 20:293, 1962.
4. Higgins, C. C. Ureteral injuries during surgery. J.A.M.A. 199:118, 1967.
5. Solomons, E., Levin, E. J., Bauman, J., and Baron, J. A pyelographic study of ureteric injuries sustained during hysterectomy for benign conditions. Surg. Gynecol. Obstet. 111:41, 1960.

Bladder and Urethra

1. Conolly, W. B. and Hedberg, E. A. Observations on fractures of the pelvis. J. Trauma 9:104, 1969.
2. DeWeerd, J. H. Management of injuries to the bladder, urethra and genitalia. Surg. Clin. N. Am. 39:973, 1959.
3. Friend, C. R., Sonda, L. P., and Glas, W. W. Investigative studies of bladder extravasation of urine. J. Trauma 2:451, 1962.
4. Kaiser, T. F. and Farrow, F. C. Injury of the bladder and prostatomembranous urethra associated with fracture of the bony pelvis. Surg. Gynecol. Obstet. 120:99, 1965.

5. McGowan, A. J., Jr. and Waterhouse, K. Mobilization of the anterior urethra. Bull. N. Y. Acad. Med. 40:776, 1964.
6. Morehouse, D. D. and MacKinnon, K. J. Urological injuries associated with pelvic fractures. J. Trauma 9:479, 1969.
7. Myers, R. P. and DeWeerd, J. H. Incidence of stricture following primary realignment of disrupted proximal urethra. J. Urol. 107:265, 1972.
8. Peltier, L. F. Complications associated with fractures of the pelvis. J. Bone Joint Surg. 47-A:1060, 1965.
9. Quinby, W. C., Jr. Pelvic fractures with hemorrhage. N. Engl. J. Med. 284:668, 1971.
10. Seitzman, D. M. Repair of the severed membranous urethra by the combined approach. J. Urol. 89:433, 1963.
11. Turner-Warwick, R. T. The repair of urethral strictures in the region of the membranous urethra. J. Urol. 100:303, 1968.
12. Waterhouse, K., Abrahams, J. I. Gruber, H., Hackett, R. E., Patil, U. B., and Peng, B. K. The transpubic approach to the lower urinary tract. J. Urol. 109:486, 1973.
13. Uhlenhuth, E., Smith, R. D., Day, E. C., and Middleton, E. B. A re-investigation of Colles' and Buck's fasciae in the male. J. Urol. 62:542, 1949.
14. Weens, H. S., Newman, J. H., and Florence, T. J. Trauma of the lower urinary tract—a roentgenologic study. N. Engl. J. Med. 234:357, 1946.

9

Calculi

ARTHUR W. WYKER, JR.

Calculi, or stones, frequently form in the urinary tract and each year one person per 1,000 population is hospitalized because of stone. Calculi may occur at any age but are rare in children under 10 or in adults over 65, the peak incidence being in the 20 to 40 age group. Men are affected more commonly than women, and white people more commonly than black.

WHAT IS A CALCULUS

Calculus = Crystals + Organic Matrix

The organic matrix, present in *all* calculi, is a sticky, sugar-protein combination called mucoprotein. In most stones, the matrix averages 2.5% by weight, but in "matrix" stones this may reach 60%. The significance of this matrix portion of the calculus *has not been definitely established.* Boyce[3] emphasized the importance of the matrix and believed it determines the crystal orientation within the calculus and may be the cause of some renal calculi. Vermeulen,[26] on the other hand, emphasized the importance of the crystalloid component (97% by weight) and he considered calculi as matricized mineral rather than mineralized matrix.

Composition of Urinary Calculi

1. Calcium oxalate only or calcium oxalate-calcium phosphate mixture 75%
2. Calcium phosphate-magnesium ammonium phosphate   15%
3. Uric acid   7%
4. Cystine   2%
5. Miscellaneous   <u>1%</u>
                                            100%

Pathogenesis

The cause of calculus formation is *not known*. Attention has been focused on the renal papilla since Randall[22] in 1937 reported finding calcified plaques beneath the epithelium of the papilla in 17% of autopsied kidneys. Recent microscopic examination of apparently normal kidneys has revealed small deposits of calcium in the renal pyramids of *every kidney*, and these deposits were more numerous in the renal segments from recurrent stone formers. Carr,[4] using microradiographs, noted calcified bodies in the renal substance of normal kidneys lying especially at the fornices, along the blood vessels, and underneath the capsule. He believed that precipitation of calcium salts in the renal papilla is probably a normal process with normally functioning lymphatics draining off the salts. He suggested that the renal calculi develop when this *lymphatic drainage mechanism is overloaded or inefficient*. The primary stone thus starts as a small calcified body adjacent to the fornix and separated from the calyceal urine by only a thin layer of mucosa. It eventually erodes away the overlying epithelium exposing it to the calyceal urine, and it now may grow by crystallization. It should be remembered that this theory is as yet *unproven*.

Factors Which Favor the Formation of a Stone

Although the mechanism of stone formation is unclear, we do have some understanding of the factors which encourage stone formation.

1. Increased *concentration* in the urine of the stone-forming crystalloid.

A. This may be due to decreased urine volume or to a high rate of excretion of the crystalloid component into a normal volume of urine.

B. Decreased urine volume occurs when there is inadequate intake of H_2O or excessive loss of H_2O via the skin (hot climate) or bowel (ileostomy).

1) With less urinary H_2O, the concentration of *all* urinary solutes increases including those that can crystallize into stones.

C. Cystine stones, unlike calcium and uric acid stones, form *only* when there is increased concentration of the stone-forming crystalloid in the urine.

1) Cystine stone formers have 8 to 40 times as much cystine in their urine as do normal people.

D. Excess calcium, uric acid, or oxalate in the urine is associated with an increased incidence of stone formation, but excess phosphate is not.
2. Abnormally low or high urine pH (normal mean urine pH is 5.85).
   A. Uric acid stones form only in acid urine, and the more acid the urine, the greater the chance of uric acid stone formation.
   1) In solution, uric acid exists in two forms—the relatively insoluble free uric acid and the relatively soluble urate ion, and urine pH determines the ratio of these two forms (Table I).
   2) This means that with normal urinary excretion of 500 mg of uric acid per day, the amount of relatively insoluble free uric acid would be only 30 mg at pH 7 (500 × 0.06) but 425 mg at pH 5 (500 × 0.85).
   3) The solubility of this uric acid varies greatly with urine pH.
      a. At pH 5, 70 mg of uric acid are soluble in 1 liter of urine, whereas, at pH 7, 1,580 mg are soluble.
      b. This 20-fold increase in solubility of uric acid over the physiological range of urine pH, 5 to 7, emphasizes the *critical nature of urine pH in uric acid stone formation.*
   B. Calcium phosphate and magnesium ammonium phosphate calculi form only in relatively alkaline or alkaline urine.
   1) With a rise in urine pH and urinary ammonium excretion, the solubility of calcium phosphate and magnesium ammonium phosphate decreases greatly, and the urine is supersaturated so that crystal formation may occur.
   2) Calcium phosphate stones form only when the urine pH is greater than 6.6, and magnesium ammonium phosphate stones occur only when the urine pH is greater than 7.1.
   3) $Mg\text{-}NH_4\text{-}PO_4$ stones are known as "infection stones," for urinary infection with a urea-splitting organism (Proteus) is the usual cause of alkaline urine.
3. Protective substances in the urine.
   A. Pyrophosphate, magnesium, and citrate *increase calcium solubility* in the urine and may be considered calcification inhibitors.
   1) However, it has not been demonstrated that deficiencies of any one of these three substances in the urine cause stone formation.
4. Urinary tract obstruction with stasis of urine.

TABLE I

Effect of Urine pH on the Percentage of Relatively Insoluble Free Uric Acid

Urine pH	Free Uric Acid	Urate Ion
	%	%
7	6	94
6	37	63
5.75	50	50
5.0	85	15

A. Stasis, or sluggish flow of urine, may be a factor in stone formation in three ways:

1) It allows time for precipitation of crystals from normally super-saturated urine.

2) Lacking any flushing action, beginning stones are not washed away but instead may grow.

3) It encourages infection which plays a role in stone formation chiefly by its effect on urine pH.

a. Urea-splitting organisms alkalinize the urine decreasing the solubility of $Mg-NH_4-PO_4$.

CLINICAL CAUSES OF STONES

Calcium Stones—90% of All Stones

Unlike cystine and uric acid stones, which probably result from simple precipitation from a supersaturated solution and can therefore be explained in simple solubility terms, calcium stone formation is more complex and less well understood. The following four factors increase the probability of calcium stone formation.

1. Increased urinary concentration of calcium due to hypercalciuria or dehydration.

2. Alkaline urine.

3. Excess oxalate in the urine.

4. Structural abnormalities with resultant stasis of urine.

Hypercalciuria

1. Despite wide variations in calcium intake, most normal people excrete 50 to 200 mg of calcium per day in their urine, so that hypercalciuria is commonly defined as more than 300 mg/day in males and more than 250 mg/day in females.

A. Using these criteria, 30 to 40% of calcium stone formers have hypercalciuria as compared to 5 to 10% of normal people.

2. Urinary calcium is affected by the amount of calcium, phosphate, and sodium in the diet.

A. Dietary calcium has only a minimal effect on urinary calcium with large changes in dietary calcium producing very slight changes in the urinary calcium.

TABLE II

Relationship of Dietary Sodium to Urinary Calcium

Dietary Sodium	Urinary Calcium
mEq/day	*mg/day*
25	180
350	580

B. Calcium excretion varies inversely with the phosphate intake, so that a high phosphate intake tends to lower urinary calcium.

C. Calcium excretion varies directly and significantly with sodium intake (Table II).

3. The chief determinant of urinary calcium is the amount filtered by the glomeruli.

A. Sixty to 70% of calcium is not bound to the plasma proteins and is therefore filtered at the glomerulus.

1) Normally, 9,000 to 10,000 mg of calcium are filtered daily with 98% being reabsorbed.

B. When renal insufficiency is associated with a decreased glomerular filtration rate, the urinary calcium decreases.

4. Metabolic acidosis, but not respiratory acidosis, causes hypercalciuria probably by bone dissolution.

5. Clinical causes of hypercalciuria.

A. Hypercalcemia + hypercalciuria.

1) Primary hyperparathyrodism—cause of 5 to 10% of all calcium stones.

2) Immobilization.

3) Excessive ingestion of calcium + calcium-containing antacids.

4) Metastatic bone disease—although the most common cause of hypercalcemia, rarely leads to stone formation.

5) Boeck's sarcoid.

6) Vitamin D intoxication.

B. Hypercalciuria with normal or low serum calcium.

1) Idiopathic hypercalciuria—this is the most common cause of hypercalciuria and therefore the most common metabolic cause of urinary stones.

2) Renal tubular acidosis.

Alkaline Urine

1. Calcium salts are relatively insoluble in alkaline media.

2. The usual cause of alkaline urine is an infection with a urea-splitting organism such as Proteus, and the resultant stone is always composed of magnesium ammonium phosphate.

Excess Oxalate in the Urine

1. This is a *rare* cause of calcium oxalate stones but may occur after excessive ingestion of high oxalate foods, during pyridoxine deficiency, or in the genetic disorder, primary hyperoxaluria.

2. Normal urine oxalate is 10 to 50 mg/day, whereas, patients with primary hyperoxaluria excrete more than 100 mg/day.

Structural Abnormalities with Resultant Stasis of Urine

1. Medullary sponge kidney is often accompanied by tiny calculi in the dilated collecting ducts.

A. Although stasis is a factor here, about half of these patients also have hypercalciuria.

SPECIFIC DISORDERS ASSOCIATED WITH CALCIUM STONE FORMATION

Primary Hyperparathyroidism

This endocrine disorder is the most common cause of *persistent hypercalcemia* and accounts for 5 to 10% of all calcium stones. Parathyroid hormone raises the level of ionized calcium in the blood by increasing reabsorption of calcium from the bones, intestinal tract, and kidney. Hypercalcemia increases the filtered load of calcium to such a degree that this effect overbalances the increased tubular reabsorption of calcium by the kidney, the net result being *hypercalciuria*. Hypercalcemia and hypercalciuria may affect the kidney in three ways:

1. Stone formation—calcium oxalate or calcium phosphate stones may form in the renal calyces or pelvis.

2. Nephrocalcinosis—calcium deposits occur in the substance of the kidney, chiefly in the medullar portions.

3. Impaired ability to concentrate urine.

Renal Tubular Acidosis

In this disorder, there is a defect in the renal ability to excrete acid so that the urine is *consistently* relatively alkaline or alkaline (pH > 6). The retained acid causes metabolic acidosis which mobilizes calcium from the bones with resultant hypercalciuria. Calcium salts are relatively insoluble in an alkaline media, so the *combination of hypercalciuria and relatively alkaline urine* almost invariably causes nephrocalcinosis and nephrolithiasis. In less severe forms of RTA (incomplete RTA), metabolic acidosis and hypercalciuria may be absent, but urine pH is greater than 6.0 and nephrocalcinosis and nephrolithiasis often occur.

Immobilization

Normally, bone formation and absorption are taking place concurrently at an equal rate. The chief stimulus for bone formation is *longitudinal stress on the bone*, and when this is lacking, as with a leg in a cast, the bone of the leg in the cast becomes thin and decalcified while the other bones remain thick and normally calcified. With immobilization or the prolonged weightlessness of space travel, this stimulus is lacking and there is an imbalance between bone formation and absorption with resultant hypercalcemia and hypercalciuria. Immobilized patients tend to have relatively alkaline urine with resultant decrease in solubility of calcium phosphate and magnesium ammonium phosphate, and this factor may be more important than hypercalciuria in the genesis of "immobilization stones."

Idiopathic Hypercalciuria

This disorder is believed to be the cause of 30 to 40% of all calcium stones, and since calcium stones make up 90% of the total, *idiopathic hypercalci-uria is the most common cause of stone formation.* The cause of the excess calcium in the urine appears to be increased absorption of calcium from the gut. The majority of these patients have normal serum calcium levels.

URIC ACID STONES—7% OF ALL STONES

All humans are in constant danger of forming a uric acid stone owing to two defects in our handling of uric acid.

1. The normal end product of purine catabolism is allantoin, but due to a species-wide inborn error of metabolism, we lack the enzyme uricase and are unable to convert the relatively insoluble uric acid to the very soluble allantoin.

A. As a result, we constantly have relatively high levels of uric acid in the plasma and urine, and whenever our urine pH drops below 5.5, it is saturated or supersaturated with respect to uric acid, and we run the risk of uric acid stone formation.

2. Uric acid is an inert waste product of no value to the body, but unfortunately our kidneys treat it as if it were a very valuable substance and reabsorb over 90% of it.

Causes of Uric Acid Stone Formation

Most uric acid stones result from simple precipitation from a super-saturated solution and therefore can be explained in simple solubility terms. Supersaturation may result from an increased rate of uric acid excretion into a normal volume of urine, normal rate of uric acid excretion into a decreased volume of urine (dehydration), or hyperacid urine. Uric acid stones form only in acid urine, and the more acid the urine, the greater the chance of uric acid stone formation. The solubility of uric acid varies greatly with urine pH and going from pH 5 to 7, there is a 20-fold increase in uric acid solubility.

There are four clinical disorders which significantly increase the risk of uric acid stone formation—primary gout, secondary gout, hyperacid urine former, and ileostomy.

Primary Gout

In primary gout, there is overproduction of uric acid, impaired renal excretion of uric acid, or both, with resultant hyperuricemia, but *excess uric acid in the urine occurs in a surprisingly small portion of this group*—25%. The frequency of uric acid stone formation does reflect the serum and urinary uric acid levels, for the higher the levels, the greater the incidence of stone formation (Table III).

All patients with primary gout tend to have more acid urine than most normal subjects owing to a defect in ammonia production by the kidney, and the associated decrease in uric acid solubility plays a greater role in uric acid stone formation than does the excess uric acid in the urine which is present in only one-fourth of these patients.

Secondary Gout

Secondary gout is due to an accelerated rate of cell turnover with resultant hyperuricemia and hyperuricosuria. All tissue cells contain nucleoprotein, a precursor of uric acid, and in the lymphomas and certain hematological disorders, the increased formation and destruction of cells raises the level of uric acid in the blood and urine. Hematological disorders which are prone to cause secondary gout include—leukemia, polycythemia vera, lymphosarcoma, and the chronic hemolytic anemias. Unlike primary gout, the urine pH is not unduly acid in secondary gout, so that uric acid stone formation is due to the increased concentration of uric acid in the urine.

The levels of uric acid in the blood and urine tend to be higher than those in primary gout, accounting for the greater prevalence of uric acid stones (Table IV).

Cytolytic therapy with irradiation or chemotherapeutic agents, particularly when successful, releases a large quantity of uric acid into the general circulation, causing an acute fulminating hyperuricemia and hyperuricosuria which may produce anuria due to obstruction of the nephrons by uric acid crystals.

Hyperacid Urine

Over 50% of the patients with uric acid stones are not overproducers of uric acid (primary gout) nor do they have a disorder which causes an

TABLE III
Relationship of Uric Acid Levels to Stone Formation in Primary Gout

Uric Acid Levels	Uric Acid Stone Formation in Primary Gout
	%
Serum: 7–8 mg%	17
Serum: 13–14 mg%	50
Urine: normoexcretor	15
Urine: overexcretory	40

TABLE IV
Prevalence of Uric Acid Stones in Gout

Type	Prevalence of Uric Acid Stones
	%
Primary gout	20
Secondary gout	40

accelerated turnover of cells (secondary gout), but they tend to form uric acid stones because their urine is *constantly* hyperacid with pH less than 5.5.

Despite normal amounts of uric acid in the urine, it is *continuously supersaturated* with respect to uric acid owing to the relative insolubility of uric acid in acid urine.

Ileostomy

These patients also have normal amounts of uric acid in their urine but 10% of them form uric acid stones owing to decreased urine volume and hyperacid urine.

1. Decreased urine volume increases the uric acid concentration in the urine.

A. Normal people lose 100 ml of water in the stool each day whereas patients with ileostomies lose 500 to 1,000 ml/day with resultant chronic hypohydration.

B. With decreased body water, these patients excrete only 400 to 800 ml of urine per day with specific gravity greater than 1.015.

2. Hyperacid urine decreases the solubility of the uric acid present.

A. Normal people lose 5 mEq sodium in the stool each day whereas patients with ileostomies lose 75 to 100 mEq.

B. Loss of fixed base results in excretion of an acid urine with pH less than 5.5.

CYSTINE STONES—2% OF ALL STONES

Cystine stone formation is due to precipitation of cystine from a supersaturated urine, and stone formers excrete 8 to 40 times as much cystine in their urine as do normal people. Cystinuria is due to a *genetic renal tubular defect* which results in excretion in the urine of excessive amounts of four aminoacids—arginine, ornithine, lysine, and cystine. Cystine alone is poorly soluble in urine, and stones may form when the urinary cystine exceeds 300 mg/day or the cystine concentration exceeds 0.3 mg/cc (300 mg/liter).

This hereditary trait occurs in 0.2% of the population, but only 3% of these cystinurics form stones (Table V).

TABLE V
Relationship of Amount of Cystine in Urine to Incidence of Stone Formation

	% of Cystinurics	Urinary Cystine	Stone Formation
		mg/day	*%*
Normal		40-80	0
Heterozygotes	97	100-300	< 1
Homozygotes	3	300-3,000	> 50

Notice the direct relationship between the amount of cystine in the urine and the incidence of stone formation.

These patients have an associated defect in intestinal absorption of their four amino acids as well, but this is of no clinical significance.

Clinical Points of Interest

1. Stone formation may begin in childhood, and for this reason cystine stones account for about 6% of all calculi in children but only 2% of all calculi in adults.
2. These calculi, which tend to form a cast of the renal collecting system (staghorn), are radiopaque as are calcium stones, but they have a homogeneous structure, whereas calcium stones tend to have a non-homogeneous structure.
3. Most cystinurics have cystine crystals in their urine and these crystals are unique, being perfect hexagons, translucent, and almost white.
4. The solubility of cystine does not change significantly over the physiological range of urine pH, 5 to 7 being about 350 mg/1,000 cc, but raising the urine pH to 7.8 doubles the solubility of cystine.
5. Five to 10% of stones passed by cystinurics *do not contain cystine*.

CLINICAL

Signs and Symptoms

A stone may remain silent and undetected until it becomes arrested at some point in the urinary tract and obstructs the flow of urine causing pain, or it lacerates the urinary wall causing hematuria. Therefore, small stones may pass through the entire urinary tract and large stones may reside in the renal pelvis—both without producing any symptoms.

Pain, Often Severe, Is the Common Presenting Complaint

1. The mechanism of pain is *distension* of the ureter or renal pelvis proximal to the site of obstruction.
    A. The severity of the pain is determined not by the degree of obstruction or distension, but by the rapidity with which it takes place.
        1) Sudden acute distension causes severe pain, whereas gradual slow distension causes little or no pain.
2. Pain may be steady, but about 50% of the time it is spasmodic or colicky.
3. The distribution of the pain depends upon the location of the obstructing stone.
    A. Renal pelvis or calyces → pain in the costovertebral angle (CVA) region.
    B. Ureteropelvic junction and upper ureter → pain adjacent to the anterior superior iliac spine.
        1) Referred pain to the ipsilateral testis or vulva may also be present.
    C. Mid ureter → pain adjacent to mid-Poupart's ligament.

D. Ureterovesical junction and lower ureter → pain in the suprapubic region.

1) Referred pain to the ipsilateral scrotum or vulva may also be present.

Other Signs and Symptoms

1. Hematuria.

A. Gross hematuria occurs in only about 5 to 10% of cases, but microscopic hematuria occurs in more than 90% of all patients with stones.

2. Urgency of urination and defecation with associated urinary frequency.

A. These symptoms may be present when the stone is in the lower ureter close to the bladder.

B. When present, they are very helpful clinically because they not only indicate the presence of a stone but they also define its location.

3. Infection.

A. Associated infection is common with renal stones (50%) but uncommon with ureteral calculi (5 to 10%).

B. An obstructing stone encourages infection because it causes stasis of urine, damages the adjacent urinary wall, and acts as a foreign body.

C. Some stones are secondary to urinary infection.

1) Urea-splitting organisms such as Proteus alkalinize the urine decreasing the solubility of calcium salts thereby encouraging the formation of $MgNH_4PO_4$—$CaPO_4$ stones.

4. Anorexia, nausea, and vomiting.

A. These symptoms are reflex in nature and vary directly with the degree of pain experienced by the patient.

1) Anorexia accompanies mild pain, vomiting, severe pain.

B. Since pain is largely responsible for these gastrointestinal (GI) symptoms, there is usually a close time relationship between the two symptoms.

1) Vomiting commonly occurs soon after the patient experiences severe pain, not 1 to 2 hours later.

Physical Findings

In contrast to patients with acute appendicitis who tend to lie still, these patients often are hyperactive and change position frequently. Tenderness may be completely absent, but more commonly there is slight deep tenderness in the lateral abdomen, flank, or CVA region. Marked point tenderness, rebound, and muscle guarding are absent. Abdominal distension is often present, and bowel sounds are usually hypoactive. Lower ureteral calculi cannot be reached in males, but they can often be detected on pelvic examination in females.

Laboratory Studies

1. Blood count.

A. A mild leukocytosis is often present, but white blood cell (WBC) counts do not go over 15,000/cu mm unless there is associated infection.

2. Urinalysis.

A. Red blood cells (RBC)—microscopic hematuria is present in more than 90% of cases.

1) Hematuria may be present, but red blood cells may not be seen in the urinary sediment if they have been lysed by hypotonic (< 1.007) or alkaline (pH > 7) urine.

2) To detect the presence of lysed RBC, always perform a dipstick test for hemoglobin.

B. WBC—mild pyuria may be present.

1) The excess WBC in the urine represent the body's response to inflammation by the stone.

C. Bacteria—usually absent in ureteral stone cases but often present in renal stone cases.

1) When greater than 5 rod-like bacteria per high power field are detected in fresh urinary sediment, infection is present.

2) Pyuria without bacteriuria does *not* indicate infection.

D. pH.

1) A single determination is of little value since the normal range of urine pH is 4.8 to 7.4.

2) Uric acid and cystine calculi form in acid urine whereas calcium phosphate and magnesium ammonium phosphate form in relatively alkaline or alkaline urine.

a. Formation of calcium oxalate stones is unrelated to urine pH.

E. Crystal.

1) Crystals in the urinary sediment are of no diagnostic importance *unless they are cystine.*

2) Cystine is the only crystal which is never seen in normal urine, and its presence indicates cystinuria.

3. Intravenous urogram.

A. Flat plate.

1) Calcium stones (90%) and cystine stones (2%) are radiopaque, but uric acid stones (7%) are radiolucent.

2) Since uric acid stones are radiolucent, they can only be detected by filling the urinary tract with radiopaque contrast medium and noting a persistent filling defect.

B. Urographic phase.

1) With an obstructing stone in the ureter, there is usually delayed appearance of the contrast medium with dilation of the ureter down to the obstructing stone.

Diagnostic Evaluation of a Patient with Stone

1. History.

A. Is there a family history of urinary stones?

1) Genetically related stones include *all* cystine stones (cystinuria),

rare calcium oxalate stones (primary hyperoxaluria), and some uric acid stones (hereditary hyperacid urine former).

B. Does the patient have any disorder which predisposes to stone formation?

1) All stones.

a. Decreased urine volume due to excessive loss of H_2O via skin (live in a hot climate or have an occupation which causes excessive sweating) or via GI tract (chronic diarrhea).

2) Calcium stones.

a. Excessive milk, alkali, or vitamin D intake.

b. Bone disease.

c. Immobilization.

d. Diamox (diuretic which alkalinizes the urine).

e. Proteus urinary infection.

f. Urinary tract obstruction.

3) Uric acid stones.

a. Primary gout.

b. Secondary gout due to hematological disorders (leukemia, polycythemia, hemolytic anemia) or neoplasms (lymphoma) especially after cytolytic therapy.

c. Ileostomy.

C. Does the patient have any symptoms suggesting hypercalcemia?

1) Hypercalcemia decreases neuromuscular conduction causing *weakness and constipation*.

2) It decreases the kidney's ability to concentrate urine, causing *urinary frequency and nocturia*.

2. Identification of the type of stone.

A. This is the most important step in the diagnosis.

B. All stones should be analyzed by crystallographic techniques, polarizing microscopy or x-ray diffraction.

1) When stones contain more than one crystal type, the nucleus portion is more significant than the outer layer, since it is the "original" stone and treatment is aimed at the disorder responsible for its formation.

2) Chemical techniques do not permit identification of the nucleus.

C. If no stone is available, try to identify the stone by its appearance on a flat plate.

1) Radiopaque stones include all calcium stones, all cystine stones, and some uric acid stones with a calcium shell.

2) Calcium oxalate stones—most dense of all stones—tend to have a granular structure.

3) Calcium phosphate stones—moderately dense stones often showing laminations.

4) Cystine stones—may be almost radiolucent or as dense as calcium stones, the variable radiopacity apparently being related to the density of sulfur atoms in the crystal lattice.

a. They have a smoother homogeneous internal structure.

3. Urine examination.

A. pH.

1) Using nitrazine paper, check each fresh urine specimen voided during the first 2 days.

2) Less than 5.5 consistently—stone is probably uric acid, and patient may be a *hyperacid* uric acid stone former.

3) From 5.5 to 6.6—stone is probably calcium oxalate.

4) Greater than 6.5 consistently—stone is probably calcium phosphate and patient may have renal tubular acidosis.

5) Greater than 7.0 consistently—stone is probably magnesium ammonium phosphate and patient may have a urea-splitting urinary infection.

B. Is cystinuria present?

1) Most, *but not all*, patients with cystinuria have cystine crystals in the urine.

a. To increase the chances of finding these typical hexagonal crystals, bring the urine pH down to 4 to 5 level by adding a few drops of glacial acetic acid and then cool in a refrigerator for a few hours.

2) Nitroprusside test for cystinuria should be performed on the first specimen voided in the A.M.

a. It gives an approximation of the cystine content in any given specimen and is positive when the cystine concentration is greater than 75 mg/1,000 cc.

C. Is infection present?

1) Look for rodlike bacteria in *fresh* urinary sediment and obtain a urine culture.

D. 24-hour urine for calcium, uric acid, oxalate, creatinine, sodium, and cystine (Table VI).

4. Blood chemistry.

A. Serum calcium should be determined three times.

1) Total serum calcium measures ionized calcium (Ca^{++}), calcium bound to protein and the almost negligible calcium complexes.

2) *Ionized calcium* is the biologically active form and in true hypercalcemia, it is this fraction that is elevated.

TABLE VI
Twenty-four-hour Urine Output of Common Stone-forming Substances

Normal Values on a Regular Diet		Excess
	mg	*mg*
Calcium in males	50–300	> 300
Calcium in females	50–250	> 250
Uric acid	300–600	> 600
Oxalate	10–50	> 100
Cystine	40–80	> 100

a. It can be measured directly using a calcium-selective electrode, but more commonly it is measured indirectly.

b. If the total serum calcium, serum albumin, and globulin values are plotted on a triside nomogram, one can get a fairly accurate estimate of the ionized calcium level.

3) Since total serum calcium varies directly with the serum proteins, it is possible to have true hypercalcemia (increased level of ionized calcium), yet the total serum calcium may be normal or even subnormal.

B. Serum uric acid, phosphorus, Na, CO_2, Mg, Cl, and creatinine should be determined two times.

1) $CO_2 < 20$ mEq/liter in association with urine pH consistently > 6.0 suggests renal tubular acidosis.

TREATMENT

Surgery

The mere presence of a stone in the urinary tract is not an indication for surgery, since 80% of ureteral calculi and 20% of renal calculi are passed spontaneously. In addition, some small stones may reside in a renal calyx for many years without causing any symptoms and without significantly damaging the kidney.

There are two primary indications for surgery:

1. The stone is too large to pass spontaneously (> 1 cm in diameter), and it is producing enough obstruction to cause renal damage or repeated episodes of pain.

2. The stone is associated with infection.

A. When a stone obstructs any portion of the urinary tract and there is infection *proximal* to this stone, septicemia may occur so this stone *should be removed immediately* or a ureteral catheter should be passed above the obstructing stone to neutralize the obstruction and provide adequate drainage.

1) Treating the infection vigorously with high-powered antibiotics is *not* adequate treatment—the obstruction must be relieved!

Lower ureteral calculi may sometimes be removed via cystoscopy using special stone extractors which, when passed up the ureter, may entrap the stone and pull it into the bladder.

Medical

All Stones

1. Force fluids throughout the 24-hour period.

A. The resulting increase in urine volume decreases the urine concentration of *all* crystalloids, lessening the probability that small crystals will combine with others to form a stone.

B. The high flow rate of urine tends to flush out any embryo stones.

2. Urinary infections, particularly those due to urea-splitting organisms, should be treated vigorously with appropriate bactericidal antibiotics.

Calcium Stones

1. If hypercalciuria is present and the cause is known, treat the responsible disorder.

    A. Primary hyperparathyroidism—surgically remove hyperfunctioning parathyroid tissue.

    B. Renal tubular acidosis—give alkali to counteract the systemic acidosis and thereby eliminate the hypercalciuria.

    C. Boeck's sarcoid—low calcium, low vitamin D diet to counteract the hyperabsorption of calcium by the gut.

2. To reduce urine calcium concentration (Ca^{++}/ml urine).

    A. High fluid intake.

        1) Doubling the daily urine output from 1,500 ml to 3,000 ml cuts the critical urine calcium concentration in half.

    B. Low calcium intake.

        1) This has only a modest effect on urine calcium levels.

    C. Thiazides.

        1) These commonly used diuretic agents prevent the formation of calcium stones by causing a marked and *sustained lowering of the urinary calcium.*

        2) Although equally as effective as orthophosphates in inhibiting calcium stone formation, thiazides are less commonly used because of a higher incidence of side effects.

    D. Low sodium diet.

        1) Since the urinary calcium level parallels the urinary sodium level, a low sodium intake invariably lowers both the urinary sodium and calcium levels, thereby inhibiting calcium stone formation.

        2) This diet has limited usefulness but is particularly effective in those hypercalciuria patients who normally have a high salt intake.

    E. Orthophosphates.

        1) In most but not all patients, a high intake of phosphates decreases urinary calcium levels.

3. To inhibit crystallization of calcium salts.

    A. Orthophosphates.

        1) This is the regimen of choice for recurrent calcium stone formers.

        2) They effectively prevent the formation of both calcium oxalate and calcium phosphate stones by increasing the urinary excretion of pyrophosphate, a potent inhibitor of crystallization.

        3) In addition, there is an increase in urinary orthophosphate and a decrease in urinary calcium, but both these effects probably play a minor role in inhibiting calcium stone formation.

4. To reduce urine phosphorus concentration.

    A. The Shorr regimen, a low phosphorus diet plus aluminum gel, effectively prevents formation of calcium phosphate and magnesium ammonium phosphate stones by decreasing the urinary phosphorus to less than 200 mg/day.

1) It works even in the presence of urea-splitting infection and impaired renal function so is ideal for the patient with recurrent phosphatic calculi with history of multiple operations for stone.

2) Many patients will not stick to this regimen because the diet is restrictive, not very palatable, and GI dysfunction (usually constipation) is common.

5. To reduce urine oxalate concentration.

A. Despite the fact that 60 to 70% of all stones contain oxalate, urine oxalate levels are usually normal and hyperoxaluria is rare.

B. Low oxalate diet.

1) This is of no value, since only 5% of ingested oxalate is absorbed.

C. Pyridoxine.

1) This vitamin reduces urinary oxalate levels to a modest degree in patients with primary hyperoxaluria, but it does not return them to normal.

Uric Acid Stones

1. Since uric acid stones form *only* in acid urine, they can be prevented by keeping the urine dilute and at a pH around 6.5.

A. Alkalinization of the urine decreases the solubility of calcium salts so a restricted calcium intake is necessary to minimize the risk of calcium stone formation.

2. Allopurinol.

A. This drug is a very valuable one because it lowers both serum and urinary uric acid levels by inhibiting the formation of uric acid.

B. Hypoxanthine $\xrightarrow[\text{Oxidase}]{\text{Xanthine}}$ Xanthine $\xrightarrow[\text{Oxidase}]{\text{Xanthine}}$ Uric Acid

$\uparrow$ Allopurinol $\qquad$ $\uparrow$ Allopurinol

1) Allopurinol inhibits xanthine oxidase so that less uric acid is formed and hypoxanthine and xanthine quantities increase in a roughly 50:50 ratio.

2) Hypoxanthine is quite soluble at all pH levels, but xanthine has low solubility in acid urine, so there is some risk of xanthine stone formation.

C. Indications.

1) Gout and uric acid stones.

2) Primary or secondary uric acid nephropathy.

3) Recurrent uric acid stone former.

4) For pretreatment of patients with leukemia or lymphoma undergoing cytolytic therapy.

D. Side effects are infrequent—6%.

1) In the early stages of allopurinol administration, there is an increased incidence of acute attacks of gout, so give maintenance doses of colchicine during this period.

2) Chief side effect is skin rash, often with drug fever.

Cystine Stones

1. High fluid intake throughout 24-hour period.

A. All patients who form cystine stones have excess cystine in their urine and the higher the cystine concentration, the greater the probability of stone formation (Table VII).

B. Knowing the solubility of cystine, it is possible to prevent the formation of cystine stones in many patients merely by having them drink enough water to lower the cystine concentration to safe levels (Table VIII).

1) Hydration alone may be feasible for patients excreting up to 800 mg per day but is impractical for patients excreting 1,000 mg per day or more.

2) Safe concentrations must be maintained *all the time*, so 2 glasses of water must be taken at bedtime and again at 3 A.M.

2. Alkalinization.

A. Increasing the urine pH increases the solubility of cystine, but no significant effect occurs until the pH reaches 7.5; raising it to 7.8 only doubles the solubility of cystine.

B. This degree of alkalinization markedly decreases the solubility of calcium salts, and, in order to prevent calcium stone formation, alkalinization must always be combined with a high fluid, low calcium intake.

C. This is usually instituted when hydration alone is inadequate.

3. Low methionine diet.

A. Methionine is the principal dietary precursor of cystine and a

TABLE VII

		Stone Formation		
	Normal	Unlikely	Possible	Probable
Cystine concentration	< 0.1 mg/cc < 100 mg/1000 cc	0.3 mg/cc 300 mg/1000 cc	0.4 mg/cc 400 mg/1000 cc	> 0.5 mg/cc > 500 mg/1000 cc

TABLE VIII
Effect of Urine Output on Cystine Concentrations

Cystine Output	Urine Volume			
	1,000 cc	2,000 cc	3,000 cc	4,000 cc
mg		*mg/cc*		
300	*0.3*[a]	*0.15*[a]	*0.1*[a]	*0.075*[a]
500	0.5	*0.25*[a]	*0.17*[a]	*0.13*[a]
800	0.8	0.4	*0.27*[a]	*0.2*[a]
1000	1.0	0.5	*0.33*[a]	*0.25*[a]
2000	2.0	1.0	0.67	0.5

[a] Safe levels of cystine concentration are italicized.

consistently low methionine diet will decrease the urinary cystine to safe levels.

B. Although effective, patient acceptance is low, since it requires elimination of dairy products and meats.

4. D-Penicillamine.

A. This drug combines with cystine to form two complexes which are 100 times as soluble as cystine, and this subtraction lowers urinary cystine to safe levels.

B. Because of antipyridoxine effect, it is necessary also to administer pyridoxine daily.

C. This drug is reserved for those patients who excrete unusually large amounts of cystine in their urine or who are unable to adhere to the high fluid-alkali regimen.

D. One-third of all patients treated have significant side effects, chiefly skin rash, proteinuria, and granulocytopenia.

1) Blood count and urinalysis should be checked at frequent intervals.

REFERENCES AND SUGGESTED FURTHER READING

1. Allen, T. D. and Spence, H. M. Matrix stones. Trans. Am. Assoc. Genitourin. Surg. 57:77, 1965.
2. Bartter, F. C., Lotz, M., Thies, S., Rosenberg, L. E., and Potts, J. T. Cystinuria: Combined Clinical Staff Conference at the National Institutes of Health. Ann. Intern. Med. 62:796, 1965.
3. Boyce, W. H. Organic matrix of native human urinary concretions. Renal Stone Research Symposium. Edited by A. Hodgkinson and B. E. C. Nordin, p. 93. J. A. Churchill, Ltd., London, 1969.
4. Carr, R. J. Aetiology of renal calculi: micro-radiographic studies. Proceedings of the Renal Stone Research Symposium held at Leeds, April, 1968. Edited by A. Hodgkinson and B. E. C. Nordin, p. 123. J. A. Churchill, Ltd., London, 1969.
5. Clark, P. B. and Nordin, B. E. C. The problem of the calcium stone. Renal Stone Research Symposium. Edited by A. Hodgkinson and B. E. C. Nordin, p. 1. J. A. Churchill, Ltd., London, 1969.
6. Cope, O. Hyperparathyroidism: diagnosis and management. Am. J. Surg. 99:394, 1960.
7. Crawhall, J. C. and Watts, R. W. E. Cystinuria. Am. J. Med. 45:736, 1968.
8. Dent, C. E., Friedman, M., Green, H., and Watson, L. C. A. Treatment of cystinuria. Br. Med. J. 1:403, 1965.
9. DeVries, A., Frank, M., and Estman, A. Inherited uric acid lithiasis. Am. J. Med. 33:880, 1962.
10. Frei, E., Bentzel, C. J., Rieselbach, R., and Block, J. B. Renal complications of neoplastic disease. Am. J. Child. Dis. 16:757, 1963.
11. Herring, L. C. Observations on the analysis of 10,000 urinary calculi. J. Urol. 88:545, 1962.
12. Hodgkinson, A. and Pyrah, L. N. The urinary excretion of calcium and inorganic phosphate in 344 patients with calcium stone of renal origin. Br. J. Surg. 46:10, 1958–59.
13. Howard, J. E. Tried, true and new ways to treat and prevent kidney stones. Resident Staff Phys. 16:67, 1970.
14. Howard, J. E. and Thomas, W. C., Jr. Control of crystallization in urine. Am. J. Med. 45:693, 1968.
15. Kreel, L. Radiological aspects of nephrocalcinosis. Clin. Radiol. 13: 218, 1962.
16. MacDonald, W. B. and Fellers, F. X. Penicillamine in the treatment of patients with cystinuria. J.A.M.A. 197:396, 1966.
17. Marshall, V. F., Langengood, R. W., Jr., and Kelley, D. Longitudinal nephrolithotomy and the Shorr regimen in the management of staghorn calculi. Ann. Surg. 162:366, 1965.
18. Mogg, R. A. Matrix calculi. Proc. R. Soc. Med. 57:935, 1964.
19. Myers, N. A. A. Urolithiasis in childhood. Arch. Dis. Child. 32:48, 1957.

20. Myers, W. P. L. Hypercalcemia in neoplastic disease. Arch. Surg. 80:308, 1960.
21. Prien, E. L. and Frondel, C. Studies in urolithiasis I. The composition of urinary calculi. J. Urol. 57:949, 1947.
22. Randall, A. The origin and growth of renal calculi. Ann. Surg. 105:1,009, 1937.
23. Reiss, E. Primary hyperparathyroidism: a simplified approach to diagnosis. Med. Clin. North Am. 54:131, 1970.
24. Russell, R. G. G. and Fleish, H. Pyrophosphate and stone formation. Renal Stone Research Symposium. Edited by A. Hodgkinson and B. E. C. Nordin, p. 163. J. A. Churchill, Ltd., London, 1969.
25. Seegmiller, J. E. Toward a unitary concept of gout. Hosp. Prac. 1:33, 1966.
26. Vermeulen, C. W. and Lyon, E. S. Mechanisms of genesis and growth of calculi. Am. J. Med. 5:684, 1968.
27. Vermeulen, C. W., Miller, G. H., and Sawyer, J. B. Some nonsurgical aspects of urolithiasis. Med. Clin. North Am. 39:281, 1955.
28. Wilmore, D. W. and Gots, R. E. The etiology of uric acid urolithiasis following ileostomy. Arch. Surg. 99:421, 1969.
29. Yendt, E. R. Renal calculi: Can. Med. Assoc. J. 102:479, 1970.
30. Yendt, E. R., Gagne, R. J. A., and Cohanim, M. The effects of thiazides in ideopathic hypercalciuria. Trans. Am. Clin. Climatol. Assoc. 77:96, 1965.
31. Yu, T. and Gutman, A. B. Uric acid nephrolithiasis in gout-predisposing factors. Ann. Intern. Med. 67:1,133, 1967.

10

Disorders of the Kidney

JAY Y. GILLENWATER

GLOMERULONEPHRITIS

Bright originally described an association between diseased kidneys, anasarca, and albuminuria. Now glomerulonephritis is used to describe a variety of acute and chronic processes affecting the glomerulus related to a disturbance in the immunological system.

1. Pathogenesis. Experimental studies have shown two major immunological mechanisms responsible for glomerulonephritis—first the soluble antigen-antibody complexes in the blood stream that become trapped in the glomerulus, and second the development of glomerular injury from antiglomerular basement membrane antibodies.

A. Soluble antigen-antibody complexes. The renal lesion is caused by deposition of circulating antigen-antibody complexes in the glomerulus. This is seen with serum sickness glomerular nephritis, acute poststreptococcal glomerulonephritis, and systemic lupus erythematosus. Figure 1 shows a diagrammatic representation of glomerular injury from soluble antigen-

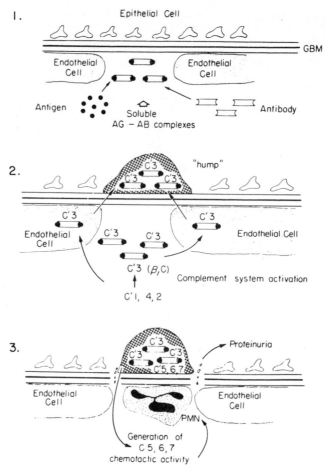

Fig. 1. Steps in development of glomerular injury by soluble antigen-antibody complexes. *Step 1*, antibody is released into the circulation in an environment of antigen excess, and soluble complexes are formed; *Step 2*, soluble complexes activate the complement system, pass through the glomerular capillary endothelium, and localize as discrete subepithelial humps; *Step 3*, generation of chemotactic factor results in polymorphonuclear leukocyte (PMN) migration and further damage. (Reproduced with permission from Fish, A. J., Michael, A. F., and Good, R. A.: Pathogenesis of glomerulonephritis, in *Diseases of the Kidney*, edited by Strauss, M. B., and Welt, L. G., p. 375, Little, Brown and Co., Boston, 1971.)

antibody complexes. The soluble antigen-antibody complexes and complement pass through the glomerular membrane and are trapped between the membrane and the epithelial cells. Complement generates a chemotactic factor that attracts polymorphonuclear leukocytes which become attached to the basement membrane. These leukocytes produce further damage including the stripping of endothelial cells from the basement membrane. This leads to aggregation of platelets with release of factors and the deposition of fibrinogen and fibrin.

B. Specific antiglomerular basement membrane antibodies. The lesion is caused by antibodies specific to the glomerular basement membrane which, along with complement, attaches to the glomerular capillary near the basement membrane. Subsequently a chemotactic factor is released which attracts polymorphonuclear leukocytes with subsequent damage to the glomerular basement membrane (Fig. 2).

2. Classification. The classification shown below is from Merrill's article in the 1974 *New England Journal of Medicine* and seems simpler and clearer than most.

Diffuse   Focal
Proliferative & exudative glomerulonephritis
Extracapillary glomerulonephritis
Membranous glomerulonephritis
                                                    Chronic (sclerosing)

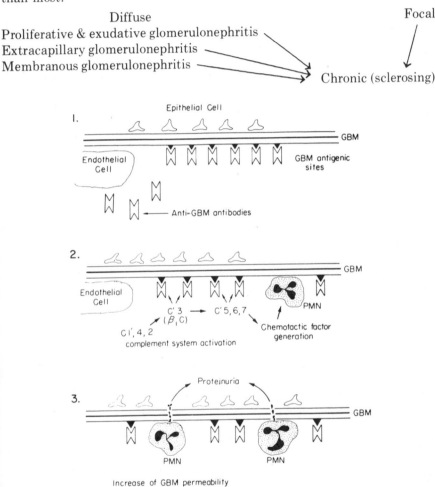

Increase of GBM permeability

Fig. 2. Steps in the development of glomerular injury by antiglomerular basement membrane (antiGBM). *Step 1*, fixation of antiGBM antibodies to antigenic sites on the GBM; *Step 2*, activation of the complement system follows with $\beta_1 C$ deposition and generation of chemotactic factor; *Step 3*, release of enzymes from polymorphonuclear leukocytes (PMN) contributes to GBM damage and increased permeability (Reproduced with permission from Fish A. J., Michael, A. F., and Good, R. A.: Pathogenesis of glomerulonephritis, in *Diseases of the Kidney*, edited by Strauss, M. B., and Welt, L. G., p. 383, Little, Brown and Co., Boston, 1971.

A. Focal glomerulonephritis refers to those cases with few glomeruli involved as opposed to the chronic case with most glomeruli involved.

B. Diffuse proliferative and exudative glomerulonephritis is seen with poststreptococcal nephritis. Proliferation of mesangial cells and endothelial cells with infiltration of the glomeruli by variable numbers of polymorphonuclear leukocytes is seen pathologically. Healing is seen in most patients.

C. Extracapillary glomerulonephritis is seen clinically as rapidly progressive glomerulonephritis and is seen with periarteritis, Goodpasture's syndrome, or Henoch-Schonlein purpura. Pathologically, it is characterized by multiplication of the cells of Bowman's capsule, with the formation of large crescents, and the compression of capillary tufts. The prognosis is poor because of rapid loss of glomeruli.

D. Membranous glomerulonephritis is characterized by thickening of the basement membrane as in patients with systemic lupus erythematosus.

3. Clinical aspects of acute poststreptococcal glomerulonephritis. Acute poststreptococcal glomerulonephritis is seen at all ages, but it is found more commonly in children, with a higher incidence in males. Classically, the disease begins with a sore throat or impetigo which disappears in a few days. Several weeks later the patient develops weakness, anorexia, tea-colored urine with decreased 24-hour volume, edema, hypertension, and anemia.

A. Epidemiology. Types 12 and 4 of beta-hemolytic streptococci have been shown to have nephrogenic qualities. Acute glomerulonephritis is more commonly seen in preschool and early school years. In the northern climate, acute glomerulonephritis is most commonly preceded by a streptococcal upper respiratory infection, while in the south, streptococcal skin infections act as the major etiological factor.

B. Immunology. Various antibodies (antistreptolysin-O (ASO), antistreptokinase, antihyaluronidase, antidesoxyribonuclease) usually increase 1 to 3 weeks after the streptococcal infection. An elevated ASO titer helps to establish clinically the existence of a preceding streptococcal infection. The ASO titer is normal in 6 months in about 50% of patients. The ASO response has no prognostic significance. With patients having sore throats who are treated with antibiotics, an elevated ASO titer is seen in only 10 to 15% of patients with acute glomerulonephritis. Serum complement levels are low in acute glomerulonephritis and return to normal in about 1 month after the acute illness.

4. Chronic Glomerulonephritis.

A. Incidence. Studies from autopsies in the United States have shown that around 1% of patients have chronic glomerulonephritis and 15% have pyelonephritis. When expressed as death caused by renal disease, chronic glomerulonephritis causes 45% and pyelonephritis 36%.

B. Natural history. There is a wide variability in the natural history of glomerulonephritis which does not readily fit into a classification. In 1942, Ellis classified chronic glomerulonephritis into two categories.

    1) Type 1. About 10% begin in childhood as acute poststreptococcal glomerulonephritis with a latent period and then hypertension and uremia.

    2) Type 2. Begins insidiously in adult life with hypertension, edema, and sometimes nephrotic syndrome seen early in life.

  C. Signs and symptoms.

    1) Proteinuria. An increased protein excretion is seen in most patients with chronic glomerulonephritis. The total 24-hour protein excretion will vary from 100 mg to over 20 g.

    2) Urinary sediment.

      a. Hematuria. The degree of hematuria varies as the degree of activity of the glomerulonephritis.

      b. Double refractile fat bodies. The renal epithelial cells may undergo fatty degeneration which can be seen under polarized light.

      c. Casts. Casts of hyaline, granular, or red blood cells are frequently seen.

    3) Hypertension. Most patients with chronic glomerulonephritis have hypertension, and in many, it is the initial sign; in many others, it indicates an advanced stage.

    4) Peripheral edema.

  D. Prognosis. It is difficult to predict the prognosis accurately because of the variability in the course of the disease. In some, there is a rapid progression of disease, while in many others, there is stabilization, and in others, a slowly progressive deterioration of renal function. This persistence of activity as measured by proteinuria, hematuria, casts, or hypertension suggests continued active inflammatory changes.

  E. Treatment. There is no known therapy to arrest the progression or restore the damaged nephrons. Symptomatic treatment is usually directed toward the edema, hypertension, congestive heart failure, and symptoms of uremia. If the patient has the nephrotic syndrome, steroids are of some value. Diet and physical activity usually are not restricted.

5. Nephrotic syndrome. The nephrotic syndrome is defined as proteinuria usually accompanied by edema, hypoproteinemia, and hyperlipemia.

  A. Etiology. The nephrotic syndrome is associated with a variety of systemic diseases: glomerulonephritis, amyloidosis, diabetes, systemic lupus erythematosus, and other collagen vascular diseases, circulatory diseases such as renal vein thrombosis, heart failure, and insect bites. It is believed to involve an immunological mechanism as discussed under acute glomerulonephritis.

  B. Pathophysiology.

    1) Glomerular permeability. Proteinuria is the hallmark of the nephrotic syndrome and may be the initiating event. An increased glomerular permeability is thought to cause the proteinuria.

2) Hypoproteinemia. A decrease in serum total protein, albumin, and gamma-globulin with an increase in alpha-2-globulin, beta-globulin, and fibrinogen is often seen in patients with the nephrotic syndrome. The primary pathophysiological mechanism seems to be excessive urinary losses of protein.

3) Lipiduria. The observation of fat bodies (double refractile fat bodies) is seen early in the nephrotic syndrome and accounts for the name "lipoid nephrosis" commonly given to it.

4) Lipidemia. Serum of patients with nephrotic syndrome usually has an increase in all lipid constituents (lipoproteins, triglycerides, and cholesterol). The exact etiology is not known, but it appears to be due in part to the urinary loss of protein causing inability to convert from the large to small lipoprotein fractions.

5) Edema. Most patients with nephrotic syndrome have related to the hypoalbuminemia causing lower serum oncotic pressure.

C. Prognosis. Children with nephrotic syndrome had an expected survival of 50% in 5 years prior to steroid therapy. With recent therapy, 75% of children with recent onset nephrosis are alive at 4 years.

D. Treatment. Specific therapy is based on the etiological classification determined from the history, clinical findings, and renal biopsy. Steroids, immunosuppressive drugs, and diuretics are used.

RENAL TUBULAR ACIDOSIS

Renal tubular acidosis (RTA) is a disorder in which, under an appropriate stimulus, the kidney is unable to acidify the urine. It is important to the urologist, not only because of its interesting medical and physiological aspects, but because renal tubular acidosis is the third most frequent cause of nephrocalcinosis (first is primary hyperparathyroidism, and second is chronic pyelonephritis).

1. Normal hydrogen ion excretion. Sixty milliequivalents of hydrogen ion are produced daily from the metabolism of proteins and organic acids. Normally, the hydrogen ions are excreted through the kidney as titratable acid (30 mEq/24 hours) and ammonium (31 mEq/24 hours). Total hydrogen ion excretion is measured by the sum of ammonia excretion and titratable acid less urinary bicarbonate.

2. Pathogenesis. Inability to maintain a normal maximal hydrogen ion gradient is the fundamental abnormality in renal tubular acidosis. The etiological factors causing the tubular disorders have not been identified. Clinically, the cases have been divided into proximal and distal nephron types.

A. Proximal-type RTA. In the proximal type, fewer hydrogen ions are secreted and less bicarbonate is reabsorbed. Because of the absolute decrease in bicarbonate reabsorption in the proximal tubule, the distal bicarbonate reabsorptive mechanism is exceeded, causing bicarbonate wastage with resultant systemic acidosis. Plasma bicarbonate then stabilizes at a low plasma level. Under these conditions, the urine becomes acidic with normal amounts of ammonia and titratable acid. In order to secrete hydrogen ion into the urine, filtered bicarbonate must be reabsorbed. Thus even in the proximal type of RTA, there is insufficient net secretion of hydrogen ions, since the loss of filtered bicarbonate into the urine is equivalent to retention of hydrogen ion in the blood.

B. Distal RTA. In distal renal tubular acidosis, the primary defect is inability of the distal tubule to establish a hydrogen ion gradient. Thus the excretion of titratable acid and ammonia remains low. The patient is unable to excrete the normally produced acid with resultant acidosis. Bicarbonate reabsorption is normal.

3. Clinical characteristics.

A. Distal renal tubular acidosis. This occurs both in infants and adults, with 70% occurring in females.

   1) Infants. Infants present with failure to thrive, muscular weakness, constipation, nephrocalcinosis, and many have rickets and osteomalacosis.

   2) Adults. Adults usually present with nephrocalcinosis and infection. Since excess cation is lost in the urine, the patients may have hypokalemia from the secondary hyperaldosteronism.

B. Proximal renal tubular acidosis. This was first described in children with the only sign being acidosis and growth failure. These children have a good prognosis with many being able to do without therapy after a few years.

4. Diagnosis. Investigation of both bicarbonate reabsorption and hydrogen ion excretion by timed urine excretion studies after an acid load is required to diagnose renal tubular acidosis. Distal RTA is demonstrated by the inability to lower urine pH below 5.5 with a metabolic acidosis. A clue to proximal RTA is the requirement of large doses of bicarbonate to maintain normal plasma bicarbonate levels. Diagnosis of proximal RTA is made by performing a bicarbonate titration or withdrawing bicarbonate on an already treated patient and following urine plasma pH while he becomes acidotic.

5. Treatment. Therapy is sufficient administration of alkali to balance the metabolic needs and urinary losses. This usually is given as the sodium and potassium salts of either bicarbonate or citrate.

RENAL CYSTS

Cystic disorders of the kidney are common and can be perplexing if the student does not approach the problem using an orderly classification. Such a classification was proposed by Spence and is shown below. The student is referred to Spence's two fine articles for a more detailed discussion of the various conditions.

*Spence's Classification of Cystic Disorders of the Kidney**

A. Renal dysplasia
  1. Congenital unilateral multicystic kidney
  2. Segment and focal renal dysplasia
  3. Renal dysplasia associated with congenital lower tract obstruction
B. Congenital polycystic kidney disease
  1. Infantile type
  2. Adult type
C. Cystic disorders of the renal medulla
  1. Renal cystic disease with congenital hepatic fibrosis
  2. Medullary cystic disease
  3. Sponge kidney
D. Simple cyst
E. Calyceal cyst
F. Cysts associated with neoplasm
  1. Cystic degeneration of parenchymal tumors
  2. Malignant change occurring in wall of simple cyst
  3. Cystadenoma and multilocular cysts
G. Cysts secondary to nonmalignant renal pathology
H. Peripelvic cysts
I. Perinephric cysts
J. Miscellaneous

---

* Spence, H. M. and Singleton, R. Urol. Survey 22:131, 1972.

EMBRYOLOGY

Before discussing the clinical aspects of cystic disorders of the kidney, it seems appropriate to explore the theories on embryological development as proposed by Osathanondh and Potter.†

Type 1: Hyperplasia of interstitial portion of dividing tubules,
  example—infantile polycystic kidney
Type 2: Inhibited ampullary activity with failure to induce nephrons from metanephric blastema,
  examples—renal dysplasia, congenital multicystic kidney
Type 3: Abnormality of both interstitial and ampullary portions plus defective response by metanephric blastema,
  examples—adult polycystic disease, sponge kidney, medullary cystic disease
Type 4: Lower urinary tract obstruction with resultant abnormality of ampullae and nephrogenic elements,
  example—urethral valves with associated dysplastic kidneys

Osathanondh and Potter described the development of the renal pelvis, calyces, and collecting tubules as arising from successive dichotomous branching (each division going into two new buds) of ureteric bud after it arises from the lower mesonephric duct. Two areas are described in each successive bud: 1) an interstitial or tubular segment, and 2) an ampullary

---

† Osathanondh, V. and Potter, E. L. Arch. Pathol. 77:459, 1964.

portion which is the advancing end of the bud. The first 5 generations form the renal pelvis; the major calyces come from the 5th to the 10th; the minor calyx from the 10th to the 15th; and the collecting ducts from the last generations. The last generations of buds pick up a cap of metanephric blastema to form the upper nephron. Ultimately 12 to 15 glomeruli attach to each of the terminal branches. The renal cystic disorders ascribed to developmental errors in the interstitial or ampullary portions of the collecting tubules are shown in the above table.

A brief discussion of the clinical aspects of the various cystic disorders of the kidney will be presented.

1. Renal dysplasia.

A. Renal dysplasia. This refers to abnormal development of the kidney with abnormal differentiation of embryonic structures. Typically, tissue such as cartilage is seen. A preceding obstruction to the lower urinary tract is seen in many cases.

B. Multicystic kidney. This is an entity different from infantile polycystic kidney. Grossly, these kidneys consist of 10 to 20 large cysts, typically presenting as an abdominal mass during the first few months of life. There is no normal parenchyma, and usually an atretic renal pedicle and ureter. The diagnosis is suspected in a child with a nonfunctional abdominal mass on an intravenous urogram, and atresia of the ureter on cystoscopic studies. Surgical exploration usually is necessary for definitive diagnosis. It is important to study carefully the opposite kidney to rule out any associated congenital anomalies, since it is this kidney which will have to sustain life (Fig. 3).

2. Polycystic kidney disease.

A. Infantile polycystic kidney disease. Osathanondh and Potter described the abnormality as uniform dilation of the tubules from hyperplasia of the interstitial portions of the dividing tubule. Incidence reported in newborns is 1:6,000 to 1:14,000, with an incidence of 1:200 in infant autopsies. The inheritance is autosomal recessive. Diagnosis is usually suspected by palpation of bilateral upper abdominal masses and a large kidney with multiple filling defects on an intravenous urogram and nephrotomograms. Prognosis usually is poor although some children do fairly well (Fig. 4).

B. Adult polycystic kidney disease. Embryologically, this is described as type 3, with abnormalities of interstitial and ampullary portions of the tubules. The incidence in adults is 1:3,500. The cysts have been demonstrated to be continuous with the nephrons, and inulin filters into them. The inheritance is autosomal dominant with high penetrance. The children of those affected average an equal proportion of normal and affected with polycystic kidney disease. Adult polycystic kidney disease usually presents in the 4th or 5th decade as an abdominal mass or with signs and symptoms of hematuria, infection, hypertension, or renal failure. Surgical intervention is indicated for stones, abscesses, or occasionally because of severe pain.

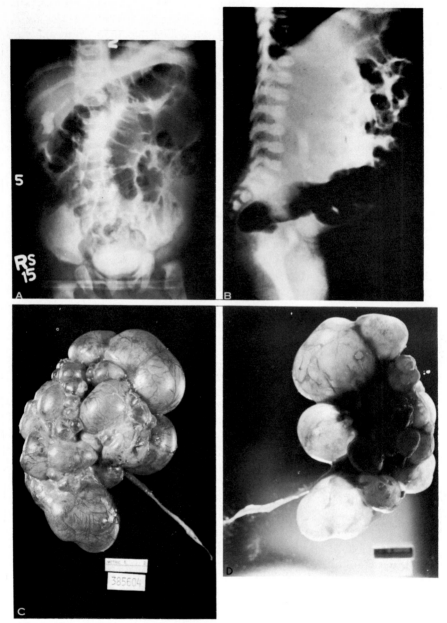

Fig. 3. Multicystic kidney of the newborn. *A* and *B*, the IVP in A-P and lateral projections. Nonfunction of the left kidney is shown, and on the lateral film, a large mass is shown. *C* and *D*, the operative specimen which is composed of large cysts.

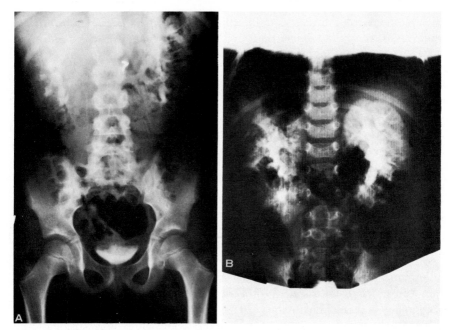

Fig. 4. Polycystic kidney of the newborn. *A*, the large kidneys bilaterally; *B*, a tomographic cut taken of these same kidneys showing the multiple small cysts throughout the kidney.

Patients with polycystic kidneys have associated anomalies of hepatic cysts and aneurysms of the basal artery of the brain.

3. Cystic disorders of the renal medulla.

A. Medullary cystic disease. This is a rare disorder of small cystic lesions confined to the medulla and is usually seen in children. These children most often present in renal failure with anemia, polyuria, low urine specific gravity, normal blood pressure, acidosis, and renal salt loss. The salt loss is not responsive to desoxycorticosterone acetate (DOCA) nor is the concentrating defect responsive to antidiuretic hormone (ADH). Retrogrades show a small kidney with normal calyces. The prognosis usually is poor.

B. Sponge kidney. Sponge kidneys have dilations of the collecting duct which appear as small cysts in the medulla. Grossly, these cysts appear as porous structures on cut surfaces. In most patients, the diagnosis is made from an incidental intravenous urogram. Some patients present with hematuria or symptoms of infection or stone. Radiologically, one sees dilated collecting tubules with or without medullary calcifications. The prognosis usually is good. Treatment is directed toward the infection or stones.

4. Simple cyst. As do many other organs, the kidney may develop a cyst of uncertain etiology. Simple cysts are the most common cystic disorders of the kidney. These may be multiple and may vary in size from a few

millimeters to very large. Usually simple renal cysts are asymptomatic. When large, they may cause pain or discomfort. Hematuria is rare. Most simple cysts are diagnosed as incidental findings on an intravenous urogram.

Clinically, the problem is deciding whether the space-occupying mass is a malignant tumor or a simple cyst. In patients who have *any* stigmata of renal malignancy (hematuria, anemia, calcification, etc.), surgical renal exploration is desirable. Nephrotomography is reported to be 95% accurate in differentiating cysts from tumors. Selective renal arteriography is reported to be more accurate. Cysts are nonopacified while tumors show neovascularity, arteriovenous fistula, venous laking, and opacification. Renal intra-arterial norepinephrine causes spasms of normal vessels, but the pathological tumor vessels, because of absence of their internal muscular layer, do not constrict. Percutaneous puncture, aspiration, and injection of the mass have been advocated by some. The presence of clear cyst fluid, normal cytology, and normal x-ray after injection of the cyst with radiopaque media have been taken to indicate a simple cyst with the connotation that no surgical procedure is necessary if no evidence of malignancy is seen. The obvious criticism is that tumor cells may be seeded or bleeding may be caused. It has been our policy to explore surgically all space-occupying masses in the kidney in patients under 60 to 65 years of age without medical diseases, rather than perform the percutaneous needle puncture. Cysts in some age groups are reported to be as much as 8 to 20 times more common than malignant tumors. If at surgery the lesion is found to be a simple cyst, the cyst is incised and its lumen is carefully inspected to rule out malignancy. The cyst wall is excised flush with the kidney surface and the edges oversewn. It must be stated that some urologists would not explore an asymptomatic space-occupying renal lesion if either the arteriogram, nephrotomogram, or aspiration studies show that it is a simple cyst. The reasoning is that the operative mortality may be as great as the chance of missing a malignancy. Support for this was found in a series of patients reported by Plaine and Hinman, who had a 2.4% serious complication or mortality (3 patients of 123 with ages of 68, 72, and 75, in which 2 had a cerebral vascular accident and 1 other died). We have had no deaths or serious complications, and we would think that the operative mortality in an under 65 age group, with no serious medical problems, should be the negligible mortality and morbidity of living donor kidney transplant patients.

5. Calyceal cysts. Dilations and cyst formation of a calyx have been called hydrocalxy, pyelogenic cyst, and calyceal diverticulum. The significant clinical feature is that the "cyst" cavity communicates with the calyx. Many are associated with stones and infections and, in some, surgical excision of the lesion is indicated.

6. Cysts associated with tumors. In certain benign tumors such as

cystadenoma, multilocular cyst, or hamartoma, the lesion is benign, but preoperative studies will not be diagnostic, and renal exploration is usually done to make the diagnosis.

A. Cystadenoma. This literally means cyst associated with an adenoma.

B. Multilocular cysts. These are very rare cysts that are solitary, unilateral, and multiloculated without communication between the epithelial lined cavities or the renal pelvis.

C. Hamartomas. These may be associated with tuberous sclerosis. They may be difficult to differentiate from a malignancy on diagnostic studies or gross inspection. Cysts and tumors can coexist under certain circumstances.

1) Cysts and tumors arising separately and independently.

2) Cystic degeneration of malignant tumor that has outgrown its blood supply.

3) Carcinoma may rarely arise on a cyst wall.

4) Papillary cystadenoma—these are rare tumors in which the cyst has papillary projections into the lumen. Blood clots are usually seen in the cyst. The prognosis is good.

7. Pararenal and perirenal cysts. The Greek prefix *para* means beside, and *peri* means around or surrounding.

A. Parapelvic cyst. Cysts may develop near the hilum of the kidney and cause compression deformities of the renal pelvis. These cysts are thought to arise from blocked lymphatics. They are benign.

B. Perinephric cyst or "hydrocele renalis." In this condition, urine accumulates beneath the renal capsule, usually as a result of renal trauma. Similar findings may be seen with subcapsular bleeding from the renal cortex (trauma or tumor). Surgical intervention is usually necessary.

CANCER OF THE KIDNEY

1. Adenocarcinoma (hypernephroma).

A. Historical aspects. Adenocarcinoma of the kidney was described both as a medullary sarcoma and as a lipoma of the kidney. In 1883, Grawitz described this tumor which was thought to arise from adrenal rests, usually in the upper pole of the kidney, giving rise to the name hypernephroma.

B. Experimentally induced. Estrogens administered to male hamsters or ovariectomized females will induce adenocarcinoma of the kidney. The animals are protected by progesterone. Lucke induced kidney tumor with a virus in the tree frog. Wrapping the kidney of rats in cellophane causes sarcomas. Large doses of lead acetate administered to rats induces renal tumors. A virus known to cause leukemia in fowls can also cause cancer of the kidney in young fowls.

C. Pathogenesis. Adenocarcinoma of the kidney begins in the renal tubular epithelium. It is unknown whether the adenocarcinoma progresses through a stage of adenomatous hyperplasia and renal cortical adenoma which have been found in 14% of patients with renal adenocarcinoma.

These tumors metastasize readily by the blood stream, most commonly to the lungs, brain, and bones. About 24% of patients have lymph node involvement. Renal carcinomas and simple cysts have been reported to coexist in 2 to 3% of patients.

D. Fate of untreated patients. In any one patient, the natural history is very difficult to predict. Examples have been reported of patients living for many years with an unresected primary tumor or of distant metastasis developing many years after nephrectomy. However, the prognosis of the unoperated renal adenocarcinoma is usually poor. Riches reported on a series of 443 patients who were unoperated for a variety of reasons and had a survival rate of 4.4% at 3 years and 1.7% at 5 years. About one-third of the patients have distal metastasis when first diagnosed.

E. Presenting signs and symptoms.

1) Classical triad. Hematuria, pain, and a renal mass are often called the "classical triad" of renal cancer. All of these findings are found in only 10 to 15% of patients at the time of diagnosis. A history of intermittent hematuria is reported in 60% of patients. A history of loin pain is found in 50%, and a renal mass is palpable in one-third of the patients.

2) Systemic effects. Renal adenocarcinoma is one of the most active tumors metabolically and endocrinologically. This tumor has so many toxic systemic effects that it is called the "internist's tumor."

a. Fever occurs in about 17% of patients and is the sole presenting complaint in 2%. No circulating pyrogens have been demonstrated, although pyrogen activity has been demonstrated in renal tumor tissue in febrile patients and not in the afebrile patients.

b. Erythrocytosis occurs in about 4%. This is thought to occur from erythropoietin production by the tumor. There is no elevation of the white blood cell count, platelet count, or splenomegaly as seen in polycythemia vera.

c. Anemia occurs in about 40%. The etiology is not known. It is not due to excessive blood loss, hemolysis, or shortened red blood cell life.

d. Hepatopathy with reversible hepatic dysfunction occurs in about 15% of patients. Abnormal liver tests unassociated with hepatic metastasis which have been reported are: elevated serum, alpha-2-globulin, alkaline phosphatase, bilirubin, bromosulphthalein (BSP) retention, and prolonged prothrombin time.

e. Hypercalemia occurs in about 6% of patients. Secretion of a parathormone-like material by renal adenocarcinoma has been demonstrated.

f. Hypertension occurs in about 37%. It is thought to be due to renin secretion, although this has not been demonstrated yet.

g. Elevated erythrocytic sedimentation rate (ESR) has been reported in 56%.

h. Amyloidosis occurs in about 3 to 5% of patients with renal cell carcinoma.

i. Neuromyopathy appears in about 4% of patients with renal cell carcinoma.

j. Enteropathy with steatorrhea, intestinal malfunction, and abnormal radiological changes has been reported in patients with renal cell carcinoma.

k. Gonadotropin production with diminished libido, gynecomastia, and areolar pigmentation has been reported in one patient with metabolic renal cell carcinoma.

l. Leukemoid reactions in patients with renal cell carcinomas have been reported.

m. Low output heart failure due to obstruction of the vena cava by tumor or high output heart failure from arteriovenous fistulae are seen in patients with renal cell carcinoma.

n. Cushing's syndrome associated with renal cell carcinoma has been reported.

o. Lindau-Von Hipple syndrome, which is angioma of the cerebellum associated with hemangioma of the retina, has been reported to be associated with renal cell carcinoma.

F. Diagnosis. Renal cell carcinoma should be suspected with any of the previously mentioned signs and symptoms. An intravenous urogram should then be requested and will show a space-occupying mass in which the differential diagnosis should be between a cyst and tumor. If calcification is seen within the mass, malignancy is reported to occur in 87%. Peripheral eggshell calcification usually is associated with cysts, but the risk of malignancy is still 20%.

Nephrotomography is reported to differentiate tumors versus cysts in 95% of cases. Renal angiography is thought to be slightly more accurate. Tumors have pathological vessels which do not have an internal muscular layer, giving an irregular and tortuous appearance with no response to epinephrine. There are also arteriovenous fistulae, venous laking, and capillary filling. Needle puncture of the mass, if it has the radiological appearance, has been advocated by some. It usually is not done in our institution since in the younger individual most solitary renal masses are explored surgically, and the mass is examined to determine if it is cyst or tumor. The pros and cons of this are discussed in the section on renal cysts.

G. Management.

1) Surgery. Radical surgical excision is the treatment of choice and has been reported to give a 10-year survival rate as high as 66%. Long-term survival has also been reported with excision of solitary metastasis. Renal vein involvement without positive lymph nodes does not seem to decrease survival. Extension into perinephric fat does not significantly alter the prognosis. Positive lymph nodes do decrease the survival rate. Better differentiated tumors have a better prognosis than the very anaplastic ones. Survivals have been reported after pulling long tumor emboli out of the vena cava.

2) Irradiation. Renal cell carcinoma is relatively radio-resistant. Postoperative irradiation has been suggested when there has been incomplete local excision of the tumor or lymph node invasion. The routine use of postoperative irradiation in every case is not recommended. The role of preoperative irradiation has not been adequately assessed.

3) Chemotherapy. Renal cell carcinomas respond poorly to all tested cytotoxic drugs. Better results have been reported with hormonal therapy. In the largest series of 80 patients, a subjective response rate of 55% was reported; 14% had marked tumor regression, and in 2.5%, the tumor was stationary for 1 year. It is recommended that patients be started on large doses of progesterone (Provera—oral), 100 mg t.i.d., or 800 mg I.M., weekly. If there is no response by 6 to 10 weeks, then testosterone, 100 mg I.M., should be given daily for 5 days, then 100 mg I.M. 3 times a week. With no response, stilbestrol, 30 to 40 mg/day, or prednisone, 40 mg/day, can be tried.

H. Spontaneous regression. Spontaneous regression of metastasis after removal of the primary tumor, although rare, can occur and over 30 have been reported. Prospective studies have shown, however, that regression of metastasis is seldom seen after excision of the primary renal cell carcinoma.

I. Metastatic neoplasm to the kidney. In malignancies, renal metastases are seldom seen clinically because most patients with widespread metastases do not survive long enough for the renal metastasis to give any symptoms. At autopsy, however, renal involvement by metastatic tumor is twice as common as primary renal cell carcinoma. Tumors of the lung and breast are those most commonly reported to metastasize to the kidney. The reported radiological studies on metastatic renal tumors show a solid density on nephrotomograms and no tumor vessels on arteriography.

2. Transitional cell tumor of the renal pelvis. Transitional cell carcinomas of the renal pelvis and ureter are uncommon. Histologically, these tumors are similar to bladder cancer and are assumed to be caused by similar etiological factors. Prognosis is good for low stage and grade tumors and very poor for high stage and grade tumors. Over 40% of these patients are reported to have associated ureteral or vesical neoplasms. The tumor usually is first suspected from intermittent painless hematuria. This tumor has none of the toxic systemic symptoms that are associated with renal adenocarcinoma. Treatment is nephroureterectomy.

3. Nephroblastoma (Wilms' tumor). Nephroblastoma is the most common genitourinary tract tumor in children, but it is still not seen often (500 each year in the U.S.). Nephroblastoma is the most common abdominal malignancy in children. Neuroblastoma is seen more frequently if the total body incidence is counted.

Most Wilms' tumors occur before the age of 3, although an occasional case in adults has been reported. Bilateral involvement has been reported in 2%, with some of these being cured. Metastasis by local extension or by the blood stream is found in 25 to 50% of cases when they are first diagnosed.

A. Pathology. Wilms' tumors usually are quite large, light colored tumors. Histologically, one sees tubules and primitive glomeruli, sometimes with connective tissue, cartilage, bone, and adipose tissue and muscle tissue.

B. Symptoms. Forty to 50% of these tumors are accidentally discovered by the child's mother as an abdominal mass. Hematuria is seen in less than one-third and is thought to represent a poorer prognosis. Fever is present in 30%, and hypertension has been reported in as high as 75% of cases. Pain is present in only about one-fourth of the cases.

C. Diagnosis. Differential diagnosis is that of an abdominal mass in childhood. The most common causes of abdominal masses are hydronephrosis, polycystic kidneys, Wilms' tumors, multicystic kidneys, and neuroblastomas. An intravenous urogram in Wilms' tumor shows gross distortion of the calyceal pattern with a large renal mass. Arteriography usually is not performed because of the danger of thrombosis in the femoral artery, and because it is not always diagnostic. Neuroblastomas are more often calcified and usually displace the kidney downward. Hydronephrosis is usually distinguishable on the x-rays.

D. Management. Surgery, radiation, and chemotherapy all are of value in the treatment of Wilms' tumor. Major advances have been made in chemotherapy during the past several years. In one study group, a combination of dactinomycin and vincristine (88% 2-year survival) was superior to either drug used alone (61 to 67% 2-year survival). Radiation usually is not given preoperatively unless the surgeon feels the mass requires shrinkage to be excised completely. Postoperative irradiation is given in many medical centers.

The child should be evaluated with a chest x-ray, intravenous urograms, and blood count and should be operated on within 48 hours. Transabdominal incisions are made, and the other kidney and abdomen are carefully examined for tumor. Wide excision of the tumor is then accomplished. Postoperatively, most centers would use chemotherapy and/or radiation.

REFERENCES AND SUGGESTED FURTHER READING

1. Melicow, M. M. and Uson, A. C. Palpable abdominal masses in infants and children: report based on review of 653 cases. J. Urol. 81:705, 1959.
2. Merrill, J. P. Glomerulonephritis. (1) N. Engl. J. Med. 290:257, 1974; (2) N. Engl. J. Med. 290:313, 1974; (3) N. Engl. J. Med. 290:374, 1974.
3. Osathanondh, V. and Potter, E. L. Arch. Pathol. 77:459, 1964.
4. Plaine, L. I. and Hinman, F., Jr. Malignancy in asymptomatic renal masses. J. Urol. 94:342, 1965.
5. Riches, E. W. Monographs on neoplastic disease. In *Tumors of the Kidney and Ureter*, edited by E. Riches, Vol. V, p. 127. Williams & Wilkins Co., Baltimore, 1964.
6. Spence, H. M. Cystic disorders of the kidney—classification, diagnosis and treatment. J.A.M.A. 163:1466, 1957.
7. Spence, H. M. and Singleton. Urol. Survey 22:131, 1972.
8. Strauss, M. B. and Welt, L. G., eds. *Diseases of the Kidney*, Vol. 1, Ed. 2. Little, Brown and Co., Boston, 1971.

11

Endocrine Function of the Kidney

E. DARRACOTT VAUGHAN, JR.

1. Introduction. Elucidation of the complex excretory role of the kidney in health and disease has been the prime concern of investigators and clinicians who have studied this organ. However, expansion of the early observation in 1898 by Tigerstedt and Bergman that the kidney contained a pressor substance has clearly demonstrated that the kidney is a potent endocrine organ producing a number of chemical substances with biological activities.

The list of humoral substances elaborated is as yet incomplete but includes:

A. Renin.

B. Erythropoietin (renal erythropoietic factor).

C. Prostaglandins.

   1) PGE_2.

   2) $PGF_2\alpha$.

D. Antihypertensive neutral renomedullary lipids (ANRL).

E. Kallikrein.

F. Enzyme for synthesis of 1,25-dihydroxyvitamin D_3.

2. Renin. Renin is a proteolytic enzyme made and secreted by the juxtaglomerular cells of the afferent arterioles in the kidney. In itself it has no known physiological actions and has not been structurally defined or isolated.

A. The induction of renin release involves at least four major mechanisms.

   1) A pressure receptor in the renal afferent arteriole (baroreceptor mechanism).

     a. Increased renin release with decreased mean pressure.

     b. Decreased renin release with increased mean pressure.

   2) A distal tubular macula densa receptor sensitive to changes in sodium delivery.

     a. Increased renin release with decreased sodium delivery.

     b. Decreased renin release with increased sodium delivery.

   3) Changes in autonomic nerve activity.

     a. Increased renin release with α- or β-adrenergic stimulation.

     b. Decreased renin release with β-adrenergic blockade.

4) Changes in potassium balance.
   a. Increased renin release with decreased plasma potassium.
   b. Decreased renin release with increased plasma potassium.

In addition, there are both systemic and intrarenal feedback mechanisms to retard further renin secretion.

B. Renin-angiotensin-aldosterone system. When renal perfusion is threatened, the kidney secretes renin into the blood stream where it acts enzymatically on a circulating plasma globulin, renin substrate, or angiotensinogen to release the decapeptide angiotensin I. This decapeptide has neurogenic activity on the central nervous system and adrenal medulla. It is rapidly hydrolyzed by converting enzymes in the lung, plasma, and kidney which remove the terminal histidyl-leucine dipeptide, liberating into the circulation the physiologically active octapeptide, angiotensin II. Angiotensin II has three actions: 1) it is by weight the most potent arteriolar constrictor known; 2) it acts directly on the kidney to cause sodium retention with low dose and natriuresis with larger amounts; 3) it acts on the adrenal cortex to increase aldosterone secretion. Aldosterone is an adrenal corticosteroid formed in the glomerulosa which acts primarily on the distal renal tubule to increase the reabsorption of sodium and to promote the excretion of potassium and hydrogen ions.

Thus angiotensin II and aldosterone act in concert by causing both vasoconstriction and sodium retention to raise blood pressure and restore renal perfusion, thereby inhibiting further renin release (Fig. 1).

The system plays a vital role in both the regulation of sodium and potassium homeostasis and in control of blood pressure.

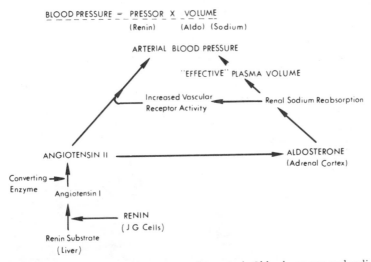

Fig. 1. Renin-angiotensin-aldosterone system for control of blood pressure and sodium and potassium balance. (Reproduced with permission from Laragh, J. H. (editor): *Hypertension Manual.* Yorke Medical Books, Dun-Donnelley Publishing Corp., New York, 1974.)

C. Measurements. Determination of the activity of the renin-angiotensin-aldosterone system involves precise measurement of plasma renin activity and urinary or plasma aldosterone levels related to the concurrent state of sodium balance. An accurate way of assessing the state of sodium balance is to relate the plasma renin activity or aldosterone excretion to the concurrent 24-hour urinary sodium excretion. For both hormones, a similar dynamic hyperbolic relationship has been found in normal subjects (Fig. 2). Because of influences of antihypertensive drugs and diuretics on the system, all patients must be off these agents for at least 3 weeks prior to measurement.

Most recently, plasma renin activity has been determined by methods which utilize a radioimmunoassay to quantitate generated angiotensin I. Plasma and urinary aldosterone levels are also measured by radioimmunoassay.

D. Abnormalities of the renin-angiotensin-aldosterone system.

1) Malignant hypertension. This disease is clinically defined by severe hypertension, neuroretinopathy, neurological signs, and rapidly progressive

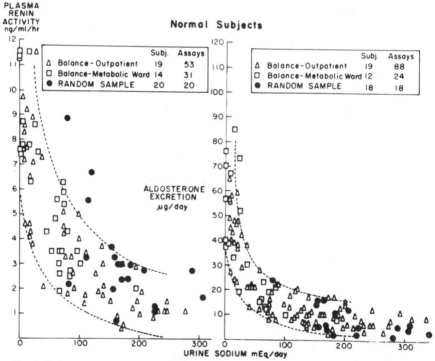

Fig. 2. Relation of plasma renin activity in plasma sample obtained at noon and corresponding 24-hour urine excretion of aldosterone to the concurrent daily rate of sodium excretion (urinary sodium mEq/day) in normal subjects. (Reproduced with permission from Laragh, J. H. (editor): *Hypertension Manual*, Yorke Medical Books, Dun-Donnelley Publishing Corp., New York, 1974.)

renal impairment. Pathological studies reveal fibrinoid necrosis of arterioles. In the majority of patients, both plasma renin activity and aldosterone excretion are elevated above the normal range. It has been postulated that the severe renal disease impairs normal feedback mechanisms that should serve to shut off the system, thus establishing a vicious cycle with more renin, angiotensin, aldosterone, vascular injury, and renal damage (see Fig. 1).

   2) Hyperaldosteronism.

   a. Primary hyperaldosteronism—excessive secretion of aldosterone by an adenoma of the zona glomerulosa of the adrenal leads to sodium retention, mild hypertension, hypokalemia, and alkalosis (see Chapter 19). Thus in this setting, the aldosterone is inappropriately high when the patient is sodium loaded, and the renin, suppressed by the sodium expansion induced by the autogenous aldosterone-secreting tumor, is inappropriately low when the patient is on a low sodium diet.

   b. Pseudoprimary hyperaldosteronism—excessive aldosterone secretion in this entity is secondary to bilateral adrenal hyperplasia. The disease is also characterized by the stigmata of hypermineralocorticism: hypokalemia, alkalosis, hypertension, and suppressed plasma renin activity. Differentiation from primary aldosteronism is mandatory because these patients are not cured of their hypertension by bilateral adrenalectomy. Recent data suggest that the [131]I-19-iodocholesterol adrenal scan may be useful in making this difficult differential diagnosis.

   3) Essential hypertension. In the past, this designation has been applied to all patients in whom no overt cause of the hypertension has been found. More recently, classification of patients with essential hypertension into 3 major subgroups according to elevated, normal, or subnormal plasma renin activity as related to the daily sodium excretion has allowed the definition of different epidemiological, pathophysiological, and mechanistic characteristics of each subgroup.

   a. High renin essential hypertension—in a large series of 219 patients with essential hypertension, 16% were found to have high plasma renin activity and normal or high aldosterone excretion. The observation that these patients are highly responsive to the β-adrenergic blocking agent, propranolol (a potent renin-lowering agent), and to specific antiangiotensin drugs (angiotensin or converting enzyme inhibitors) strongly suggests that the mechanism of the hypertension in these patients is angiotensin II-induced vasoconstriction mediated by abnormally increased renin secretion.

   b. Low renin essential hypertension—subnormal plasma renin activity in the absence of hypersecretion of aldosterone has been demonstrated in approximately 25% of patients with essential hypertension. These patients do not exhibit hypokalemia or alkalosis which would suggest mineralocorticoid excess. These patients have been found to be more responsive to spirolactone or chlorthalidone than normal renin patients and are unresponsive to propranolol. This pharmacological evidence suggests that their hypertension is maintained primarily by volume or sodium excess which is combated by diuretic therapy.

c. Normal renin essential hypertension—the majority of patients, more than 50%, will exhibit normal values of plasma renin activity and aldosterone excretion for any level of sodium excretion. Control of the hypertension usually requires combination antihypertensive therapy, suggesting an interaction of inappropriate vasoconstriction and volume retention. Thus, here again there is inappropriate volume for the capacity of the vascular bed with alterations in both components.

4) Renovascular hypertension. This subgroup contains only patients who exhibit a renal arterial abnormality, hypertension, and proof of a causal relationship by demonstration of control of hypertension following successful renal revascularization or nephrectomy.

Animal models have shown that there are two forms of renovascular hypertension. The hypertension in the animal with one kidney removed and stenosis of the artery to the remaining kidney is maintained by excess sodium, while the hypertension in the animal with both kidneys *in situ* and one renal artery clipped is maintained by excess renin secretion and angiotensin II formation. The volume (sodium) form switches to a vasoconstriction (angiotensin II) form with sodium restriction.

Clinical studies indicate that curable unilateral renovascular hypertension in man is of the renin-dependent, vasoconstriction form. Potentially curable patients can be identified by the demonstration of three criteria based on four renin measurements.

a. Hypersecretion of renin as shown by a high peripheral renin level as related to the concurrent 24-hour sodium excretion.

b. Lateralization of renin secretion with a demonstration of contralateral suppression of renin secretion, as shown by renal venous renin minus renal arterial renin value of zero, $(V - A) = 0$, from the uninvolved kidney.

c. The finding of a $(V - A)/A > 48\%$ from the involved kidney, with the degree of elevation above 48% reflecting the degree of ipsilateral renal ischemia, is the third characteristic of renovascular hypertension.

The finding of these three criteria together in hypertensive patients with unilateral renal artery stenosis strongly suggests curability with appropriate surgical therapy.

5) Hypertension and renal parenchymal disease. The incidence of hypertension in patients with unilateral renal parenchymal disease is greater than that in the normal population. However, uninephrectomy in these patients has resulted in a disappointingly low cure rate of hypertension—only 25 to 37%.

In contrast to patients with renovascular hypertension, it has recently been shown in 63 patients with renal parenchymal disease that the peripheral plasma renin was high in only 13%, normal in 64%, and low in 23%. Accordingly, these patients did not appear to have purely renin-dependent hypertension due to unilateral renal disease. Thus treatment, of the inappropriate vasoconstriction-volume interaction found in the majority of these patients should be directed to specific antirenin or antivolume pharmacological regimens rather than to surgical intervention.

6) Hypertension and chronic end stage renal disease. The majority of patients with end stage renal disease maintained by dialysis will be hypertensive. In most cases, the hypertension can be controlled by regular dialysis and volume control alone. This type of hypertension in the bilaterally nephrectomized patient represents the purest form of volume hypertension. However, in a small fraction of patients, dialysis actually accelerates the hypertension. This hypertensive response to dialysis-induced volume depletion is characterized by a dramatic rise in renin values indicating increased renin secretion. In these patients, bilateral nephrectomy is the treatment of choice for blood pressure control.

E. Unifying concepts. Throughout the entire discussion of the actions of the renin-angiotensin-aldosterone cascade, it is apparent that there has been a unifying concept stating that hypertensive states are maintained by an inappropriate vascular volume for the capacity of the vascular bed. This state of imbalance can occur owing to abnormal volume or sodium retention (volume hypertension), to excessive arteriolar constriction (vasoconstriction), or to an inappropriate interaction of the two.

The renin-angiotensin-aldosterone system is unique, exerting major control over both vasoconstriction (via angiotensin) and volume control (via aldosterone). Thus measurements of the components of the system as related to the concurrent rate of sodium excretion allow hormonal profiling that has etiological, prognostic, and therapeutic implications.

3. Erythropoietin (erythropoieses-stimulating factor). Erythropoietin is a glycoprotein hormone primarily produced in the kidney, probably from both cortex and medulla, which stimulates the differentiation of sensitive stem cells in the bone marrow.

A. Release. Production of erythropoietin is inversely related to oxygen delivery or relative oxygen need by the erythropoietin-forming renal cell. Exact pathways of release and feedback control are not fully established.

B. System. Whether or not there exists an erythropoietin system similar to the renin-angiotensin system is controversial (see Erslev, A. J., Renal Biogenesis of Erythropoietin in reference 7), but Gordon and coworkers have presented evidence for the following scheme. They propose that hypoxia stimulates the kidney to produce a renal erythropoietic factor (EPF or erythrogen) which acts on a substrate perhaps from the liver to generate erythropoietin. Circulating erythropoietin then exerts a negative feedback on the substrate (erythropoietinogen).

C. Actions. Erythropoietin in the plasma acts on an erythropoietin-responsive cell (ERC) in the bone marrow to produce a rapid release of reticulocytes, thereby increasing red cell mass. Moreover, there is an increase in erythropoid precursor cells in the bone marrow resulting in an increase in iron incorporation into heme in the newly formed red blood cells.

D. Abnormalities. The role of erythropoietin in clinical anemias and polycythemias is beyond the scope of the present discussion (see suggested reading).

1) In anephric man, erythropoietin production is maintained at reduced levels by extrarenal organs. Thus while loss of renal erythropoietin is a partial explanation of the characteristic anemia found in chronic renal disease, its absence does not account for the multiple defects in red cell production encountered.

2) Polycythemia has been reported in association with a number of benign and malignant lesions of the kidney and diseases with extrarenal, usually neoplastic, production of erythropoietin.

    a. Renal.

        1) Renovascular hypertension.

        2) Renal cell carcinoma.

        3) Wilms' tumor.

        4) Renal cystic disease.

        5) Hydronephrosis.

    b. Extrarenal.

        1) Cerebellar hemangioblastoma.

        2) Pheochromocytoma.

        3) Hepatic carcinoma.

        4) Adrenal adenoma.

        5) Ureteri fibromyoma.

4. Prostaglandins. Prostaglandins are a group of biologically active 20-carbon, lipid-soluble, unsaturated hydroxy acids. While initially isolated from human seminal plasma, it is now clear that the renal medulla is a rich source of PGE_2 and also produces $PGF_2\alpha$.

A. Actions. Both renal prostaglandins increase heart rate and cardiac output. PGE_2 decreases vascular resistance while $PGF_2 \alpha$ increases total peripheral resistance. PGE_2 increases renal blood flow, sodium excretion, and free water clearance.

B. Abnormalities. The absence of renal antihypertensive substances, both prostaglandins and neutral antihypertensive lipids, has been postulated to play a role in renoprival hypertension (hypertension in the anephric animal). Indeed, administration of prostaglandins, renal medullary extracts, or actual medullary implants have been shown to ameliorate several forms of experimental hypertension, including renoprival and renovascular hypertension. However, the role of abnormalities of prostaglandin production in human hypertension remains poorly defined.

5. Antihypertensive neutral renomedullary lipids (ANRL). In addition to prostaglandins, the renal medulla is also the source of a low molecular

weight neutral lipid which also has been shown to have a potent antihypertensive effect.

A. Release, synthesis, and actions. The major work with this compound has been performed by injecting the purified renomedullary extract into hypertensive animals demonstrating an antihypertensive effect. Thus, clarification of this substance's normal physiological role in man, its control and release mechanisms, and the possibility of intermediates remains unresolved.

B. Abnormalities. To date, without studies of this compound in man, the demonstration of abnormalities awaits definition of its normal physiological role.

6. Kallikrein (kinin-forming enzyme). Present evidence suggests the existence of a kinin-forming system in the kidney with the kidney being the site of production of a proteolytic enzyme, Kallikrein.

A. System. Kallikrein, the renal proteolytic enzyme, acts on an α-2-globulin substrate (kininogen) to cleave off the decapeptide kallidin (lys-bradykinin). Both kallidin and its degradation product, the nonapeptide bradykinin, directly cause vasodilatation.

B. Control and actions. The role of the renal kallikrein system remains unclear at the present time, but it has been suggested that the system may play a role in the regulation of blood pressure or intrarenal vascular regulation.

C. Abnormalities. Alterations of kallikrein excretion have recently been found in both experimental and clinical hypertensions, although further studies are necessary to clarify its exact role.

7. 1,25-Dihydroxyvitamin D_3. This metabolite of vitamin D has been found to act more rapidly on both calcium mobilization from bone and upon the intestinal calcium transport system than 25-hydroxyvitamin D_3.

It is now well documented that the kidney is the site of synthesis of this metabolite.

REFERENCES AND SUGGESTED FURTHER READING

1. DeLuca, H. F. The kidney as an endocrine organ for the production of 1,25-dihydrovitamin D_3, a calcium-mobilizing hormone. N Engl. J. Med. 289:359, 1973.
2. Fisher, J. W. (Editor). Kidney Hormones. Academic Press, New York, 1971.
3. Fisher, J. W. Erythropoietin: pharmacology, biogenesis and control of production. Pharmacol. Rev. 24:459, 1972.
4. Kaufman, J. J. (editor). Management of renovascular hypertension. Urol. Clinics North Am. 2:2, 1975.
5. Laragh, J. H. (Editor). Hypertension Manual. Yorke Medical Books, Dun-Donnelley Publishing Corp., New York, 1974.
6. Margolius, H. S., Geller, R., Pisano, J. J., and Sjoerdsma, A. Altered urinary kallikrein excretion in human hypertension. Lancet 2:1063, 1971.
7. Rubin, A. L., Cheigh, J. S., and Stenzel, K. H. (editors). Symposium on the endocrine function of the kidney. Am. J. Med. 58:1, 1975.
8. Vaughan, E. D., Jr., Bühler, F. R. Laragh, J. H., Sealey, J. E., Baer, L., and Bard, R. H. Renovascular hypertension: renin measurements to indicate hypersecretion and contralateral suppression, estimate renal plasma flow and score for surgical curability. Am. J. Med. 55:402, 1973.

12

Renal Failure

JAY Y. GILLENWATER

ACUTE RENAL FAILURE*

The normal kidney is responsible for excretory and regulatory functions as well as for synthesizing certain compounds. Acute renal failure is a syndrome characterized by the rapid loss of the kidney's ability to maintain a normal physiological environment by loss of these normal excretory functions. Oliguria of less than 400 cc/24 hours and, less commonly, anuria, usually accompany this functional loss. However, recently a syndrome has been recognized of transient azotemia and decreased renal function with excretion of 2 to 3 liters of urine volume. Acute renal failure has traditionally and operationally been divided into three etiological categories: 1) prerenal, 2) renal, and 3) postrenal. This classification has been useful, since it draws attention to the prerenal and postrenal causes which may be immediately reversible.

1. Historical information. The term "acute tubular necrosis" is often used to designate the clinical syndrome of acute renal failure, although more precisely it is merely a frequent morphological finding. Acute tubular necrosis is not a new clinical entity. While World War I physicians were familiar with anuria and uremia following crushing injuries, it was the air raids on Britain in 1940 with the resultant crush injuries and oliguria that brought acute renal failure into focus. The clinical course was described by Bywaters and Beall,[3] and the renal histopathology was described by Lucke and Mallory.[9, 10] The management of acute renal failure has improved with better understanding of fluid, electrolyte, and nutritional problems, and with the availability of dialysis. However, the pathogenesis and the pathophysiological mechanisms involved in the production of oliguria remain unsolved.

2. Pathology of the kidney in acute renal failure. Two excellent reviews by Brun[2] and Heptinstall[7] recently have been published on the pathology of the kidney in acute renal failure. Necrosis of renal failure follows ingestion of nephrotoxic substances or in cases of renal cortical necrosis. In acute renal failure which is not attributed to nephrotoxic agents, there is a low

---

* Portions of this chapter first appeared in an article by Gillenwater, J. Y. and Westervelt, F. G. J. Urol. 101:433, 1969. Copyright 1969, Williams & Wilkins Co., Baltimore.

incidence of tubular necrosis. Brun stated that in the majority of cases, "The histopathologic studies of material obtained by renal biopsy or from early fixed necropsy specimens do not give the answer to the question, 'Why does the kidney in acute renal failure not produce any urine?'."

The classic studies by Oliver and associates[11] using microdissection of the nephron in acute renal failure defined two main types of lesions: the ischemic and the nephrotoxic.

A. Ischemic. The ischemic or tubulorrhexic lesion is a severe necrosis with rupture of the tubular basement membrane and destruction of tubular epithelium. This lesion is present throughout the tubule, more prominent in the proximal tubule where it enters the medulla, and in the distal convoluted tubule.

B. Nephrotoxic. In the nephrotoxic lesion, the proximal tubule is usually most affected with destruction of the tubular cells, the basement membrane remaining intact. Oliver emphasized the patchy nature of each lesion. The most characteristic finding by Brun was focal dilation and epithelial flattening of the distal convoluted tubules with pigmented casts in the distal nephron. There is no correlation between the degree of histological abnormality and the clinical severity of the disease.

3. Pathogenesis. The intrarenal mechanisms responsible for the oliguria of acute renal failure are not completely understood. The postulated mechanisms have been:

A. Hypoxia secondary to decreased renal blood flow.

B. Tubular obstruction by casts of cellular debris.

C. Tubular compression by interstitial edema.

D. Tubular backflow through defects caused by disruption of the cells.

E. A decrease in glomerular filtration by preglomerular vasoconstriction.

As described previously, there is little histological change to account for the profound decrease in renal function. Hypoxia secondary to decreased renal blood flow (RBF) was previously believed to play an important etiological role in acute renal failure.

A. Ischemia. The frequent clinical association of a major hypotensive episode resulting in acute renal failure has suggested that ischemia from a decreased renal blood flow is important in the production and maintenance of oliguria. Animal experiments have shown that renal blood flow and renal oxygen uptake are considerably reduced in acute hemorrhagic shock. This concept was supported by the early studies in 1949 and 1950 which showed a marked decrease in renal blood flow (3 to 10% of normal) in patients with acute renal failure. Their estimations were based on the direct Fick principle using *para*-aminohippuric acid (PAH) extractions for the terminations of renal blood flow. The measurement of renal function by standard clearance techniques in acute renal failure is to be criticized because the damaged tubular cell does not have normal tubular secretion or reabsorption capabilities, and there could be unselective movement of substances across the tubular epithelium. Using a new technique of infusing inert radioactive gasses which is independent of tubular secretion, Brun[2] and others have found, however, that renal blood flow in patients with acute renal failure was more than 30% of normal in both the oliguric and diuretic phases.

It has been stated that oxygen deprivation is not likely to cause the oliguria seen in acute renal failure. The decreased renal oxygen uptake in acute renal failure is believed to be the result of reduction in renal function. Renal function usually remains adequate in chronically ill patients with the severest degrees of arterial oxygen unsaturation. Renal venous oxygen saturation as low as 50% is not indicative of oxygen lack by the kidney. They pointed out that hemorrhagic shock from gastrointestinal bleeding rarely causes acute renal failure and cited experimental procedures with severe ischemia producing renal infarction or extensive cortical necrosis rather than focal lesions of tubulorrhexis seen in acute renal failure in man. Thus, it is believed that ischemia *per se* is not the principal etiological factor in acute renal failure.

B. Intrarenal tubular obstruction. Initially, the oliguria was attributed to tubular obstruction with casts or cell debris. The importance of casts causing oliguria in man has been questioned because of the relative infrequency and lack of dilated tubules proximal to them. Flanigan and Oken,[5] using micropuncture techniques, found that intratubular pressure was low rather than elevated in rats with mercury-induced renal failure. They believed that the casts and cellular debris resulted in rather than caused the decreased flow through the tubules.

However, Earley[4] pointed out that other authors have found that within the first 24 hours of experimental acute renal failure in rats, some tubules were distended with increased intratubular pressure while others were collapsed with decreased intratubular pressure. This suggests that intratubular obstruction secondary to debris may be due to the reduced glomerular filtration rate and cellular damage and could be important in the pathogenesis of the oliguria.

C. Tubular backflow. The concept of increased tubular backflow through defects in the wall of the damaged tubules was supported by the nephron dissection studies of Oliver and associates.[11] Flanigan and Oken[5] found no increased proximal tubular absorption of fluid and believed it unlikely that any passive or active factors could explain the oliguria on the basis of increased proximal tubular reabsorption without also postulating an increased permeability of the tubule, which was not found in their experiments. Other authors have found some leakage across the tubules in animals with acute renal failure.

D. Interstitial pressure. In examining the possible role of increased interstitial and intratubular pressure, Brun[2] found that the wedged renal vein pressures in the small veins were normal in patients with acute renal failure, both in the diuretic and oliguric phases, and that a reliable measure of the interstitial pressure could be obtained by the determination of the pressures in the small veins. Flanigan and Oken[5] found that the intratubular pressure was low and not elevated, and that there was no evidence of any primary tubular obstruction from casts. Experience with renal decapsulation in patients has not proved beneficial. Thus, there is no clinical or experimental evidence that oliguria is caused by increased intratubular or interstitial pressure.

E. Decreased glomerular filtration. The reduction of glomerular filtration by preglomerular vasoconstriction is currently believed to be the most important factor in the pathogenesis of oliguria in acute renal failure.[4, 8] Micropuncture studies in animals have confirmed a decrease in single nephron filtration in experimental acute renal failure. The patients with acute renal failure have been shown to have 30 to 50% of normal renal blood flow with oliguria, while patients who have chronic renal failure with similar reductions in blood flow do not have the oliguria. Hollenberg and his associates,[8] using hemodynamic and angiographic techniques, found that patients with acute renal failure had decreased or absent superficial cortical blood flow while it was present in patients with chronic renal failure. Brown et al.[1] recently reported elevated plasma renin levels in 22 of 25 patients with acute renal failure. They stated that this evidence is compatible with Goormaghtigh's proposal that an excess of renin and angiotensin may act within the kidney to produce acute renal failure. Brown and associates suggested that renin is placed in the afferent arterioles and allows the conversion of substrate to angiotensin I. This in turn is changed by a converting enzyme in the kidney to angiotensin II in time to cause constriction of the afferent glomerulus and/or glomerular capillaries to decrease glomerular filtration rate and peritubular blood flow, thus causing oliguria. While this is an attractive hypothesis, it should be stated that many investigators do not accept it and point to the frequent elevation of renin in other situations with the absence of oliguria.

F. Summary. The available clinical and experimental data do not fully explain oliguria in acute renal failure. While there is as much as 50 to 70% decrease in renal blood flow, there is much question as to the importance, if any, of hypoxia in initiating and perpetuating the clinical syndrome. Normal interstitial and intratubular pressures militate against meaningful interstitial edema or tubular obstruction. There appears to be a severe depression of glomerular filtration rate, the mechanism of which remains to be elucidated.

4. Management. Through a better understanding of acute renal failure, the mortality has been reduced from more than 90% to less than 50%. The major advancements have been through means of avoiding prolonged oliguria, better management of fluid and electrolyte problems, use of dialysis, improved general patient care, and newer forms of antimicrobial therapy. One of the most important contributions was the demonstration that

iatrogenic fluid, electrolyte, and drug overloading were frequent causes of debility and death in acute renal failure. Infection and the primary underlying diseases, rather than uremia, are now the leading causes of death. Recently, Vertel and Knochel[12] pointed out that nonoliguric acute renal failure is more common than previously believed. Early recognition of acute renal failure in the absence of oliguria depends upon clinical alertness. An essential early step in the management is to look for specifically treatable and reversible causes of acute renal failure such as urinary tract obstruction, circulatory failure, certain nephrotoxins, and electrolyte abnormalities.

5. Preventive measures. Many episodes of acute renal failure could be prevented by the avoidance of renal hemodynamic abnormalities or nephrotoxic agents. The use of appropriate intravenous fluids (including mannitol) prior to and during anesthesia with an ensuing brisk diuresis will minimize much of the decrease in renal blood flow and glomerular filtration rate that is seen during surgical procedures. Certain iatrogenic causes such as the use of distilled water as an irrigating fluid during transurethral resection or transfusion with incompatible blood must be avoided. While the prevention or prompt treatment of hypotension is stressed, the injudicious use of vasoconstrictor agents must be deplored. Certain antibiotics such as neomycin, streptomycin, kanamycin, polymixin, colistin, or gentamicin should be used with caution, especially in patients with known renal disease. In cases of acute trauma with excessive tissue destruction, a brisk diuresis should be initiated with mannitol if urine flow is not adequate with extracellular fluid volume expansion.

6. Prerenal failure. The many prerenal conditions which cause oliguria are all characterized by a contracted plasma volume with a decreased renal blood flow and glomerular filtration. Such conditions may be reversible and include hemorrhage, septicemia, myocardial infarction with congestive failure, and fluid and electrolyte depletion occurring in diarrhea, burns, surgery, or trauma. Obviously, the best procedure in these conditions would be to prevent the decrease in plasma volume by monitoring blood volume, arterial pressure, and central venous pressure, and by fluid replacement. In the evaluation of the oliguric patient, the history, physical findings, evaluation of urine and use of diuretics should point to the diagnosis of acute renal failure. The urine of patients with oliguria from prerenal causes should have a urine-to-plasma osmolality greater than 1.5, a urine sodium concentration less than 25 mEq/liter, urine urea nitrogen concentration-to-plasma greater than 12, urine-plasma creatinine ratio greater than 40:1, and increased blood urea nitrogen-creatinine ratio greater than 20:1. The latter is observed because of tubular flow: the reabsorption of urea increases, whereas creatinine excretion remains constant. Recently, helpful tests to distinguish irreversible "renal" damage from prerenal or reversible "renal" damage have made use of diuretics such as mannitol, furosemide,

or ethacrynic acid. Mannitol is infused in amounts of 12.5 to 25 g in less than 200 volume intravenously or in large intravenous doses (150 to 200 mg) of ethacrynic acid or furosemide. Recently, some clinicians have been giving mannitol and furosemide simultaneously because of possible synergistic effects. A positive response indicating prerenal or reversible "renal" disease is greater than 50 to 100 cc/hour urine output. In patients with positive responses, careful volume expansion with monitoring central venous pressure and continued diuretic therapy is indicated. Prompt relief of acute arterial obstruction is indicated when it is encountered. Return of renal function has been reported in patients with renal artery embolectomy following up to 4 days of anuria. Diagnosis is made by renal angiography and diagnosis may be indicated by extremely high serum levels of lactic dehydrogenase. Bilateral renal vein thrombosis probably is better managed conservatively.

7. Postrenal failure. Obstructive uropathy is an easily correctable cause of acute renal failure and should be looked for in any patient when another diagnosis is not clearly evident. Postrenal failure presents classically as anuria or anuria alternating with polyuria. Anuria also can be seen infrequently in acute glomerulonephritis, bilateral cortical necrosis, or renal arterial obstruction. The obstruction may be due to urethral strictures, benign prostatic hypertrophy (BPH), bilateral ureteral obstruction from tumor, stones, ligature, or inflammation, and ureteropelvic junction obstruction. Physical examination may reveal a palpable bladder, enlarged or malignant prostate, and pelvic masses. These patients should then have a plain abdominal x-ray and an intravenous urogram if the renal failure is not too severe. The iodine dyes are safe to use in renal failure. With serum creatinines of 5 to 10 mg%, adequate visualization is possible about one-third of the time, and with serum creatinine levels over 10 to 15 mg% adequate visualization usually is not seen. Occasionally, visualization is better immediately after dialysis, since the osmotic diuretic effect of urea with resultant lower urine concentration is not as pronounced. Cystoscopy and retrogrades usually are not necessary to rule out ureteral obstruction. We do not hesitate to cystoscope and perform bilateral occlusive retrogrades under local anesthesia on these patients.

8. Oliguric phase. Excellent reviews[13, 14] on the management of acute renal failure have been published, and therefore only certain points will be emphasized.

A. Management.

1) Conservative. Fluid balance is monitored best by charting daily body weights. The intake should be adjusted to allow about 0.5 pounds of weight loss per day. This usually amounts to 500 cc plus measured fluid losses. Too often, the patient with acute renal failure becomes overhydrated with resultant hyponatremia. Administration of sodium causes hypervolemia with consequent congestive heart failure and pulmonary edema. If

the physician must resort to parenteral alimentation, at least 100 g of glucose per day should be provided, so that ketosis and protein catabolism will be minimized. Oral feeding, if tolerated, is preferred. A diet containing 20 g of high quality protein (including one egg per day), 500 mg of sodium, minimal potassium, and at least 1,200 calories can be made palatable and will improve the patient's well-being and morale. Hard candy is allowed freely, and chewing gum will stimulate saliva flow and lessen thirst. Anabolic agents such as testosterone or norethandrolone will decrease negative nitrogen balance in some patients, especially postpartum women.

Extracellular electrolytes and pH should be monitored at least every 24 hours. The blood urea nitrogen usually will rise at least 20 mg/100 ml per day and more rapidly in patients with damaged tissue or infection. Acute potassium intoxication, especially in the young patients with trauma, once was one of the most important complications. If hyperkalemia develops, a cation exchange resin such as sodium polystyrene sulfonate (kayexalate) can be given as a retention enema or orally. For emergency treatment of hyperkalemia, the sodium or calcium salts (1 ampule of sodium bicarbonate, 44 mEq; 1 to 3 g of calcium gluconate) can be given intravenously under electrocardiographic control, since they are direct antagonists of potassium at the myocardium. Glucose infusion with insulin often will substantially reduce plasma potassium levels in less than 1 hour.

The underlying disease should be treated aggressively, whether by means of prompt dialysis for certain cases of poisoning or surgical correction of hemorrhage or a perforated viscus. Infection now causes more than 50% of the deaths in acute renal failure. Special attention should be given to care of surgical wounds, debridement of necrotic tissue, drainage of pus or hematoma. Indwelling urethral catheters are to be avoided if possible. Any infection should be treated promptly, preferably using one of the antibiotics that is not nephrotoxic or eliminated by the kidney. The dosage of the latter drugs must be reduced appropriately. Prophylactic antibodies are not given. Digitalis and other drugs dependent upon the kidney for excretion must be used with caution, if at all.

2) Dialysis. Peritoneal dialysis frequently is used because it is more widely available and is simpler than hemodialysis. However, if rapid fluid and electrolyte correction is needed, hemodialysis usually is employed, if available. The advent of the ion exchange resins has considerably lessened the problem of hyperkalemia. The exact indications for dialysis are not fixed, but prophylactic dialysis frequently is used in an effort to prevent rather than reverse uremia, making early referral to a dialysis center desirable.

9. Diuretic phase. The fluid replacement should be given in volumes sufficient to keep the weight stable or to allow a loss of about ½ pound per day. This usually will be close to the volume of the urinary output. The sodium lost in the urine (usually about 70 mEq/liter) should be replaced.

The potassium loss is unpredictable, and replacement may be necessary, especially if the patient is receiving digitalis. Special care should be given to prevent and control any infection, especially pulmonary infection. The patient should be as ambulatory as possible. Azotemia may continue to increase although urine volume exceeds 2 liters/day. Indeed, dialysis occasionally is necessary during the diuretic phase. The diuretic phase is not a time for complacency.

10. Prognosis. In most large series, the mortality of patients with acute renal failure is about 50%, with death usually due to infection or to the primary underlying disease. The mortality is most often highest in the post-traumatic acute renal failure or postoperative patients. Hall[6] recently followed 186 patients with acute renal failure at the Mayo Clinic. The mortality was 53%. Twenty-two of thirty-six patients (61%) who were studied more than 3 months after recovery had "incomplete" renal function recovery. The patients with impaired clearances were older at the onset of acute renal failure and had a longer period of oliguria than patients who had "complete" recovery. Recurrent urinary tract infection was found in 30%.

11. Summary. The pathogenesis of acute renal failure has not been clearly established. Histological examination of the kidney early in acute renal failure shows minimal necrosis, except in nephrotoxic lesions, and does not define the etiology of the oliguria.

With better management, the survival rates from acute renal failure have increased from 10% to more than 50%. Adequate care is best rendered by those with a full understanding of the pathophysiology of the syndrome and with ready access to dialysis facilities.

CHRONIC RENAL FAILURE

The word uremia, which means "urine in the blood," traditionally has been used to describe the symptom complex resulting from failure of renal function. It is now clear that more is involved than the retention of intoxicating substances. Chronic renal failure may be associated with loss of intoxicating substances. Chronic renal failure may be associated with loss of regulatory functions such as erythropoiesis, control of blood pressure, and loss as well as retention of many substances. "Chronic Bright's disease" is a term which also has been used to embrace all forms of chronic renal disease. The term, "chronic renal failure," would seem to be more appropriate and will be used here.

Chronic renal failure is the result of end stage renal disease from a variety of causes including pyelonephritis, glomerulonephritis, obstructive uropathy, hypertension and vascular disease, and congenital lesions. The diseases of the kidney may primarily involve the glomeruli (increased permeability or decreased volume of filtrate) or may produce various patterns of tubular insufficiency. Although the initial manifestations may vary, they tend to become similar and show both glomerular and tubular insufficiency as the renal disease progresses.

1. Functional disturbances.

A. Water metabolism. Impairment of concentrating ability is one of the most common functional defects in chronic renal failure. In pyelonephritis and obstructive uropathy, early impairment of concentrating ability is seen, presumably because of early damage to the long nephrons that go to the inner medulla causing impairment of the medullary osmotic gradient and of water reabsorption. An additional mechanism is the osmotic diuresis caused by the high solute load (urea, etc.) of the glomerular filtrate which impairs the tubular reabsorption of water. The impairment of concentrating ability leads to production of urine osmolality near that of plasma, "isosthenuria." "Polyuria" may occur but is uncommon. "Nocturia" is more common and usually is due to a reversal of the diurnal pattern rather than the polyuria. Because of the inability to concentrate the urine, the loss of even moderate amounts of water will lead to dehydration if not replaced. The ability to form a dilute urine usually is preserved until the renal failure is advanced. However, because of the reduction in total number of nephrons, the absolute volume of free water generated will be impaired. Water intoxication may be precipitated by administration of large volumes of water to patients with advanced renal failure.

B. Acidosis. Acidosis in chronic renal failure results from impairment of renal tubular mechanisms for excretion of acid and reabsorption of bicarbonate. The net excretion of acid is the sum of the urinary excretion of ammonium + titratable acid − bicarbonate, which equals 40 to 60 mEq of hydrogen ion per day in persons on an average diet. The body's acid is produced primarily by oxidation of proteins containing sulfur and phosphorus. Patients with chronic glomerulonephritis have greater quantitative reduction in excretion of ammonium ion than titratable acid or wastage of bicarbonate. Patients with chronic glomerulonephritis can lower the urine pH to normal levels with an acid load, and so the low net acid excretion reflects the loss of nephrons. The urinary titratable acid is primarily formed by combination of hydrogen with the filtered dibasic phosphate and sulphates. As glomerular filtration is reduced, less phosphate is reabsorbed to provide greater urinary excretion. However, with filtration rates below 20% of normal, the total amount of phosphates available as titratable acid is reduced, impairing the ability of the kidney to get rid of hydrogen ion, since the production of the ammonium ion usually is impaired earlier and to a greater extent. The serum electrolyte picture usually shows decreased CO_2 combining power and normal chloride concentration because of the number of anions from the various undetermined organic acids.

2. Electrolyte metabolism.

A. Sodium. With chronic renal disease, the kidney loses much of its flexibility in handling sodium and does not handle either sodium overloading or deprivation well. Under normal conditions, the chronically diseased kidney is able to excrete the intake of sodium. Since there is a reduction in the volume of filtered material in renal failure, a greater percent of filtered sodium must be excreted (*i.e.*, less percent reabsorbed) to achieve normal sodium output. This means that some patients must excrete 1 to 10% of filtered sodium instead of the normal 0.5 to 1%. This larger volume of tubular flow causes an osmotic diuresis that impairs concentrating and diluting ability. Many patients with chronic renal disease have mild (rarely severe) salt-losing tendencies. This loss of salt causes extracellular fluid contraction and decreased renal blood flow and glomerular filtration rate. On the other hand, most patients with renal failure develop systemic and pulmonary edema with excess salt. The clinician is faced with the problems of giving the patient enough sodium to keep his extracellular fluid volume up to provide maximal glomerular filtration without putting the patient in pulmonary edema.

B. Potassium. The renal excretion of potassium remains normal until the terminal stages of renal disease. Again, since there is a decrease in the number of nephrons, each nephron must excrete a proportionally greater amount of potassium. Normally, potassium is completely reabsorbed in the proximal tubule and secreted in exchange with sodium in the distal tubules. The adaptive process in renal failure is believed to represent increased distal tubular secretion of potassium rather than decreased proximal tubular reabsorption. With oliguria, excess dietary potassium, or increased body catabolism with protein breakdown, increased serum potassium levels may develop. On rare occasions, there is excess renal loss of potassium with development of potassium deficiency.

3. Calcium and phosphorus. In chronic renal failure, total and ionized plasma calcium usually are slightly reduced with elevated plasma phosphorus. Tetany due to low plasma calcium concentrations rarely occurs because total ionized calcium is increased in acidosis. Plasma phosphorus does not usually increase until there is loss of at least 80% renal function because of the compensatory increased phosphate excretion per remaining nephron. Increased fecal phosphorus and calcium loss is believed to compensate some for the impaired renal excretion. Slowly, progressive chronic renal failure is associated with a variety of bone diseases, collectively termed "renal osteodystrophy." Bone lesions of rickets, osteomalacia, osteosclerosis, and hyperparathyroidism are seen. The basic mechanisms for the bone lesions in chronic renal failure are poorly understood.

4. Anemia of chronic renal failure. Normochromic and normocytic anemia is common in chronic renal failure. The mechanisms postulated include decreased production or responsiveness of erythropoetin and reduction in life span of the erythrocyte. The anemia fails to respond to treatment by iron compounds, vitamin B_{12} and folic acid. If the anemia is symptomatic, the treatment is transfusion of packed red blood cells.

5. Excretion of drugs in renal failure. Drugs are generally divided into two

categories. The first consists of those drugs not handled by the kidney and their half-life is independent of renal function. These drugs usually are inactivated by the liver with formation of glucuronic, acetyl, or sulfonated derivates. They usually have low urine concentration in renal failure. The second group of drugs are those which are excreted primarily through the kidney. The excretion rate of these drugs usually does not change until the renal function falls below 25%. In renal failure, the dose of these drugs must be reduced to avoid accumulation and toxicity. In treating urinary tract infections in patients with renal failure, a standard starting or loading dose of the antibiotics can be given. The frequency of administration will depend on the metabolism and excretion of the drug in relation to the degree of impairment of renal function.

REFERENCES AND SUGGESTED FURTHER READING

1. Brown, J. J., Gleadle, R. J., Lawson, D. H., Lever, A. F., Linton, A. L., Macadam, R. F., Prentice, E., Robertson, J. J. S., and Tree, M. Renin and acute renal failure: Studies in man. Br. Med. J. 1:253, 1970.
2. Brun, C. Acute anuria: a study based on renal function tests and aspiration biopsy of the kidney. Ejnar Munksgaards Forlag, Copenhagen, 1964.
3. Bywaters, E. D. L. and Beall, C. Crush injuries with impairment of renal function. Br. Med. J. 1:427, 1941.
4. Earley, L. E. Pathogenesis of oliguric acute renal failure. N. Engl. J. Med. 282:1370, 1970.
5. Flanigan, W. J. and Oken, D. E. Renal micropuncture study of the development of anuria in the rat with mercury-induced acute renal failure. J. Clin. Invest. 44:449, 1965.
6. Hall, J. W., Johnson, W. J., Maher, F. T., and Hunt. J. C. Immediate and long-term prognosis in acute renal failure. Ann. Intern. Med. 73:515, 1970.
7. Heptinstall, R. H. Pathology of the Kidney. Little, Brown and Co., Boston, 1966.
8. Hollenberg, N. K., Adams, D. F., Oken, D. E., Abrams, H. L., and Merrill, J. P. Acute renal failure due to nephrotoxins. N. Engl. J. Med. 282:1329, 1970.
9. Lucke, B. Lower nephron nephrosis (renal lesions of crush syndrome, of burns, transfusions, and other conditions affecting lower segments of nephrons). Milit. Surg. 99:371, 1946.
10. Mallory, T. B. Hemoglobinuric nephrosis in traumatic shock. Amer. J. Clin. Path. 17:427, 1947.
11. Merrill, J. B. The Treatment of Renal Failure, Ed. 2, Grune & Stratton, New York, 1967.
12. Merrill, J. P. Acute renal failure. In Diseases of the Kidney, edited by M. B. Strause and L. G. Welt, Ed. 2, Chap. 17. Little, Brown and Co., Boston, 1971.
13. Oliver, J., MacDowell, M., and Tracy, A. The pathogenesis of acute renal failure associated with traumatic and toxic injury. Renal ischemia, nephrotoxic damage and the ischemuric episode. J. Clin. Invest. 30:1037, 1951.
14. Vertel, R. M. and Knochel. J. P. Nonoliguric acute renal failure. J.A.M.A. 200:598, 1967.

13

Disorders of the Ureter

E. DARRACOTT VAUGHAN, JR.

1. Introduction. Maintenance of nephron function is the prime concern of nephrologists and urologists alike. However, it is mandatory to remember that for preservation of normal nephron function, the urine must be transmitted normally from the collecting system to the bladder and then from the body. Thus, disorders involving the ureteral function must not be neglected.

2. Embryology. The embryology of the ureter is discussed in detail in Chapter 7. However, certain points of primary importance warrant emphasis.

A. The ureteral bud arises from the caudal portion of the mesonephric duct before it bends and enters the cloaca.

B. The mesonephric duct distal to the ureteral bud is called the common duct and subsequently is incorporated into the bladder, being intimately involved in the formation of the trigone and the ureterovesical junction.

C. Duplicated ureters will then empty distal to the orthotopic opening and may be distal to the external sphincter only in the female.

D. As the ureter grows in a cephalic direction, its tip forms an ampulla. Division of the ampulla and maturation of the metanephric blastema requires reciprocal induction. Thus, ureteral abnormalities can result in congenital renal lesions such as polycystic disease, renal agenesis, renal dysplasia, renal hypoplasia, or multicystic renal disease.

3. Anatomy.

A. Gross. Like the pancreas, the ureter lies silently in the retroperitoneum revealing disease only by pain due to obstruction of ureter and swelling of the renal capsule. Thus, extensive ureteral disease can occur without symptoms or signs.

The ureters are about 28 to 32 cm in length with narrow areas at the ureteropelvic junction, the area where it crosses the iliac vessels, and at the ureterovesical junction. Obstruction often occurs at these points.

B. Innervation. Nerves to the ureter are from the autonomic nervous system. Their role in ureteral function is unclear, but evidence suggests that peristalsis of the ureter is not dependent on innervation.

C. Blood supply. The blood supply is abundant with complex anastomoses of branches from the renal artery, aorta, iliac arteries, and superior and inferior vesical arteries. The vessels enter medially except near the bladder, so that exposure in the ureter is made from the lateral side. The extensive anastomoses allow total ureteral mobilization. However, the ureter cannot be transected at both ends simultaneously without risk of necrosis.

4. Histology.

A. The mucosa of the ureter is comprised of transitional epithelium, lacks a basement membrane, and lies on the lamina propria. This layer has multiple infoldings, thus allowing distension without rupture.

B. The muscularis is classically divided into a circular layer and two longitudinal layers. However, in actuality, in most portions of the ureter these layers spiral down the ureter and are interrelated in a helical fashion. The lower intramural ureter has only longitudinal muscular layers. Loss of peristalsis of these muscular layers can cause impairment of urine flow without overt mechanical obstruction (see functional obstruction, Chapter 4).

C. The adventitia, or outer fibrous coat, contains the blood vessels, lymphatics, and nerve fibers and allows movement of the ureter with peristalsis. Extrinsic disease which impairs this gliding action can also cause functional obstruction.

5. Physiology. The physiology of the ureter is solely related to the movement of the urine from the renal pelvis to the bladder. Normal and abnormal ureteral physiology is discussed in detail in Chapter 4, Obstructive Uropathy.

6. Pathology.

A. Anomalies. Anomalies of the ureter are extensively discussed in Chapter 7, Congenital Abnormalities. It is emphasized that ureteral anomalies may lead to renal anomalies. In addition, because of the common origin from the mesonephric system, associated abnormalities of the internal genital ductal system may occur concurrently with ureteral anomalies. The following brief classification of ureteral anomalies is given for review.

    1) Agenesis.

    2) Hypoplasia.

       a. With no renal tissue.

       b. With hypoplastic kidney.

    3) Partial duplication.

       a. Ureteral diverticulum.

    4) Total duplication.

       a. With ureterocele.

       b. With ectopia.

    5) Stricture.

       a. Ureteropelvic junction.

       b. Ureterovesical junction.

6) Megaloureter.
7) Ureterovesical reflux.
    a. With megacystis.
8) Abnormal position.
    a. Pelvic kidney.
    b. Crossed renal ectopia.
    c. Fused kidneys.
    d. Common renal pelvis.
9) Compression anomalies.
    a. With abnormal renal vessels.
    b. Retrocaval ureter.

B. Inflammatory disease. Infectious diseases of the ureter should be viewed within the overall context of bacterial, fungal, tuberculous, and parasitic diseases of the urinary tract as a whole (see Chapters 6 and 21).

1. Bacterial. As previously discussed, urinary tract infections are usually ascending in nature and caused by gram-negative organisms. It is well documented that bacteria in the ureter can impair ureteral peristalsis leading to stasis, thus compounding damage due to infection *per se.* Nonmechanical hydronephrosis can be associated with pyelonephritis and ureteritis and may sometimes be reversed by antibiotics alone.

The presence of ureteral involvement may sometimes be diagnosed by edema of the pelvis giving linear striations on intravenous urography or by multiple round filling defects in the ureter, indicating ureteritis cystica.

Treatment of ureteral bacterial infection follows the tenets established for bacterial upper urinary tract infection.

Ureteral and renal infection in the presence of obstruction is a urological emergency and demands immediate relief of the obstruction. Thus, intravenous urography is indicated in all patients with acute pyelonephritis to rule out obstruction.

2. Tuberculosis. Tuberculosis of the ureter is a part of the systemic disease and the genitourinary disease which is hematogenous in origin (see Chapter 21).

The ureter has the unique tendency to stricture during treatment for genitourinary tuberculosis especially toward the ureterovesical junction. Thus, interval intravenous urography is necessary during and following treatment.

3. Fungal diseases. Disseminated fungal infections are now being more commonly recognized in diabetics, patients with carcinoma on chemotherapy, and immunosuppressed patients, especially following renal transplantation. Ureteral obstruction due to fungus balls of either Aspergilla or *Candida albicans* have been reported and should be considered in the high risk patient with symptoms of obstruction and lucent filling defects and obstruction demonstrated on intravenous urography.

4. Parasitic involvement of the lower ureter, although rare in this country, is commonly seen in areas where *Schistosoma haematobium*

infestation of the bladder is found. Involvement is followed by fibrosis and ureteral stricture.

C. Calculi. Calculous disease of the urinary tract, including the ureter, has been extensively discussed in Chapter 9. The extremely high prevalence of the occurrence of ureteral calculi should be reemphasized, especially in the differential diagnosis of the "acute abdomen." Do not neglect to rule out urological pathology in this common setting.

D. Neoplasia. Ureteral tumors are rare and may be divided according to the site of origin (primary to the urinary tract or secondary from other structures) or according to their malignant potential.

1) Classification.

a. Primary ureteral tumors—either benign or malignant.

The benign are less common than malignant lesions, and are either epithelial in origin or nonepithelial. The former are most common and are usually benign papillomata (a number of authors, however, consider this lesion as a low grade malignancy). The nonepithelial tumors are mesodermal, and the most common by far is the ureteral polyp.

The malignant ureteral tumors are of two kinds. Those epithelial in origin are transitional cell in origin and may be papillary or solid and sessile. As with bladder tumors, the prognosis depends on grade (degree of anaplasia) and stage. Because of the retroperitoneal location of the ureter and the lack of a basement membrane, these tumors are often high stage (into muscle) before being recognized. Thus, although rare, these tumors have a poor prognosis. The tumors are often multiple and may seed down the ureter and into the bladder. In the patient with a low stage bladder tumor and nonvisualization of an upper system, a primary ureteral tumor should be suspected.

Malignant tumors of mesodermal origin include leiomyosarcoma and other less common sarcomas; however, these are exceedingly rare and are rapidly fatal with diffuse spread.

b. Secondary ureteral tumors may be borne to the ureter by hematogenous spread of tumor cells or by direct extension of the tumor into the urinary tract. While tumors from many primary sites have been reported, all are rare, and in 90% of patients, there will be evidence of tumor elsewhere. Direct extension from the cervix, bladder, prostate, pancreas, stomach, or from lymphomas are most common, but often the ureter is compressed and not directly involved.

2) Signs and symptoms.

a. As stated, unless there is obstruction, evidence of ureteral tumors often occurs only late in the course of the disease.

b. The most common symptom is asymptomatic hematuria. Obstructive symptoms can also occur with the passage of clots.

c. Symptoms of ureteral obstruction, due to either clot or tumor.

d. Signs and symptoms of the primary disease are predominant over ureteral symptoms in the patients with secondary tumors.

3) Diagnosis.

a. Urinalysis demonstrating gross or microscopic hematuria and the absence of pyuria and bacteriuria. Negative urinary culture for bacteria and tuberculosis.

b. Intravenous urography—there is usually function unless severe obstruction has occurred (remember to obtain delay films). Usually a radiolucent filling defect will be seen in the ureter, with or without proximal dilation.

c. Ureteral catheterization with collection of cells for cell block and/or cytology, and retrograde pyelography usually confirms the diagnosis. Cytology is positive in the majority of patients with malignant transitional cell lesions.

d. Arteriography is usually of little value.

4) Treatment. Although conservative management with local resection has been advocated by some, the most accepted management is nephrectomy and total ureterectomy down to the bladder. As stated above, prognosis is good in low grade and stage lesions but poor in high grade and stage lesions.

Differentiation of benign lesions is difficult, but if a polypoid lesion is demonstrated on intravenous urography and retrograde pyelography, and cytology is negative, open ureterotomy and local resection with frozen section pathological examination can be performed. Approach to secondary ureteral lesions depends on the extent of the primary disease, and nephroureterectomy is rarely indicated.

E. Injury. Ureteral injuries have been discussed in Chapter 8 on trauma. Injuries may be divided by etiology into blunt, penetrating, and iatrogenic. The ureter is in a protected position in the retroperitoneum and thus is rarely injured. However, its location, while protective, also makes the diagnosis of an injury difficult. A rapid intravenous urogram at the time of evaluation of penetrating abdominal injuries should not be overlooked. Unfortunately, ureteral avulsion or tear secondary to blunt trauma is often not recognized until late in the patient's course, when urinary ascites or retroperitoneal uroma or abscess occurs.

F. Extrinsic disease. The ureter with its intimate relationship with other retroperitoneal and intraperitoneal structures often becomes involved with either extrinsic constriction and obstruction (see Chapter 4, Urinary Obstruction) or fistula formation.

1) Neoplasia. The most common neoplastic diseases that cause ureteral compression are:

a. Carcinoma of the cervix.

b. Retroperitoneal tumors, most commonly lymphoma.

c. Carcinoma of the pancreas.

d. Carcinoma of the prostate.

e. Carcinoma of the bladder.

f. Carcinoma of the colon.

g. Testicular tumor with nodal involvement usually causes deviation of the ureter but not obstruction.

2) Benign disease. The most common group of diseases that cause extrinsic compression fall under the category of retroperitoneal fibrosis. Ormand first described the entity in 1948 and offers the following classification.

a. Inflammatory—secondary to diverticulitis, pelvic inflammatory disease, or other inflammatory processes.

b. Extravasation—secondary to ureteral extravasation (rare).

c. Malignant (see above).

d. Chemical—best documented with methylsergide (Sansert).

e. "Weber-Christian"—retractile mesenteritis.

f. Idiopathic—(? autoimmune).

g. Periureteral fibrosis.

The characteristics of these diseases consist of prodromal symptoms of headache, backache, weight loss, with subsequent symptoms of ureteral obstruction. The intravenous pyelogram usually shows bilateral or unilateral hydronephrosis with medial deviation of the ureters. The key to diagnosis is that ureteral catheters can easily be passed up to the renal pelves. Treatment consists of ureteral lysis and moving the ureters to an intraperitoneal position.

3) Ureteral fistulae. These communications of the ureter to the gastrointestinal tract or the female reproductive system are usually secondary to trauma, either penetrating or iatrogenic, or secondary to tumor.

a. Symptoms—usually watery diarrhea or vaginal discharge and/or pneumaturia.

b. Diagnosis—usually easy if studies are done in a systematic fashion with both contrast material and dyes.

To document that the watery fluid is from the genitourinary system, an intravenous pyelogram with Indigo carmine added can be given. The intravenous pyelogram may reveal the site of communication, while the abnormal fluid drainage will turn blue.

Definitive diagnosis—cystogram can be performed with blue dye. If there is no reflux or associated vesical fistula, the study will be normal and no dye will be present in the rectum or vagina.

Cystoscopy with retrograde pyelography can then be performed with red dye placed up the left ureter and green dye up the right ureter. The retrograde will reveal the area of the ureteral lesion, and the color of the dye will confirm the presence of the fistula and on which side it is occurring.

c. Treatment—has to be individualized, but effort should be made to preserve the involved renal unit.

G. Miscellaneous.

1) Endometriosis. Rarely involves the ureter and when it does is usually

in association with extensive pelvic disease. Involvement can be either extrinsic with compression or intrinsic with actual invasion through the mucosa. The symptoms, including hematuria, occur during menstruation when there is endometrial proliferation.

2) Leukoplakia. This is a term for squamous cell metaplasia of the ureter which occurs in association with long standing chronic irritation secondary to infection or calculous disease. Whether or not it is a premalignant lesion is controversial.

3) Malacoplakia. A poorly understood condition in which the ureteral mucosa is involved with yellow-brownish, soft areas with large phagocytic mononuclear cells on microscopic section. The etiology is unknown, but most cases have been associated with infection and/or calculi.

REFERENCES AND SUGGESTED FURTHER READING

1. Bergman, H. (Editor). *The Ureter*. Hoeber Medical Division, Harper and Row, New York, 1967.
2. Boyarsky, S., Gottschalk, C. W., Tanagho, E. A., and Zimskin, P. D. (Editors). *Urodynamics: Hydrodynamics of the Ureter and Renal Pelvis*. Academic Press, New York and London. 1971.
3. Bretland, P. M. *Acute Ureteric Obstruction: A Clinical and Radiological Study*. Appleton-Century-Crofts, New York, 1972.
4. Ross, J. A., Edmond, P., and Kirkland, I. S. *Behaviour of the Human Ureter in Health and Disease*. The Williams and Wilkins Co., Baltimore, 1972.
5. Scott, W. W. and McDonald, D. F. Tumors of the ureter. In *Urology*, edited by M. F. Campbell and J. H. Harrison, Vol. 2, Chapter 25. W. B. Saunders Co., Philadelphia, 1970.

14.

Disorders of the Bladder

ARTHUR W. WYKER, JR.

The bladder is a muscular container which retains urine until it is convenient for the individual to expel it. Its wall is designed to permit stretching. The mucosa is multilayered, transitional epithelium which is loosely attached to the underlying muscle by delicate submucosa. When the bladder is empty, the mucosa accordionates into folds, and when the bladder is full, the mucosa flattens out and becomes smooth and taut. The underlying smooth muscle contains three poorly defined layers which form a meshwork. All portions of the bladder are richly supplied with both parasympathetic and sympathetic fibers. In the following chapter on the neurogenic bladder, a detailed discussion of bladder function is presented with special emphasis on neuromuscular physiology, both normal and abnormal.

TUMORS OF THE BLADDER

Bladder tumors make up 3% of all neoplasms in the body, and they cause approximately 9,000 deaths each year. They occur most commonly in the 50 to 70 age group, primarily in men, with a male-to-female ratio of 3 to 1.

Etiology

Unlike most cancers, a specific causative agent can be identified for around 5% of all bladder tumors.

Exogenous Carcinogens

In 1895, Rehn reported an abnormal incidence of bladder cancer among aniline dye workers, and subsequent investigations showed that the causative agent was 2-naphthylamine, not aniline. Currently, there are four proven bladder carcinogens—2-naphthylamine, 4-aminodiphenyl, benzidine, and chlornaphazine. The first three were used in chemical and allied industries and the fourth in the treatment of Hodgkin's disease and leukemia. These chemical carcinogens may enter the body via the skin or respiratory tract, and they are excreted in the urine in concentrations 100 to 200 times that of the plasma. All portions of the urinary conduit are exposed to the same concentration of the chemical carcinogen but most of the tumors produced occur in the bladder owing to its more prolonged exposure.

Endogenous Carcinogens

The chemical compounds causing bladder cancer are all aromatic amines, so investigators studied tryptophan metabolism since this amino acid appears to be the major source of aromatic amines in human urine. There is some evidence that when tryptophan metabolism is disturbed, there is an increased quantity of potentially carcinogenic chemical intermediates in the urine. Smoking is thought to cause an increased incidence of bladder cancer in this fashion.

Mechanical Irritation

There is an increased incidence of bladder cancer in patients with bladder stones or long-standing indwelling catheters. Chronic irritation of the bladder mucosa causes hyperplastic changes which may progress to frank neoplasia.

Urinary Schistosomiasis

In Egypt and other countries where this parasitic infection is common, there is an increased incidence of bladder cancer. Schistosomal irritation induces squamous metaplasia which may progress to squamous cell carcinoma. Sixty percent of schistosomal carcinomas are the squamous cell type, 12 times the usual frequency in nonschistosomal bladder cancers. There is also some evidence that these patients have increased amounts of carcinogenic substances in the urine.

Exstrophy of the Bladder

In this very rare congenital anomaly, the open bladder is everted and the exposed delicate mucosa is subject to chronic irritation. If this mucosa remains exposed for a prolonged period, chronic irritation may induce glandular metaplasia which occasionally progresses to adenocarcinoma many years later.

Pathology

There are two distinct modes of carcinogenesis in the urinary bladder. 1. Tumors arise from mucosa which is almost uniformly abnormal—the so-called "restless epithelium."
   A. Random biopsies from multiple areas of the bladder reveal abnormal mucosa with preneoplastic or neoplastic changes.
      1) Epithelium is often hyperplastic and there is an abnormal arrangement and appearance of the cells.
      2) Carcinoma-in-situ may be present with cancer cells being limited to the mucosa.
   B. These tumors tend to recur frequently.
   C. The widespread changes in the mucosa suggest that this form of bladder tumor may be caused by some urinary carcinogen.
   D. Treatment of this type of bladder tumor is difficult, and many patients eventually require removal of their bladders.
2. Tumors arise from normal mucosa.
   A. Random biopsies from the bladder reveal normal mucosa.
   B. These tumors are often single and recurrences are few and far between.
   C. Treatment is usually not difficult with most tumors being easily removed by transurethral excision.

TABLE I
A Simple Classification of Epithelial Bladder Tumors

1. Benign
   A. Papilloma
2. Malignant
   A. Carcinoma-in-situ
   B. Transitional cell carcinoma
   C. Squamous cell carcinoma
   D. Adenocarcinoma
   E. Undifferentiated carcinoma

Classification

Papillomas are small fernlike growths covered by normal transitional epithelium. Delicate pink fronds can be seen waving back and forth in the bladder lumen. Approximately 30% of all papillomas are multiple at the time of initial diagnosis. Although benign, these tumors are considered malignant because they tend to recur, and 10 to 20% are followed by frank carcinoma.

Transitional cell carcinoma is the most common type of malignant bladder tumor, making up around 90% of all bladder carcinomas. The remaining 10% include squamous cell carcinoma (6%), adenocarcinoma (2%), and undifferentiated carcinoma (2%).

The earliest form of bladder cancer is carcinoma-in-situ, where the cancer cells are still confined to the mucosa. These tumors often progress to invasive cancer after a period of months or years.

Pattern of Growth

These tumors may grow into the bladder lumen (papillary) or into the bladder wall (infiltrating); some grow in both directions. Transitional cell carcinomas are usually papillary, whereas stratified squamous tumors are usually infiltrative.

Staging and Grading

The stage of a bladder tumor refers to the degree of penetration into the bladder wall, whereas the grade indicates the degree of anaplasia. It is important to classify tumors in this manner, for the prognosis of any bladder tumor is largely determined by its stage and grade (Table II).

The grade of a tumor varies from 1 to 4 with grade 1 lesions showing only slight anaplasia, whereas grade 4 lesions show marked anaplasia. Thus, if a bladder tumor is poorly differentiated and involves the deep muscle of the bladder wall, it is classified as a stage B_2, grade 3 tumor.

Clinically, there is about a 75% correlation between the stage and grade of any bladder tumor, with low grade tumors usually being of low stage and high grade tumors usually being of high stage. Low stage tumors have a

TABLE II
Stage of Bladder Tumors

Stage		Bladder Wall Penetration
0		None (carcinoma-in-situ)
A	} Low	Submucosa
B_1		Superficial muscle
B_2		Deep muscle
C	} High	Perivesical fat
D		Adjacent organs or metastases

much better prognosis than high stage tumors, with a 5% incidence of pelvic lymph node metastases, versus a 40% incidence with the high stage lesions.

Spread of Carcinoma

The primary growth of penetrating bladder tumors is into the wall beneath the mucosal lesions, but they may also send out lateral extensions under adjacent, normal appearing mucosa. Metastases occur via lymphatic and hematogenous routes, the most common first site being the pelvic lymph nodes. Other frequent sites of metastases are the liver, lungs, pelvic bones, and lumbar vertebrae. Metastases to the regional lymph nodes do not usually take place until the tumor penetrates into the midportion of the bladder muscle.

Clinical Picture

Signs and Symptoms

The primary symptom is *gross, painless hematuria.* It occurs in over 80% of patients, and in most cases it is the only symptom. Although hematuria may be persistent, it more often is intermittent with weeks to months between bleeding episodes. These blood-free intervals are treacherous, for they encourage both patient and physician alike to procrastinate with a resultant delay in diagnosis.

Diagnosis

The diagnosis of bladder carcinoma can only be made by cystoscopy and biopsy, and it is usually performed for one of the following indications.
1. Gross, painless hematuria.
2. Symptoms of an irritable bladder without a probable cause such as infection or obstruction.
3. Unexplained microscopic hematuria or pyuria.
4. Malignant cells noted on urinary sediment studies.
5. Filling defect in the bladder on an intravenous urogram.

Urinary cytology studies are particularly useful in detecting the early carcinoma-in-situ lesions. These tumors often produce no symptoms and may not be detectable on cystoscopy, but they shed malignant cells into the urine. If urine cytology reveals apparent urothelial cancer, the urinary tract must be carefully evaluated by cystoscopy and intravenous urography at regular intervals until the source of the malignant cells is identified. It is not unusual for patients to go 2 to 4 years before the tumor is identified.

Determination of Stage of the Tumor

The stage of a bladder tumor may be estimated clinically or precisely determined pathologically; 80% of the time, the clinical and pathological stages are identical. Clinical staging is accomplished by bimanual palpation of the empty bladder under general anesthesia coupled with transurethral excision of the tumor and underlying bladder muscle. Low stage tumors do not penetrate deeply into the underlying bladder muscle, and no mass is palpable. High stage tumors, on the other hand, extend deep into the bladder muscle or beyond, and a mass is often palpable.

There are additional studies which may be helpful in staging a bladder tumor.

1. Intravenous urogram.

   A. If a bladder tumor obstructs the ureterovesical junction causing hydroureter and hydronephrosis, it probably is a high stage tumor.

2. Pelvic lymphangiogram.

   A. This study is of limited value because the primary lymph nodes involved—perivesical, obturator, and internal iliac—are not filled via pedal lymphography.

   B. If pelvic lymph node metastases are demonstrable, the tumor would be classified as stage D.

3. Pelvic angiography.

   A. This technique, using triple contrast, has been reported to be the most accurate method of clinical staging.

   B. The bladder is filled with carbon dioxide, the perivesical tissues with oxygen, and the arterial supply to the bladder is outlined by injecting contrast medium into the internal iliac arteries.

   C. Abnormal tumor vessels may be demonstrated in the bladder wall only (stage B) or outside the bladder wall (stage C or D).

Treatment

Low Stage Tumors—O, A, B_1

1. These noninvasive tumors are usually treated by transurethral excision.
2. Because these tumors tend to recur, the patients must undergo cystoscopy at 4- to 12-month intervals for the rest of their lives.

High Stage Tumors—B_2, C

1. These invasive tumors cannot be controlled by local excision, and they require radical surgery, irradiation, or both.
2. The combination of preoperative irradiation to the bladder and pelvic lymph nodes followed 4 to 6 weeks later by a cystectomy has resulted in the highest survival rates reported in the literature.

   A. Only about one-third of these patients survive 5 years.

Chemotherapy

A number of drugs have been used but the most effective agent has been Thiotepa. This drug may be tried in those patients who have frequent, recurrent superficial tumors and about one-half will have some reduction in the number of tumor recurrences. This drug does not have any significant effect on the invasive high stage tumors. Thiotepa is usually instilled into the empty bladder weekly for 4 to 6 weeks, and if it has been demonstrated to have some impact on the bladder tumors, it may be used periodically afterwards. It is absorbed into the systemic circulation and may cause bone marrow depression, so blood studies are monitored during the course of treatment. Some patients note a reduced bladder capacity after treatment.

CHRONIC INTERSTITIAL CYSTITIS

This uncommon disorder of unknown etiology is characterized by pain on bladder filling and marked urinary frequency. It is extremely rare in men, occurring most often in middle-aged women. Infection is absent and urinalyses are usually normal, so that many of these unfortunate ladies are thought to be neurotic, owing to the great disparity between their disabling symptoms and their normal urine findings.

Pathology

The primary lesion is patchy fibrosis of the bladder wall involving chiefly the submucosa. Fibrosis reduces the stretchability of the bladder wall so that the bladder capacity is reduced and the patient voids frequently in small amounts, often 75 to 150 ml. The mucosa is adherent to the underlying area of fibrosis, so that with bladder distention it tends to crack and bleed; sometimes a tiny ulcer results. These lesions are responsible for the pain which occurs with bladder filling.

Diagnosis

The diagnosis is often suggested by the history, but it must be established by cystoscopy. The stimulus to void is pain rather than the usual sensation of fullness. After voiding, the pain usually goes away completely. The bladder capacity and voiding volumes are reduced often to around 100 ml. Urinalyses are consistently negative and intravenous urograms reveal normal upper urinary tracts.

On cystoscopy, one or more patches of reddened mucosa may be seen, and with bladder distension, some of these may tear, oozing a little blood. Frank ulcers are rare.

Treatment

Under general anesthesia, the bladder is hydraulically distended and the areas of fissure or ulcer are thoroughly coagulated. This form of treatment is usually effective but may have to be repeated at 6- to 12-month intervals.

DIVERTICULUM

A diverticulum is an outpouching of the bladder wall which may hold from 10 to 2,500 ml of urine. Its wall is devoid of muscle so it has no expulsive force. When voiding takes place, it balloons out like a cardiac aneurysm, and since it retains urine it predisposes to infection, stone formation, and carcinoma.

There are two chief causes of acquired diverticula—lower urinary tract obstruction and the reflex type of neurogenic bladder. Both of these conditions provoke vigorous bladder contractions which raise the pressure inside the bladder and force the mucosa between the thickened, spread apart muscle. The resulting pouch or diverticulum is really a herniation of the bladder wall. Diverticula occurring in association with the reflex type of neurogenic bladder are often located above and lateral to the ureterovesical junction. In this strategic location they effectively shorten the submucosal tunnel of the ureter, allowing reflux. Large retentive diverticula which cause significant bladder dysfunction should be excised at the same time the urinary obstruction is relieved.

REFERENCES AND SUGGESTED FURTHER READING

Carcinoma

1. Barnes, R. W., Bergman, R. T., Hapley, H. L., and Love, D. Control of bladder tumors by endoscopic surgery. J. Urol. 97:864, 1967.
2. Caldwell, W. L. Carcinoma of the urinary bladder. J.A.M.A. 229:1643, 1974.
3. Jewett, H. J. and Strong, G. H. Infiltrating carcinoma of the bladder: relation of depth of penetration of bladder wall to incidence of local extension and metastases. J. Urol. 55:366, 1946.
4. Jewett, H. J. Cancer of the bladder—diagnosis and staging. Proc. Nat. Conf. Urol. Cancer, Washington, D.C. March 29-31, 1973.
5. Kaufman, J. J. Adjunctive radiotherapy in the treatment of invasive carcinoma of the bladder. In *Current Controversies in Urologic Management*, p. 60. W. B. Saunders & Co., Philadelphia, 1972.
6. Lacy, S. S., Whitley, J. E., and Cox, C. E. Vesical arteriography: an adjunct to staging of bladder tumors. Br. J. Urol. 42:50, 1970.
7. Lerman, R. I., Hutter, R. V. P., and Whitmore, W. F., Jr. Papilloma of the urinary bladder. Cancer 25:333, 1970.
8. Marshall, V. F. The relation of the preoperative estimate to the pathologic demonstration of the extent of vesical neoplasms. J. Urol. 68:714, 1952.
9. Melamed, M. R., Voutsa, N. G., and Grabstald, H. Natural history and clinical behavior of in situ carcinoma of the human urinary bladder. Cancer 17:1533, 1964.
10. Price, J. M. Etiology of bladder cancer. In *Benign and Malignant Tumors of the Urinary Bladder*, edited by E. Maltry, Jr., Chap. 7. Medical Examination Publishing Co., Flushing, N. Y., 1971.
11. Schade, R. O. K. Some observations on the pathology and natural history of urothelial neoplasms. Beitr. Pathol. 145:325, 1972.
12. Utz, D. E., Hanash, K. A., and Farrow, G. M. The plight of the patient with carcinoma in situ of the bladder. Trans. Am. Assoc. Genitourin. Surg. 61:90, 1969.
13. Veenema, R. J., Dean, A. L., Jr., Roberts, M., Fingerhut, B., Chowhury, B. K., and Tavassoly, H. Bladder carcinoma treated by direct instillation of Thiotepa. J. Urol. 88:60, 1962.
14. Veenema, R. J., Dean, A. L., Jr., Uson, A. C., Roberts, M., and Longo, F. Thiotepa bladder instillations: therapy and prophylaxis for superficial bladder tumors. J. Urol. 101:711, 1969.
15. Whitmore, W. F., Jr. Cancer of the urogenital tract: Bladder cancer, combined radiotherapy and surgical treatment. J.A.M.A. 207:349, 1969.
16. Whitmore, W. F., Jr. The treatment of bladder tumors. Surg. Clin. North Am. 49:349, 1969.
17. Whitmore, W. F., Jr. and Marshall, V. F. Radical total cystectomy for cancer of the bladder: 230 consecutive cases five years later. J. Urol. 87:853, 1962.

Chronic Interstitial Cystitis

1. Hanash, K. A. and Pool, T. L. Interstitial cystitis in men. J. Urol. 102:427, 1969.
2. Johnston, J. H. Local hydrocortisone for Hunner's ulcer of the bladder. Br. Med. J. 2:698, 1956.
3. Oravisto, K. J., Alfthan, O. S., and Jokinen, E. J. Interstitial cystitis—clinical and immunological findings. Scand. J. Urol. Nephrol. 4:37, 1970.

15

Neurogenic Bladder

ARTHUR W. WYKER, JR.

The urinary bladder has two primary functions—passive collection and active expulsion of urine—and when one or both of these functions are impaired by lesions of the nervous system, a neurogenic bladder results.

NERVE SUPPLY TO THE BLADDER AND URETHRA

The bladder is supplied by both parasympathetic and sympathetic nerves, but for practical purposes, voiding should be viewed as a *parasympathetic activity*, since the sympathetic nerves play no role in voiding.

Parasympathetic Supply

1. The bladder is a reflex organ and the pathway for this voiding reflex is the pelvic parasympathetic nerves.

A. Afferent or sensory limb—desire to void.

B. Efferent or motor limb—detrusor muscle contraction leading to voiding.

2. The reflex center for voiding is located in the 2nd, 3rd, and 4th sacral segments of the spinal cord (conus medullaris) at the level of the L1 vertebra (Fig. 1).

3. This voiding reflex may be considered a simple reflex arc like the knee jerk, and, except during the first 1 to 2 years of life, *it is under brain control*.

A. If this were not true, every time bladder tension reached a critical degree, we would wet our pants!

4. If these pelvic nerves are damaged or diseased and the voiding reflex is lost, the bladder becomes overdistended and it loses its tone and contractile power.

A. Bladder contractions may still occur because of the stretch reflex in the bladder wall itself, but they are *small and ineffectual*. The bladder is unable to empty itself with resultant large residual urine and overflow incontinence.

5. Habib[10] studied the effects of stimulating the individual sacral nerves involved in the voiding reflex (Table I).

A. Stimulation of both S3 and S4 nerves in man caused powerful detrusor contractions, but stimulation of S4 caused better voiding because of less sphincter resistance.

NERVE PATHWAYS FOR VOIDING

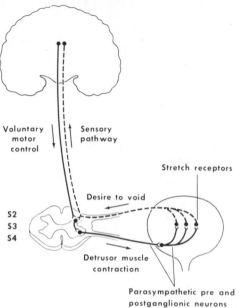

Fig. 1.

TABLE I

Stimulation of Sacral Nerves in Man (after Habib[10])

	Detrusor Contraction	Increased Sphincter Resistance	Erection
S2	0	0	0
S3	++++	++++	Yes
S4	++++	++	Yes

Sympathetic Supply

1. The sympathetic nerve supply to the bladder originates from the lower thoracic and upper lumbar segments of the spinal cord, T10 to L3.

   A. These fibers form a compact plexus over the sacral promontory, hypogastric plexus, which breaks up into a right and left hypogastric nerve.

   B. These hypogastric nerves terminate in the pelvic plexus on the lateral aspect of the rectum and then continue on to the bladder as the vesical plexus.

2. These sympathetic nerves play *no role in voiding*, but they do play a vital role in the emission of semen.

   A. Division of the hypogastric nerves has no effect on voiding but does prevent ejaculation of semen.

B. Stimulation of the hypogastric nerves has no apparent effect on the detrusor muscle of the bladder, but it does have other effects.

1) The trigone muscle contracts, closing the internal vesical orifice, thereby preventing semen from entering the bladder.

2) The smooth muscle of the prostate, seminal vesicle, and ejaculatory ducts contracts with resultant emission of semen.

Somatic Supply

1. The pudental nerves and the pelvic parasympathetic nerves emanate from *a common spinal cord source*, the S2, 3, 4 segments or conus medullaris.

2. The pudental nerves carry sensory fibers from the perineum, scrotum, and posterior urethra and motor fibers to the pelvic floor muscles and the external urinary and external anal sphincter.

3. These nerves, via their control of the external urinary sphincter, allow a person to voluntarily shut off his urinary stream.

4. Division of these pudental nerves has no significant effect on voiding although interruption of urination is less precise.

A. Loss of pudental function causes loss of erections and physiological ejaculations.

MUSCLES INVOLVED IN VOIDING

1. Detrusor muscle of the bladder.

A. The bladder is a meshwork of smooth muscle with each fiber being traceable through all three layers—inner longitudinal, middle circular, and outer longitudinal.

B. The bladder and urethra are *anatomically and functionally a single unit*, for the detrusor muscle extends without interruption as the muscular wall of the urethra.

1) These muscle fibers are so arranged that when bladder wall tension increases with passive filling or with active detrusor contraction, they tend to pull open the bladder neck, creating a funnel between the bladder and the urethra, facilitating voiding.

C. Normal voiding cannot occur without sustained contraction of the detrusor muscle, and this is dependent on an intact parasympathetic nerve supply.

D. The other function of the bladder, the passive collection and storage of urine, is myogenic and non-neurogenic and is due to the ability of the smooth muscle to resist passive stretch.

1) This muscle capability is called bladder tonus, and it is present even in a completely denervated bladder.

E. Whether a bladder is normotonic, hypotonic, or hypertonic depends primarily on the status of the bladder wall muscle.

1) Overstretching the bladder wall → hypotonicity.

2) Inflammation of the bladder wall → hypertonicity.

3) The degree of bladder tonus may be determined by the bladder pressure-volume curve on the cystometrogram.

2. Urinary sphincters and pelvic muscles.

A. There is no true internal urinary sphincter, and the external urinary sphincter plays only a minor role in maintaining passive continence.

B. Urine is normally retained in the bladder, *not* by an intact ring of circular muscle fibers at the bladder neck (internal sphincter), as was once thought, but by the tone of the smooth muscle and elastic tissue of the prostate and membranous urethra in the male and of the entire urethra in the female.

1) The striated external urinary sphincter lightly invests the outer wall of the urethra, contributing slightly to this closure mechanism.

2) The internal vesical orifice and the urethra are passively closed by this mechanism, permitting the bladder to accommodate a large volume of urine without leaking.

C. The external urinary sphincter is a *voluntary*, *striated* muscle which, when contracted, can pinch closed the urethra.

1) It can maintain continence for only the short time that it is being contracted, so that it plays no significant role in maintaining continence in the relaxed state.

2) The external urinary sphincter, external anal sphincter, and levator ani muscle, all innervated by the pudental nerve, *contract or relax simultaneously.*

3) This muscle complex is voluntarily contracted when a person wants to shut off his urinary stream and it is reflexly contracted when he coughs or sneezes, thereby helping to prevent stress incontinence.

4) These muscles are reflexly relaxed during normal voiding.

3. Diaphragm and recti muscles.

A. These muscles are not essential for normal voiding, but most people fix their diaphragms and tighten their recti muscles slightly during urination.

B. Contraction of these muscles increases intra-abdominal pressure which compresses the bladder, increasing intravesical pressure and facilitating urination.

C. When the voiding reflex is lost, detrusor muscle contraction cannot take place, so these muscles indirectly squeeze the bladder and are the driving force for voiding.

BLADDER SENSATION AND BLADDER FUNCTION

Sensation

1. When urine accumulates in the bladder, there is no sensation of any kind until about 150 ml are present and the patient first experiences a desire to void. When 300 to 400 ml accumulate, the patient experiences the sensation of a full bladder coupled with an intense desire to void.

A. These sensations are due to stimulation of tension receptors in the bladder wall, and they are carried by the pelvic parasympathetic nerves (afferent limb of voiding reflex).

2. Further distension of the bladder causes a sensation of uncomfortable urgency, and this sensation often arises just prior to voiding.

A. This sensation originates in the urethra and is carried by the pudental nerves.

1) It may be temporarily abolished by deliberate contraction of the pelvic floor muscles.

3. The awareness of urine passing through the urethra is also carried via the pudental nerves.

4. Pain is a *nonphysiological* stimulus of receptors in the bladder wall and may be carried by any one of the three nerves supplying the bladder and the urethra.

A. Mucosal receptors in the trigone—pelvic nerves.

B. Overdistension of the bladder wall—hypogastric nerves.

C. Posterior urethra—pudental nerves.

Function—Passive Storage of Urine

1. As the bladder slowly fills with urine, the tension in the bladder wall steadily increases but the intravesical pressure remains low.

A. This capacity, called bladder tonus, depends upon the physical state of the bladder wall (elasticity) and is nonreflex, non-neurogenic, persisting even after complete denervation of the bladder.

1) Overstretching the bladder wall reduces bladder tonus (hypotonic), whereas inflammation of the bladder wall, cold weather, anxiety, and diversion of the urine from the bladder all increase bladder tonus (hypertonic).

B. The explanation for this persistence of low intravesical pressure despite bladder filling is found in Laplace's law.

1) This law states that the hydrostatic pressure in a hollow sphere is two times the tension in its wall divided by the radius.

$$P = \frac{2T}{r}$$

2) As long as bladder wall tension and the radius of the bladder increase equally, the intravesical pressure remains constant.

2. When the elastic limits of the bladder wall are reached, both bladder wall tension and intravesical pressure rise precipitously.

Function—Active Expulsion of Urine

1. Voiding usually follows activation of the voiding reflex by a critical degree of bladder filling, but this is not essential, for *man alone can void at any degree of bladder filling.*

2. The voiding reflex is operational and results in effective bladder emptying only when the following conditions are present.

A. The pelvic parasympathetic nerves and spinal cord are intact.

B. The bladder is not overdistended.

C. There is no mechanical obstruction to urine flow.

3. In infancy, this reflex is not under brain control, so that voiding is *involuntary and automatic*.

4. Around the age of 2, this reflex comes under brain control and voiding becomes *voluntary*.

A. Facilitation and inhibition centers in the brain modify this simple reflex by their action on the internuncial neuron interposed between the afferent and efferent neurons.

5. When the detrusor muscle of the bladder contracts completing the voiding reflex, the opposing urinary sphincter muscles relax owing to *reciprocal innervation* between the pelvic and pudendal nerves.

A. All muscular movement involves reciprocal activity of opposing muscles, for without this coordination, there could be no effective muscular contraction.

1) Flexion of the biceps muscles causes simultaneous relaxation of the triceps muscles, permitting flexion of the arm.

B. Clinical examples where muscle action is blocked by simultaneous contraction of opposing muscles:

1) When a hypnotized person is told that he cannot flex his arm, he is unable to do so despite vigorous efforts.

a. Muscle action here is blocked by involuntary contraction of the arm extensors, so that both flexors and extensors are contracting vigorously with the net result—no movement.

2) Individuals with psychogenic retention are unable to void because contraction of the external urinary sphincter muscle opposes the contraction of the detrusor muscle of the bladder.

6. Voiding of small volumes of urine takes place without activation of the voiding reflex and without detrusor muscle contraction.

A. The Valsalva maneuver (straining) increases both the intra-abdominal and intravesical pressures.

B. Deliberate relaxation of the pelvic muscles decreases urethral resistance.

C. When intravesical pressure is greater than intraurethral pressure, urine is squeezed out.

CLINICAL

There is no uniform way of classifying neurogenic bladder dysfunction. The interrelationship and the bases for the proposed schemes of classification follow (Table II).

I will use the classification of McLellan based on the behavior of the bladder.

TABLE II
Classification of Neurogenic Bladder

Site of Neurological Lesion	Behavior of Bladder		Bladder Muscle Tone
Upper motor neuron	Incomplete	Uninhibited	Spastic
	Complete	Reflex	
Lower motor neuron	Incomplete	Hypotonic	Flaccid
	Complete	Autonomous	

CYSTOMETRICS

Any measurement of the neuromuscular function of the bladder may be included in a cystometric study. Initially, it was designed primarily to measure changes in bladder activity and bladder pressure during gradual filling. There are four major components of bladder function which are assessed—sensation, reflex voiding, tonus, and rhythmic contractions. Sensation and reflex voiding are *neurogenic;* tonus and rhythmic contractions are *myogenic.* Myogenic changes may indirectly alter both sensation and reflex voiding, and neurogenic changes may indirectly alter both tonus and rhythmic contractions so that *cystometrics may fail to distinguish* clearly between neurogenic and myogenic changes (Fig. 2).

Cystometric Study

1. Observe the patient voiding if feasible.
   A. When the patient's bladder is comfortably full, watch him void noting

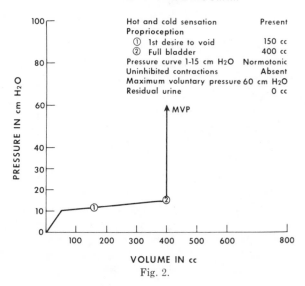

NORMAL CYSTOMETROGRAM

Fig. 2.

his method of initiating urination and the size, force, and continuity of his urinary stream.

    1) Normally, voiding is initiated without any hesitancy or straining, and the urinary stream is uninterrupted and of good size and force.

2. Determine the residual urine by passing a catheter after the patient has voided.

    A. Significant residual urine is common in all forms of neurogenic bladder except the uninhibited type.

    B. Other non-neurogenic causes of residual urine include:

        1) Bladder outlet obstruction with bladder decompensation.

        2) Vesicoureteral reflux.

3. Bladder sensation.

    A. The awareness of fluid within the bladder is determined at two points.

    1) First desire to void—the patient normally is unaware of fluid within the bladder until 100 to 150 ml have been instilled.

    2) Full bladder—the patient normally becomes uncomfortably full when 350 to 600 ml have been instilled.

    B. Temperature sensation is tested by instilling hot and cold water.

4. Bladder tonus.

    A. This is determined by pressure-volume curve on a cystometer, allowing sterile water to enter the bladder at a rate of about 1 ml/sec.

    B. The bladder may be classified as hypotonic, normotonic, or hypertonic.

    1) The degree of bladder tonus depends *primarily on the state of the bladder wall.*

    C. Hypotonicity results from overstretching of the bladder wall.

    1) Neurogenic—in the hypotonic neurogenic bladder, the loss of perception of bladder fullness permits overstretching of the bladder muscle.

    2) Myogenic—long standing bladder outlet obstruction may eventually cause fatigue of the bladder muscle with resultant overstretching.

    D. Hypertonicity results from increased irritability of the bladder wall.

    1) Neurogenic—in the uninhibited and reflex neurogenic bladders, the irritability results from the hyperactive voiding reflex.

    2) Myogenic causes of increased irritability.

        a. Inflammation of the bladder wall due to cystitis, stone, or tumor.

        b. Hypertrophied bladder secondary to bladder outlet obstruction.

        c. Diversion of urine away from the bladder.

5. Uninhibited contractions of the detrusor muscle.

    A. These are abnormal and do not occur in the normal bladder.

    B. Neurogenic—in the uninhibited and reflex neurogenic bladders, the absence of central inhibition of the voiding reflex *commonly* results in uninhibited contractions.

    C. Myogenic—inflammation of the bladder wall may occasionally cause uninhibited contractions.

6. Maximal intravesical pressure.

A. This is determined by asking the patient with a full bladder to attempt voiding.

1) The resultant rise in pressure may result solely from the increase in intra-abdominal pressure caused by straining, or it may result from the summation of abdominal straining and detrusor muscle contraction.

2) With detrusor muscle contraction, fluid usually escapes alongside the catheter, and the intravesical pressure falls in slow, steplike drops.

3) With abdominal straining, the elevated intravesical pressure drops immediately to prestraining levels and no urine escapes alongside the catheter.

B. The normal pressure required to void is 30 to 80 cm of water.

C. The presence of a voluntary detrusor muscle contraction indicates an intact voiding reflex arc.

7. Denervation supersensitivity test for neurogenic bladder.

A. Lapides *et al.*[14] introduced this urecholine test to help in the detection of neurogenic bladder dysfunction.

1) It is based on the fact that an organ chronically deprived of its motor or sensory nerves develops an increased sensitivity to its neurohumoral transmitter.

a. The bladder being stimulated by acetylcholine becomes supersensitive to urecholine on denervation.

B. Test.

1) One hundred milliliters of fluid are instilled into the bladder two or three times to determine a baseline response to stretch.

a. Normally this is 5 to 20 cm of water.

2) Inject 1 mg in a child, 2.5 mg in an adult, of urecholine subcutaneously, and again instill 100 ml of fluid 10, 20, and 30 min after injection.

C. Results.

1) Normal—bladder pressure rises 5 to 15 cm of water over control.

2) Hypotonic or autonomous neurogenic bladder—bladder pressure rises more than 15 cm of water over control, often 40 to 60 cm of water.

3) Uninhibited neurogenic bladder—uninhibited contractions develop at smaller volume than control.

4) Reflex neurogenic bladder—reflex contractions occur at smaller volumes than control.

NEUROGENIC BLADDER DYSFUNCTION DUE TO LESIONS ABOVE THE SACRAL VOIDING CENTER
Uninhibited Neurogenic Bladder

This is the most common type of neurogenic bladder with the least variation from normal (Figs. 3 and 4).

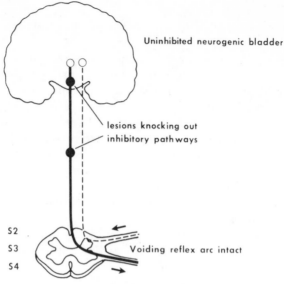

Uninhibited neurogenic bladder

lesions knocking out
inhibitory pathways

S2
S3
S4

Voiding reflex arc intact

Fig. 3.

UNINHIBITED NEUROGENIC BLADDER

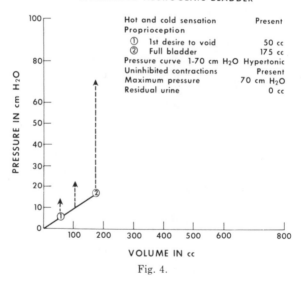

Hot and cold sensation	Present
Proprioception	
① 1st desire to void	50 cc
② Full bladder	175 cc
Pressure curve 1-70 cm H₂O	Hypertonic
Uninhibited contractions	Present
Maximum pressure	70 cm H₂O
Residual urine	0 cc

VOLUME IN cc

Fig. 4.

1. Neurological lesion.

A. The lesion or lesions involve inhibitory fibers in the brain or spinal cord.

B. The sacral voiding center is constantly under cortical regulation via both stimulatory and inhibitory fibers, so that loss of inhibition permits sensory impulses from the bladder *freely* to activate the voiding reflex, causing uninhibited bladder contractions.

2. Etiology.
   A. Cerebral vascular accident (stroke).
   B. Brain tumors involving the frontal lobe.
   C. Arteriosclerosis of the spinal cord.
   D. Multiple sclerosis.
   E. Anxiety.
   F. Unknown.
3. Bladder sensation.
   A. Usually this is limited to urgency, often accompanied by urgency incontinence.
      1) Some patients are able to avoid incontinence by voluntary contraction of their pelvic floor muscles.
   B. Less commonly, sensation is normal.
4. Voiding pattern.
   A. Voiding is *reflex and involuntary*.
   B. The voiding reflex, lacking higher center control, is hyperactive so that smaller than normal volumes of urine may trigger this reflex.
      1) This results in urinary frequency with decreased volume per voiding.
   C. Since only the inhibitory pathways are interrupted, *voluntary* voiding is still possible because of the presence of intact stimulatory pathways.
      1) Voluntary voiding must take place *before* there is sufficient urine in the bladder to trigger the voiding reflex.
5. Urinary symptoms.
   A. *Urgency* is the chief complaint, and this is often accompanied by incontinence and urinary frequency.
6. Neurological examination.
   A. Most of these patients have *no neurological abnormalities except for the characteristic finding on cystometrogram*.
   B. Characteristic neurological findings will be present if the neurogenic bladder is the result of a cerebral vascular accident, brain tumor, or multiple sclerosis.
7. Urological studies.
   A. Intravenous urogram, cystourethrogram and cystoendoscopy are normal although bladder capacity is often reduced, and trabeculation of the bladder wall is common.
   B. Cystometrogram.
      1) The diagnostic finding is the presence of *involuntary bladder contractions*.
      2) The pressure-volume curve is hypertonic and the bladder capacity is reduced.
      3) Sensation is often normal.
8. Differential diagnosis.
   A. This type of neurogenic bladder often goes undetected for two reasons.
      1) Neurological examination is frequently normal.
      2) The presenting symptoms of urgency and urgency incontinence are

often attributed to prostatic obstruction or to inflammatory lesions in or adjacent to the bladder.

B. The diagnosis of uninhibited neurogenic bladder may be made when urgency results in involuntary bladder contractions and there is no inflammatory process in or near the bladder.

9. Management.

A. The aim is to decrease the irritability of the voiding reflex.

1) Anticholinergic agents accomplish this by blocking parasympathetic transmission at both the neuromuscular junction and the ganglia of the vesical plexus.

2) Probanthine, 30 mg orally every 3 hours, usually prevents urgency incontinence and increases bladder capacity.

Reflex Neurogenic Bladder

This is potentially the most serious type of neurogenic bladder (Fig. 5).

1. Neurological lesion.

A. The lesion or lesions are located in the brain or spinal cord, and they interrupt *all* the spinal cord pathways to the sacral voiding center.

B. Conscious, voluntary control of the voiding reflex is completely lost.

2. Etiology.

A. Traumatic transection of the spinal cord above the sacral voiding center is the most common cause.

B. Cerebral vascular accident (stroke).

C. Brain or spinal cord tumor located above the sacral voiding center.

D. Widespread multiple sclerosis.

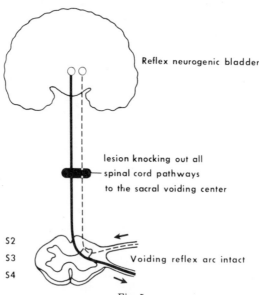

Fig. 5.

3. Bladder sensation.

A. The normal sensation of a full bladder with a desire to void is abolished, but a vague sensation of fullness in the lower abdomen is present if the lesion is T6 or below.

1) This is due to the sympathetic nerve fibers from the bladder reaching the intact thoracolumbar cord.

B. Lesions above T5 cause autonomic dysreflexia manifested by paroxysmal hypertension, bradycardia, headache, sweating, clogging of nasal airways, and flushing of the face and neck.

4. Pathophysiology of voiding pattern.

A. The voiding reflex is intact, but it is completely divorced from higher center control.

1) Voiding is therefore *reflex and involuntary*, and the patient is unable to postpone, initiate, or arrest voiding at will.

B. This unregulated voiding reflex differs from normal.

1) It is hyperactive so that smaller than normal urine volumes may trigger it.

2) It may be activated by nonurological sensory stimuli reaching the isolated lower segment of the spinal cord.

C. The bladder tends to be *spastic* when it is bombarded by frequent, erratic nervous impulses, each of which produces a spastic contraction of the detrusor muscle.

1) The degree of spasticity is increased when the bladder wall is inflamed by infection, stones, or an inlying catheter.

D. Spastic bladder has the following characteristics.

1) Spastic bladder contraction is sudden and forceful but unsustained.

a. Isolated spinal cord is capable of phasic but not sustained discharges.

2) Reduced capacity.

3) Thickened wall—trabeculation.

4) Increased intraluminal pressure.

E. Individual voiding patterns depend on the irritability of the voiding reflex.

1) In a minority of patients, voiding approximates normal except for the lack of voluntary control. Bladder capacity is 200 to 300 cc, and the reflex voiding contraction is activated only by a critical degree of bladder filling.

2) Most patients have a more irritable voiding reflex with some degree of spasticity of the bladder. In the most severe cases, bladder capacity is less than 50 cc, and involuntary bladder spasms occur every 15 to 30 min.

5. Urinary symptoms.

A. Frequent involuntary voiding is the chief complaint.

6. Neurological examination.

A. The nature and extent of the underlying neurological disorder determine the neurological findings.

1) Look for characteristic findings—cerebral vascular accident, multiple sclerosis, tumor of the brain or spinal cord, traumatic transection of the cord.

B. With complete transection of the spinal cord, there is loss of all sensation and voluntary movement *at and below* the level of the lesion.

1) There is a flaccid paralysis at the level of the lesion due to destruction of the anterior horn cells and anterior roots, and a spastic paralysis below the level of the lesion.

C. Tests for sacral reflex activity.

1) Anal sphincter tone is hypertonic or normal.

2) Bulbocavernosus reflex is positive.

7. Urological studies.

A. The changes in the urinary tract parallel the degree of spasticity of the reflex bladder.

1) A severely spastic bladder is the *most abnormal of all neurogenic bladders* and causes the greatest damage to the upper urinary tracts.

B. Intravenous urogram.

1) Hydronephrosis and hydroureter develop when the neurogenic induced changes in the bladder wall are sufficient to disrupt the function of the ureterovesical junction causing obstruction or permitting reflux.

2) If infection has been present, changes of chronic pyelonephritis are often seen.

C. Cystourethrogram.

1) Bladder capacity tends to be small and the margins of the bladder are grossly irregular because of trabeculation, cellules, and diverticula.

2) Vesicoureteric reflux is common, occurring in about 50% of reflex neurogenic bladders.

3) The bladder neck may be permanently open because of the chronic overactivity of the detrusor muscle.

4) There is usually a significant amount of residual urine postvoiding, but in the more spastic bladders it may be zero.

5) A urethral stricture or fistula may be present if the patient has been on prolonged urethral catheter drainage.

D. Cinefluorography.

1) Voiding is initiated by an involuntary detrusor contraction, but, unlike the normal individual, there is no simultaneous descent of the bladder base.

2) The external sphincter, normally relaxed during voiding, often contracts intermittently, temporarily pinching off the urinary stream and causing a ballooning out of the posterior urethra.

3) Both abnormal findings on voiding—lack of descent of the bladder base and intermittent contraction of the external sphincter—reflect the spasticity of the pelvic musculature.

E. Cystoendoscopy.

1) Trabeculation is present, often of a severe degree, and may be accompanied by cellules and diverticula.

2) A diverticulum is often located above and lateral to the ureterovesical junction.

a. Hutch showed how this strategically located diverticulum shortened the effective length of the intravesical ureter, permitting vesicoureteric reflux.

3) Bladder capacity is usually reduced, and involuntary bladder contractions often make visualization difficult.

4) Bladder stones may be present.

5) Inflammatory changes in the mucosa are common because of infection or presence of foreign bodies such as a catheter or stone.

F. Cystometrogram.

1) Involuntary bladder contractions and a hypertonic pressure-volume curve are the most characteristic findings.

a. In the mildly spastic bladder, the capacity may exceed 200 ml, and involuntary bladder contractions may occur only at the time of voiding.

b. In the severely spastic bladder, the capacity may only be 50 ml, and repeated involuntary bladder contractions may occur during the study.

2) The normal sensation of a full bladder and the accompanying desire to void are absent (Figs. 6 and 7).

8. Differential diagnosis.

A. The diagnosis of reflex neurogenic bladder is easily made when a patient with an obvious and characteristic neurological deficit e.g., cerebro-

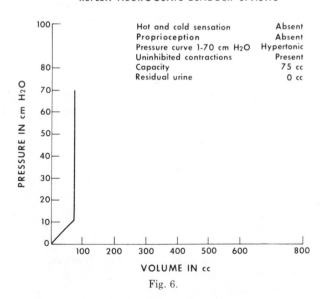

REFLEX NEUROGENIC BLADDER- SPASTIC

Hot and cold sensation	Absent
Proprioception	Absent
Pressure curve 1-70 cm H2O	Hypertonic
Uninhibited contractions	Present
Capacity	75 cc
Residual urine	0 cc

Fig. 6.

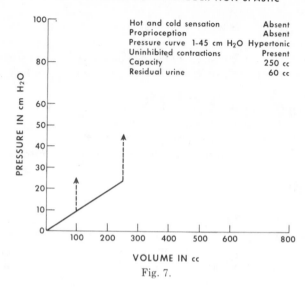

REFLEX NEUROGENIC BLADDER-NON-SPASTIC

Hot and cold sensation	Absent
Proprioception	Absent
Pressure curve 1-45 cm H₂O	Hypertonic
Uninhibited contractions	Present
Capacity	250 cc
Residual urine	60 cc

Fig. 7.

vascular accident) lacks the sensation of bladder fullness and voids suddenly and involuntarily.

B. Bladder outlet obstruction as seen in benign prostatic hypertrophy may mimic this form of neurogenic bladder when it causes compensatory hypertrophy of the bladder wall with resultant trabeculation, cellules, and diverticula.

1) With obstruction, one would expect to find an obstructing lesion on cystoendoscopy, normal bladder sensation, and a nonhypertonic anal sphincter.

C. The ice-water test is positive in reflex neurogenic bladders but is negative in normal and nonspastic forms of neurogenic bladder.

9. Management of nontraumatic reflex bladder.

A. Since voiding must take place by *involuntary* detrusor contraction via the intact *voiding reflex*, an attempt is made to bring this voiding reflex under reasonable control.

B. Reduce the irritability of the voiding reflex.

1) Avoid factors which cause inflammation of the bladder wall—infection, inlying catheter, stones.

2) Inhibit parasympathetic transmission with anticholinergic drugs such as Probanthine.

C. Try to gain control over the voiding reflex so that voiding is more or less voluntary.

1) Teach the patient to recognize abnormal sensations which warn of impending voiding.

2) Teach him to find "trigger areas" which, when stimulated, can activate the voiding reflex.

3) Success of this training depends primarily on the bladder capacity.

a. Trainable bladders usually have a capacity of over 200 ml, whereas untrainable bladders have a capacity of less than 100 ml.

b. When the bladder capacity is only 50 to 100 ml, involuntary voiding must occur at frequent intervals and is best managed by having the patient wear a condom external drainage apparatus (male).

D. Eliminate any obstruction to urine flow.

1) The most common cause is a *spastic external sphincter.*

a. This muscle, normally relaxed throughout voiding, tends to be spastic in these patients, and when it contracts during voiding, urethral resistance is greatly increased and the urinary stream may be completely shut off.

b. Division or resection of this sphincter transurethrally is better than division of the pudental nerves because it does not cause any loss of potency.

2) Contracture of the bladder neck, benign prostatic hypertrophy, or urethral stricture should be corrected by the appropriate surgical procedure.

E. Patients with severe, spastic neurogenic bladders may require elimination of the voiding reflex via appropriate nerve destruction.

1) This is indicated primarily for those patients with deteriorating upper urinary tracts.

2) Spastic bladder is converted to a flaccid bladder.

3) Dividing the third and fourth sacral roots bilaterally increases the bladder capacity, eliminates reflex bladder contractions, and improves the appearance and function of the upper urinary tracts.

4) More extensive neurectomies or subarachnoid alcohol injections are indicated if there are severe reflex spasms of the lower extremities.

a. Muscles become atrophic and pressure sores are more prone to occur.

b. Complete impotence develops.

c. Some spasticity of the lower extremities is good metabolically, for muscle pull maintains bone integrity and decreases calcium mobilization.

F. Urinary diversion, usually via an ileal conduit, is necessary in some patients with deteriorating upper urinary tracts.

10. Management of acute transection of the spinal cord above the sacral voiding center.

A. Spinal shock phase.

1) Immediately after injury, there is loss of *all* sensation and movement at and below the level of the lesion.

a. Despite an intact voiding reflex arc, the bladder is areflexic and flaccid because of interruption of the stimulatory fibers from the higher centers.

2) This phase lasts 3 days to 8 weeks, during which time reflex activity gradually returns to the isolated cord.

3) During this waiting period preceding the return of the voiding reflex arc, the aim should be the retention of the muscle capability of the bladder and the avoidance of factors which cause inflammation of the bladder wall with resultant increased irritability of the voiding reflex.

4) Both these goals are best achieved by *intermittent catheterization*.

a. Overdistension of the bladder is avoided and the infection rate is very low.

b. Unfortunately, it may not always be feasible since it requires specially trained personnel and sterile techniques.

5) If intermittent catheterization is not feasible, use a small, nonirritating urethral catheter for continuous drainage.

a. Angulation at the penoscrotal junction encourages development of a stricture or fistula at this site, so straighten out the urethra by taping the catheter to the lower abdomen.

b. Minimize infection by using closed drainage, periodic cleansing of the penis and catheter, high fluid intake, and small doses of urinary antiseptics.

c. Change the catheter every 1 to 2 weeks. Use this opportunity to determine bladder function by removing the catheter in the morning and reinserting a new catheter in the evening.

B. When the voiding reflex returns, urological management is quite similar to that for nontraumatic reflex bladder.

NEUROGENIC BLADDER DYSFUNCTION DUE TO LESIONS OF THE VOIDING REFLEX ARC

Hypotonic Neurogenic Bladder

This type of neurogenic bladder often goes undetected when neurological examination is normal (Figs. 8 and 9).

1. Neurological lesion.

A. The lesion is located on the *sensory side* of the voiding reflex arc.

2. Etiology.

A. Diabetes mellitus.

B. Tabes dorsalis.

C. Herniation of a lumbar intervertebral disk.

D. Multiple sclerosis.

3. Bladder sensation.

A. Loss of bladder sensation is the primary cause of bladder dysfunction.

B. The patient experiences no sensation of bladder filling and no desire to void even when the bladder holds over 1,000 ml.

4. Pathophysiology of voiding pattern.

A. With loss of the sensory limb, the voiding reflex cannot be activated so that voiding must take place *without detrusor muscle contraction*.

B. Loss of perception of bladder fullness allows the detrusor muscles to be

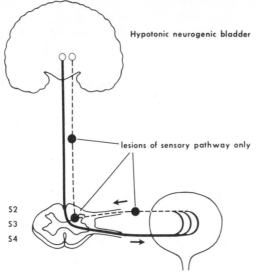

Hypotonic neurogenic bladder

lesions of sensory pathway only

S2
S3
S4

Fig. 8.

HYPOTONIC NEUROGENIC BLADDER

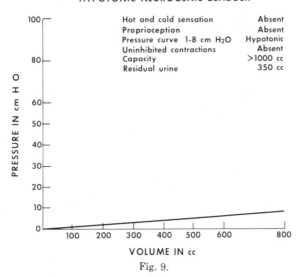

Hot and cold sensation	Absent
Proprioception	Absent
Pressure curve 1-8 cm H_2O	Hypotonic
Uninhibited contractions	Absent
Capacity	>1000 cc
Residual urine	350 cc

PRESSURE IN cm H_2O

VOLUME IN cc

Fig. 9.

overstretched, producing a hypotonic bladder incapable of efficient contractions.

    1) The hypotonia of the bladder is on a mechanical basis but is caused by the neurological deficit.

    C. Voiding is by *extrinsic pressure*, not by bladder contraction.

    1) The bladder is mechanically squeezed indirectly by straining (Valsalva) or directly by compressing it manually (Crede).

2) These manipulations increase the intravesical pressure, and when this pressure overcomes urethral resistance, urine escapes.

3) The urinary stream shuts off when the extrinsic pressure is discontinued.

5. Urinary symptoms.

A. The patient often notes a loss of the desire to void accompanied by difficulty in emptying the bladder.

1) Excessive straining may be necessary and this is sometimes accompanied by passage of flatus per rectum.

B. Stress incontinence may occur.

6. Neurological examination.

A. Sensory changes may be present in the lower extremities and there may be absent or hypoactive knee and ankle jerks.

B. Diabetic neuropathy involving the bladder may be suspected if the sweat test shows loss of sweating in the lower extremities.

C. The anal sphincter tone is usually normal.

D. Bulbocavernosus reflex is usually positive.

E. Some patients may have no neurological deficit.

7. Urological studies.

A. Intravenous urogram.

1) The upper urinary tracts are usually normal but may show mild degrees of hydroureter and hydronephrosis.

2) The bladder is larger than normal in size, often filling the pelvis, and the postvoiding film reveals a high residual urine.

B. Cystourethrogram.

1) The bladder is large and smooth walled, and the bladder neck often has a funnel shape.

2) Reflux is uncommon.

C. Cinefluorography.

1) Voiding is accomplished by abdominal straining or by manual compression of the bladder.

2) The bladder base descends, the bladder neck opens, and contrast medium is forced down the urethra.

3) In some patients there is a temporary holdup of the contrast medium at the level of the external sphincter.

4) The bladder contour is asymmetrical during voiding, and the urinary stream shuts off abruptly when the extrinsic pressure is discontinued.

D. Cystoendoscopy.

1) The urethra and bladder appear normal except for the large bladder capacity.

2) The bladder is usually smooth walled but may have fine trabeculations.

E. Cystometrogram.

1) All bladder sensation is *absent*.

2) Bladder capacity is large with low pressure-volume curve.

a. Intravesical pressure often remains less than 10 cm of water despite over 500 cc in the bladder.

3) There are no involuntary bladder contractions.

4) Residual urine is *invariably high*, usually over 150 cc.

8. Differential diagnosis.

A. Prolonged overdistension of the bladder, whether neurogenic or non-neurogenic in origin, results in a hypotonic bladder with large capacity, low pressure-volume curve, and high residual urine.

B. Primary myogenic hypotonicity (non-neurogenic) is likely if:

1) The patient has any sensation of bladder filling.

2) An obstructive lesion is detected at the bladder outlet.

3) The bladder capacity decreases and bladder tone increases after a period of catheter drainage.

C. Appropriate tests for diabetes mellitus, tabes dorsalis, or a herniated intervertebral disk may be rewarding.

9. Management.

A. The aim of all treatment is *improved bladder emptying*.

B. Nonsurgical measures.

1) The patient should void every 2 to 3 hours in the sitting down position via abdominal straining, Crede maneuver, or a combination of the two.

2) A parasympathetic nerve stimulant such as urecholine may be helpful.

C. Surgical measures.

1) These are usually reserved for the more difficult cases.

2) Division or transurethral resection of the external sphincter.

3) Transurethral resection of the bladder neck and prostate.

4) Unilateral pudental neurectomy.

5) Implanted detrusor muscle stimulator.

D. To decrease the chances of infection when the residual urine is significant, urinary antiseptics are valuable.

1) A combination of Mandelamine, 1 g, and vitamin C, 1 g, both given 4 times a day, is a good regimen.

Autonomous Neurogenic Bladder

When the bladder is cut off from outside nervous control, it is self-governing or autonomous (Figs. 10 and 11).

1. Neurological lesion.

A. The lesions knock out *both* the sensory and motor limbs of the voiding reflex arc leaving no neural bridge between the bladder and the central nervous system (brain and spinal cord).

B. Location.

1) Voiding center in the sacral segments of the spinal cord.

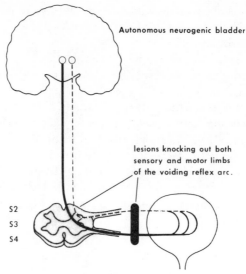

Fig. 10.

AUTONOMOUS NEUROGENIC BLADDER

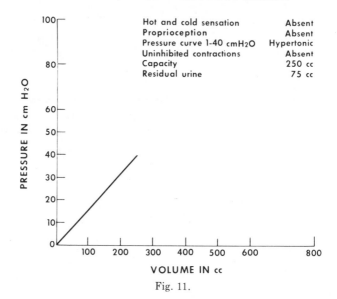

Hot and cold sensation	Absent
Proprioception	Absent
Pressure curve 1-40 cmH$_2$O	Hypertonic
Uninhibited contractions	Absent
Capacity	250 cc
Residual urine	75 cc

Fig. 11.

    2) Cauda equina.

    3) Pelvic parasympathetic nerves.

2. Etiology.

    A. Meningomyelocele of the lumbosacral cord.

    B. Extensive pelvic surgery with destruction of pelvic nerves.

C. Trauma or tumor involving the sacral segments of the spinal cord or the cauda equina.

3. Bladder sensation.

A. *All* bladder sensation is usually lost, although some patients may experience a vague sense of abdominal fullness when the bladder is distended.

4. Pathophysiology of voiding pattern.

A. Since the voiding reflex arc is out, voiding is via extrinsic pressure either by straining (Valsalva) or by manual compression of the bladder (Crede).

1) The effectiveness of extrinsic pressure in emptying the bladder depends chiefly upon the state of the *external urinary sphincter.*

2. In the majority of patients, the external sphincter is relaxed so that urine can be expressed easily and the bladder emptied satisfactorily.

b. In the minority of patients having some sphincter resistance, urine can be expressed only with strong pressure, the resultant urinary stream is weak, and the bladder cannot be emptied satisfactorily.

B. In the complete form, the bladder muscle, lacking central nervous system control and completely dependent upon its intrinsic neural mechanism, *contracts ineffectually or not at all.*

5. Urinary symptoms.

A. *Dribbling of urine* is common, particularly in children with meningomyelocele.

1) Overflow incontinence occurs when accumulated urine in the bladder raises the intravesical pressure sufficiently to overcome the lower than normal urethral resistance.

2) Stress incontinence may occur at any degree of bladder filling when a sudden increase in intra-abdominal pressure follows coughing, sneezing, lifting, or just bending.

B. Difficulty in emptying the bladder despite straining is a common complaint in adults.

6. Neurological examination.

A. The somatic internal pudental nerves and the autonomic pelvic parasympathetic nerves take origin from the *same* spinal cord segments so that assessment of internal pudental nerve function gives an accurate reflection of the integrity of the voiding reflex arc.

1) Both sets of nerves are usually involved in these cases.

B. Findings due to dysfunction of the internal pudental nerves.

1) Anal canal is often patulous and there is little or no tone in the anal sphincter.

2) Manual compression of the bladder causes escape of urine—expressibility.

3) Perineal anesthesia of the saddle type is present.

4) Bulbocavernosus reflex is absent.

C. If the neurological lesion involves the lumbar nerves, there may be sensory and motor changes in the lower extremities.

7. Urological studies.

A. Intravenous urogram and cystourethrogram.

1) The upper urinary tracts may be normal in early or incomplete lesions, but in most cases there are varying degrees of hydroureter and hydronephrosis.

2) The bladder neck is often funnel-shaped and the bladder outline is usually irregular because of trabeculation, cellules, and diverticula.

B. Cinefluorography.

1) This is described under hypotonic neurogenic bladder.

C. Cystoendoscopy.

1) The bladder neck is often patulous, and the bladder is usually trabeculated with cellules and diverticula being found in the more severe cases.

D. Cystometrogram.

1) Bladder sensation is *absent*.

2) The pressure-volume curve is hypertonic and there are no uninhibited contractions.

3) Bladder capacity is usually in the normal range.

4) Residual urine depends largely on the degree of sphincter resistance, varying usually from 50 to 150 ml.

8. Differential diagnosis.

A. The most characteristic finding is a *lax anal sphincter* with loss of both tone and voluntary contractility.

B. Other findings suggesting an autonomous neurogenic bladder.

1) Bladder expressibility.

2) Perineal anesthesia of the saddle type.

3) Presence of both urinary and rectal incontinence.

4) Motor changes in the lower extremities or sensory changes in the saddle area and lower extremities.

5) Abnormalities of the lumbosacral spine.

   a. Spina bifida occulta.

   b. Sacral agenesis.

C. Bulbocavernosus reflex is negative.

D. Cystometrics reveal a hypertonic curve, absent bladder sensation, no uninhibited contractions, and significant residual urine.

E. Ice-water test is negative.

9. Management.

A. Patients are taught to void every 2 hours by straining, augmented by manual compression of the bladder, hoping to empty the bladder sufficiently to prevent incontinence and infection secondary to residual urine.

1) In a minority of patients, this is successful and these patients are continent, have no significant residual urine and no infections, and their upper urinary tracts remain normal.

2) The majority of patients have urinary incontinence, recurrent urinary infections, and slow but progressive deterioration of the upper urinary tracts.

B. To facilitate bladder emptying, urethral resistance may be decreased in the follwing ways.

1) External sphincterotomy.

2) Transurethral resection of the bladder neck and/or prostate when appropriate.

C. Because of incontinence, repeated infections, and deterioration of the upper urinary tracts, the majority of these patients require urinary diversion.

1) Ileal conduit is the most common type used today.

2) Urethral transposition is excellent for girls with meningomyelocele.

SPECIAL PROBLEMS IN NEUROGENIC BLADDER (TABLE III)

1. Urinary incontinence.

A. In the uninhibited and reflex type, the voiding reflex is *intact* and hyperactive, and it may be activated involuntarily.

1) The detrusor muscle contracts with little or no warning, with resultant escape of urine.

B. In the hypotonic and autonomous types, the voiding reflex is absent, but overflow and stress incontinence occur whenever accumulated urine or a vigorous cough raises the intravesical pressure sufficiently to overcome the lowered urethral resistance.

2. Inability of the bladder to evacuate its urine.

A. Normal voiding requires *sustained* contraction of the detrusor muscle of the bladder with reciprocal relaxation of the pelvic muscles.

B. The uninhibited neurogenic bladder is the only one that is able to evacuate its contents.

C. In the reflex type with intact voiding reflex arc, you would think that the strong detrusor contractions would empty the bladder, but two factors tend to prevent this.

1) The detrusor muscle contraction is *not sustained.* Apparently excitatory impulses from the brain are necessary for sustained contractions.

2) The external urinary sphincter may not reciprocally relax during voiding, thereby causing obstruction.

D. In the hypotonic and autonomous types, bladder emptying is also inefficient but for different reasons.

1) Detrusor power is reduced or absent owing to the loss of the voiding reflex. Bladder contractions, if present, are due to the stretch reflex in the bladder wall itself and they are weak and ineffectual, usually raising the intravesical pressure less than 10 cm of water.

2) When these patients void by extrinsic pressure, the pressure head created is transmitted *equally* to the bladder and to the intra-abdominal urethra.

TABLE III

Summary of Findings in Neurogenic Bladder

	Bladder Sensation	Voiding Pattern	Urinary Incontinence	Anal Sphincter	Perineal Anesthesia	Bulboca-vernosus Reflex	Express-ibility of Bladder	Bladder Capacity	Residual Urine	Involun-tary Bladder Contrac-tions
Normal	Normal	Normal	Absent	Normal tone and con-tractility	Absent	Present	Absent	350-650 ml	0	Absent
Uninhibited	Present	Precipitous, involuntary, via detrusor contraction	Urgency in-continence	Normal or hypertonic	Absent	Present	Absent	Reduced	0	Present
Reflex	Absent	Precipitous, involuntary, via detrusor contraction	Urgency in-continence	Hypertonic	Present	Present	Absent	Reduced, often drastically	Present	Present
Hypotonic	Absent	Voluntary, via extrinsic pressure (strain or Crede)	Overflow and stress in-continence	Normal	Variable	Present	Present	Increased, often up to 1,000 ml	Present	Absent
Autonomous	Absent	Voluntary, via extrinsic pressure (strain or Crede)	Overflow and stress in-continence	Lax	Present	Absent	Present	Variable	Present	Absent

a. This impedes bladder emptying by reducing the pressure gradient between the bladder and the urethra.

3) The bladder neck may offer resistance during voiding since it is pulled open *only* when the bladder is sufficiently distended with urine.

a. The normal bladder neck opening mechanism—active detrusor muscle contraction—is absent.

4) In about one-third of cases, the pelvic muscles do not relax sufficiently during voiding, and this further increases urethral resistance.

3. Infection.

A. This is common in neurogenic bladders for two reasons.

1) The inability of the neurogenic bladder to empty itself results in residual urine, an excellent culture medium for the common uropathogens.

2) Use of an indwelling catheter for more than a few days *invariably* causes infection.

B. The incidence of infection has been drastically reduced when *intermittent catheterization* (q 8 hours) has been substituted for continuous catheter drainage during the spinal shock phase following spinal cord injury.

1) There has been a parallel reduction in the complications of infection—reflux, stones, hydroureter, and hydronephrosis.

2) The chief drawback is the number of skilled personnel necessary to carry out these catheterizations.

C. Urea-splitting organisms render the urine alkaline, decreasing the solubility of calcium and predisposing to stone formation.

4. Hydronephrosis with accompanying loss of renal function.

A. This may occur in any type of long standing neurogenic bladder.

1) The incidence is highest in the spastic reflex and autonomous neurogenic bladders, lowest in the hypotonic and uninhibited types.

B. Upper urinary tract changes tend to parallel those in the bladder.

1) The greater the degree of bladder trabeculation, the greater the likelihood of hydroureter and hydronephrosis.

2) The ureterovesical junction is decompensated by these changes in the underlying bladder wall with resultant obstruction or reflux.

C. Infection causes loss of renal function by direct effects of bacteria on the ureter and kidney and also indirectly by effects on the bladder wall.

1) Inflammation of the bladder wall may cause hypertonicity and trabeculation, reflux, and stenosis of the bladder neck.

REFERENCES AND SUGGESTED FURTHER READING

1. Abramson, A. S. Advances in the management of the neurogenic bladder. Arch. Phys. Med. Rehabil. 52:143, 1971.
2. Caine, M. and Edwards, D. The peripheral control of micturition: a cine-radiographic study. Br. J. Urol. 30:34, 1958.
3. Claridge, M. Intravesical pressure and outflow resistance during micturition. Acta Neurol. Scand. Suppl. 20, 42:95, 1966.

4. Comarr, A. E. The practical urological management of the patient with spinal cord injury. Br. J. Urol. 31:1, 1959.
5. Currie, R. J., Bilbisi, A. A., Schiebler, J. C., and Bunts, R. C. External sphincterotomy in paraplegics—technique and results. J. Urol. 103:64, 1970.
6. Davidson, A., Morales, P., and Becker, M. Micturition patterns in paraplegia: a cinefluorographic study. J. Urol. 96:189, 1966.
7. Enhörning, G. Simultaneous recording of intravesical and intra-urethral pressure. Acta Chir. Scand. Suppl. 276, 1961.
8. Gibbon, N. O. K. Urinary incontinence in disorders of the nervous system. Br. J. Urol. 37:624, 1965.
9. Guttman, L. Clinical Symptomatology of spinal cord lesions. In *Handbook of Clinical Neurology*, chap. 9, edited by P. J. Venken and G. W. Bruyn, North-Holland Publishing Co., Amsterdam, 1969.
10. Habib, H. N. Experience and recent contributions in sacral nerve stimulation for voiding both human and animal. Br. J. Urol. 39:73, 1967.
11. Hofman, P. Bladder and sphincter functions and their disorders. In *Handbook of Clinical Neurology*, Vol. I, chap. 9, edited by P. J. Venken and G. W. Bruyn, North-Holland Publishing Co., Amsterdam, 1969.
12. Juel-Jensen, P. Neurological bladder dysfunction, cystometry in diagnosis and treatment. Acta Neurol. Scand. Suppl. 3, 38:113, 1962.
13. Lapides, J. Cystometry. J.A.M.A. 201:618, 1967.
14. Lapides, J., Friend, C. R., Ajemian, E. P., and Reus, W. S. Denervation supersensitivity as a test for neurogenic bladder. Surg. Gynecol. Obstet. 114:241, 1962.
15. McLellan, F. C. *The Neurogenic Bladder*. Charles C Thomas, Springfield, Ill., 1939.
16. Plum, F. Bladder dysfunction. Mod. Trends Neurol. 3:151, 1962.
17. Rose, D. K. Cystometric bladder pressure determinations—their clinical importance. J. Urol. 17:487, 1927.
18. Ross, J. C., Gibbon, N. O. K., and Damanski, M. Division of the external urethral sphincter in the treatment of the paraplegic bladder. Br. J. Urol. 30:204, 1958.
19. Smith, E. D. The urinary tract in myelomeningocele. In *Spina Bifida and the Total Care of Spinal Myelomeningocele*, Chap. 9. Charles C Thomas, Springfield, Ill., 1965.
20. Straffon, R. A. The neurogenic bladder. In *Clinical Neurosurgery*, Chap. 21. Williams & Wilkins, Baltimore, 1970.
21. Tang, P. and Ruch, T. C. Non-neurogenic basis of bladder tonus. Am. J. Physiol. 39:249, 1967.
22. Turner, R. D. and Bors, E. History and physical examination in neurologic urology. In *The Neurogenic Bladder*, edited by S. Boyarsky. Williams & Wilkins Co., Baltimore, 1967.

16

Disorders of the Prostate

ARTHUR W. WYKER, JR.

PROSTATE

The prostate gland is clinically important primarily for two reasons. 1) Benign prostatic hyperplasia (BPH) occurs in 50 to 75% of men over 50 years of age and produces urinary tract obstruction, often requiring surgery. 2) Carcinoma of the prostate is the third most common cancer in adult men, accounting for approximately 17,000 deaths each year.

Embryology and Development

The entire prostate is formed by five epithelial outgrowths from the prostatic urethra creating five separate lobes; but with further growth, the only clearly definable lobe is the posterior lobe (Figs. 1 and 2). The posterior lobe differs from the remaining prostate in the following ways.
1. Embryology. The posterior lobe develops from endoderm, the rest of the prostate from mesoderm.
2. Anatomical location. The posterior lobe is a wedge-shaped portion of prostate below the ejaculatory ducts and is clearly separated from the rest of the prostate by these ducts and a connective tissue septum.
  A. Occupying most of the posterior surface adjacent to the anterior rectal wall, it is readily and totally palpable.
3. Carcinoma *commonly* originates in the posterior lobe, but benign prostatic hyperplasia *never* does.
4. In the usual "prostatectomy" for BPH, the posterior lobe is not removed.
  A. This accounts for the bewilderment of patients when told that they have cancer of the prostate despite having had a "prostatectomy."

Anatomy and Histology

Strategically surrounding the urethra at the bladder neck, the adult prostate resembles a large chestnut with its apex near the urogenital diaphragm. It averages 3 cm in length, width, and thickness and is roughly a 50-50 mixture of glandular tissue and fibromuscular stroma (Fig. 3).

On rectal examination, the prostate is a bilobar structure with a shallow sulcus between the two lateral lobes, extending about 1 finger-breadth on either side of the median sulcus. The entire posterior lobe and the

225

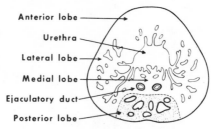

Anterior lobe
Urethra
Lateral lobe
Medial lobe
Ejaculatory duct
Posterior lobe

Fig. 1. Schematic cross-section of the prostate gland showing the various lobes.

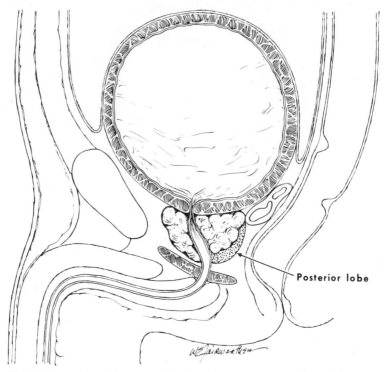

Posterior lobe

Fig. 2. Sagittal section of the male pelvis showing the relationship of the posterior lobe to the rest of the prostate gland.

intracapsular portion of the lateral lobes distal to the bladder neck can be palpated, but the median lobe and intravesical portion of the lateral lobes *cannot* be felt. This is important clinically, for although carcinoma may arise in any portion of the prostate where there is glandular tissue, nodular hyperplasia (BPH) usually originates from the median lobe (not palpable) and the lateral lobes (partially palpable).

Maturation

For the prostate to reach the adult size of 20 to 25 g, two factors are necessary—*time and testes*. At birth, the prostate is only identifiable

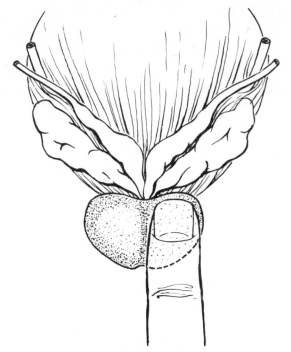

Fig. 3. Diagram showing the size of the prostate in relation to the examiner's finger.

microscopically, and at age 5, it still weighs only 1 g. But with puberty and resultant testosterone production, the prostate gradually enlarges until it reaches adult size at about the age of 20. If testosterone is not produced, as in a eunuchoid state, the prostate remains small and nonfunctional throughout life, and it is not subject to BPH or carcinoma.

Function

The prostate gland secretes about 1 ml of cloudy fluid each day which exits via the prostatic ducts into the prostatic urethra and is carried out with the urine. When ejaculation takes place, about one-half of the semen volume is prostatic fluid. When the spermatozoa clump together after ejaculation, the prostatic enzyme fibrinolysin liquifies the semen. In these two ways prostatic fluid *facilitates fertilization:* 1) it serves as a vehicle for spermatozoa, 2) it breaks up clumps of spermatozoa.

BENIGN PROSTATIC HYPERPLASIA

Etiology and Incidence

The cause of BPH is unknown. It is first observed in men around the age of 40, and the incidence steadily increases with age. Randall noted *gross evidence of obstructive BPH* in 20% of men at ages 50 to 60, 30% of men at ages 60 to 70, 40% of men at ages 70 to 80, and 50% of men older than 80 years of age. The incidence of microscopic prostatic hyperplasia is about 20% higher for each decade, reaching 75% in men over 80 years of age.

Pathology

In the mature prostate, there are two groups of glands: the inner periurethral group and the outer group (Fig. 4). Nodular hyperplasia (BPH) tends to originate from the inner glands, whereas carcinoma more commonly originates from the outer glands (Fig. 5).

Hyperplasia may occur in glandular or stromal tissue producing nodules which, because of their frequent origin near the urethra, often produce early obstruction. When the prostate enlarges, it may do so from side to side, superiorly to inferiorly (toward bladder or anus), it may herniate and grow inside the bladder, or any combination of these. Symptoms result, not from enlargement of the prostate *per se*, but from obstruction of the prostatic urethra or bladder neck. The enlarging nodules push the uninvolved prostatic tissue to the periphery of the prostate, and this compressed prostatic tissue is called the *false capsule* (Fig. 6).

Important Clinical Points

1. All surgical procedures employed for BPH, whether transurethral resection, suprapubic, retropubic, or perineal prostatectomy, *remove the same volume of tissue and utilize the same cleavage plane between the hyperplastic nodules and the false capsule.*

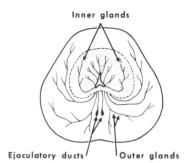

Fig. 4. Schematic cross-section of the mature prostate showing the inner periurethral glands and the outer glands.

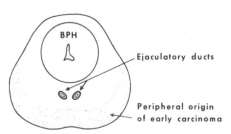

Fig. 5. Schematic cross-section of the prostate showing the sites of origin of nodular hyperplasia (BPH) and carcinoma.

2. The term "prostatectomy" as usually employed is incorrect, for the entire prostate is not removed, only the hyperplastic tissue and the prostatic urethra. Prostatic adenomectomy would be a more exact term.
3. Since prostatic tissue remains after "prostatectomy," BPH may recur at a later date or carcinoma may develop.
4. The posterior lobe is not involved in the hyperplastic process and is not disturbed when "prostatectomy" is performed, remaining behind as part of the prostatic shell.

A. Therefore, carcinoma, if present, may go undetected at the time of prostatectomy or may develop at a later date.

Pathophysiology

When nodular hyperplasia (BPH) produces bladder outlet obstruction, the bladder muscle hypertrophies because of the increased effort necessary to empty the bladder. Bladder muscle is a meshwork of interlacing muscle fibers rather than separate, intact layers. When their muscle bundles hypertrophy, irregular, gridlike ridges result. This is called trabeculation, and the degree of trabeculation as seen via cystoscopy is a good indication of the severity of bladder outlet obstruction.

The forceful bladder contractions raise the pressure inside the bladder and may force the mucosa between the thickened, spread apart muscle fibers, producing cellules and diverticula. Since a diverticulum has little or no muscle in its wall, it has no expulsive force. Therefore, when voiding occurs, it is ballooned out, not unlike a cardiac aneurysm. By retaining urine, it predisposes to infection and calculus formation (Fig. 7).

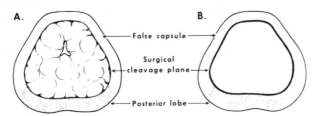

Fig. 6. Drawing showing the portion of the prostate removed by the usual "prostatectomy" for BPH.

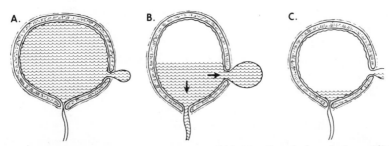

Fig. 7. Drawing showing the changes in a small bladder diverticulum during voiding.

If obstruction increases, bladder muscle eventually becomes fatigued and is unable to empty the bladder. Up to this point, the bladder was able to compensate for bladder outlet obstruction with increased muscular effort, but now it is *decompensated. Residual urine is the hallmark of decompensation.*

Bladder decompensation results from a combination of: 1) bladder outlet obstruction by BPH imposing an excessive work load on the bladder, 2) impaired bladder muscle contractility due to fatigue.

When the bladder fails to empty itself, the resting pressure within the bladder is higher than normal, disturbing the ureter-bladder pressure gradient and making it more difficult for urine to reach the bladder. Back pressure produces hydroureter and hydronephrosis with resultant loss of renal function.

Clinical Findings

Symptoms

The initial symptom of bladder outlet obstruction is *urinary frequency* with associated nocturia. This results from *decreased bladder capacity.* Normal bladder muscle can stretch without marked changes in tension, permitting accumulation of relatively large volumes of urine in the bladder before a sharp rise in intravesical pressure initiates the desire to void. Hypertrophied bladder muscle has a higher resting tonus, so that smaller volumes of urine may initiate the desire to void. A decrease in force and caliber of the urinary stream and a delay in getting the stream started (hesitancy) are often noted as well but are frequently accepted by the patient as part of the aging process. When the bladder muscle begins to become fatigued, there is a further decrease in force of the urinary stream and the patient often dribbles at the end of urination, or he may void in two stages.

With bladder decompensation, the resultant residual urine decreases the functional capacity of the bladder and increases the frequency of urination. Infection may develop at any time but is particularly prone to do so when there is significant residual urine. It further increases the urinary frequency and is usually accompanied by urgency and dysuria.

Painful urinary retention may occur at any time along the way but may be precipitated by the following:

1. Overdistension of the bladder.

A. Overstretched bladder muscle fibers *contract less effectively.*

2. Ingestion of anticholinergic drugs.

A. These belladonna-like drugs (*e.g.*, banthine) depress bladder muscle contractility.

3. Trauma to the perineum.

A. Riding in a car, jeep, or tractor over rough terrain may produce edema in the prostatic urethra, increasing the degree of obstruction with accentuation of all symptoms.

4. Drinking alcoholic beverages.

A. Some, *but not all*, patients note increased symptoms after drinking alcoholic beverages, particularly beer. This is believed to be due to congestion and edema of the prostatic urethra.

5. Acute urinary infection.

A. Resultant edema may increase the degree of obstruction.

Physical Examination

If possible, *watch the patient void.* Since the urinary flow rate varies with the amount of urine in the bladder (the higher the volume, the greater the flow rate), a more meaningful examination results when the bladder is comfortably full.

Examination of the Prostate

A careful rectal examination of the prostate is important in evaluating a patient with BPH, but *it may be misleading.*

1. BPH most commonly involves the lateral lobes and the median lobe, but rectal examination permits palpation only of the posterior lobe and *extravesical* portion of the lateral lobes. The median lobe, a frequent site of hyperplasia, cannot be palpated nor can the *intravesical* portion of the lateral lobes.

2. The size of the prostate is not directly related to the degree of obstruction.

A. When nodular hyperplasia involves *only* the lateral lobes without involvement of the median lobe, the prostate may be 5 to 8 times normal size (greater than 100 g) yet produce little or no obstruction. The bladder neck is not distorted, and when voiding occurs, the enlarged lateral lobes do not significantly obstruct the prostatic urethra.

B. The prostate gland may be one-half the normal size and still produce complete obstruction with urinary retention. This is most commonly seen with enlargement of only the median lobe which, although small in size, sits rigidly like a thumb at the posterior bladder neck, producing severe bladder outlet obstruction (Fig. 8).

3. It is difficult to estimate the actual size of the obstructing hyperplastic tissue (the portion removed at "prostatectomy") because of the great variation in the thickness of the false capsule (Fig. 9).

A. On rectal examination, both prostates are the same size, yet twice as much tissue must be removed in patient A than in patient B because of the difference in thickness of the false capsule.

Palpation and percussion of the lower abdomen after voiding may reveal a distended bladder indicating a residual urine of more than 150 ml. Pressure on this distended bladder produces a desire to void, but no urine escapes from the urethral meatus.

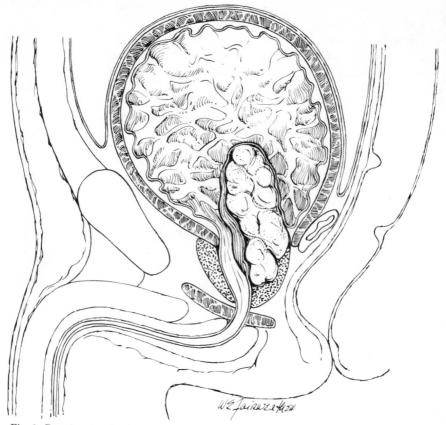

Fig. 8. Drawing showing bladder outlet obstruction due to enlargement of the median lobe.

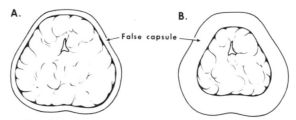

Fig. 9. Cross-section of the prostate gland showing the variation in thickness of the false capsule.

X-Ray Studies

An intravenous urogram provides a good assessment of the effects of prostatic obstruction on the urinary tract.

1. Obstructive changes may be identified and roughly quantitated.
   A. Bladder: trabeculation, diverticula, calculi, residual urine.
   B. Ureter and kidney: hydroureter and hydronephrosis.

2. Intravesical extension of the enlarged, hyperplastic prostate may be seen as a filling defect at the bladder outlet.

3. Extravesical extension of the enlarged, hyperplastic prostate may lift the bladder out of the pelvis.

Laboratory Studies

Over-all renal function should be determined by serum creatinine and urea, or more precisely, by a 12- or 24-hour creatinine clearance. The presence or absence of infection should be determined by urinalysis and urine culture.

Special Diagnostic Studies

Determination of Residual Urine

The quantity of urine remaining in the bladder after voiding gives a reasonable estimate of the degree of bladder decompensation. A normal adult man has less than 10 ml of residual urine, whereas most patients coming to "prostatectomy" have greater than 100 ml. This can be measured or roughly quantitated in the following ways.

1. If the bladder above the pubis is palpable or percussible after the patient has voided, the residual urine must be greater than 150 ml.

2. An intravenous urogram with postvoiding cystogram may be obtained.

A. This provides a rough estimate of residual urine.

B. It is painless and avoids catheterization.

3. Exact determination of residual urine may be made by gentle passage of a well lubricated, small (no. 14) red rubber catheter using sterile technique.

A. Infection may result in 1 to 2% of cases.

B. Slight edema produced in the prostatic urethra and bladder neck may aggravate obstruction and sometimes precipitate urinary retention.

Cystoendoscopy

Cystoendoscopy permits direct observation of the urethra and bladder.

1. Other causes of infravesical obstruction can be ruled out.

2. The intraurethral and intravesical portion of the prostate may be seen, so that a more accurate estimate may be made of the size of the prostate and the nature of the obstruction.

3. Most importantly, the bladder can be inspected and the changes here are the best indicator of the degree of obstruction; the greater the degree of trabeculation, the greater the obstruction.

Silent Prostatism

Five percent of men with prostatic obstruction have *no significant urinary complaints* but early decompensation results in varying degrees of hydronephrosis and renal insufficiency. These patients are usually admitted on the medical service for evaluation of weakness, vague abdominal complaints, and loss of energy. Symptoms are secondary to azotemia and accompanying anemia or to the chronically distended bladder. The key urological symptom is bedwetting or leakage of urine on bending or coughing. This overflow incontinence occurs when a slight increase in intravesical pressure overcomes the urethral resistance.

Usual Findings

1. Visibly distended bladder, often palpable and percussible to the umbilicus. Residual urine is greater than 1,000 ml and may be 2,000 to 3,000 ml.
2. The prostate gland is often surprisingly normal in size on rectal examination, but it may be enlarged.
3. There is usually no evidence of neurological disease.
4. Serum urea and creatinine are elevated, and there is moderate anemia.
5. Intravenous urogram reveals bilateral hydroureter, hydronephrosis, and a distended bladder

Prolonged bladder drainage is usually necessary before "prostatectomy" can be performed to permit maximal return of renal function and bladder tone.

Differential Diagnosis

Other causes of infravesical obstruction, such as urethral stricture, carcinoma of the prostate, contracted bladder neck, or narrow urethral meatus, can usually be excluded by the history and careful examination of the urethra and prostate. Urethrograms and cystoendoscopy are often helpful.

A neurogenic bladder is functionally obstructed and may present a somewhat similar picture. There are usually other abnormal neurological findings, so particular attention should be directed to: 1) perineal sensation, 2) tone and voluntary contractility of the anal sphincter, 3) knee and ankle jerks, 4) vibratory and position sense in toes, 5) Babinski reflex. Cystometrics should be performed if neurogenic bladder is suspected.

Treatment

Surgery is the only cure for BPH. If nodular hyperplasia, once present, invariably continued and produced progressive bladder outlet obstruction culminating in urinary retention, one would be justified in recommending a "prostatectomy" as soon as the diagnosis was definitely established. However, hyperplasia may *cease at any time*, so that surgery is reserved for those patients with evidence of bladder decompensation.

Indications for Prostatectomy

1. Inability to void (persistent urinary retention).
2. Evidence of back pressure on upper urinary tracts.

A. Hydroureter and hydronephrosis on intravenous urogram.

B. Decreasing renal function.

3. Residual urines of greater than 100 ml with recurrent infections.

Some patients have such severe symptoms that "prostatectomy" is required.

CARCINOMA OF PROSTATE

Etiology and Incidence

The cause of prostatic cancer is unknown but androgens may play a role in its development. This is the most common cancer in men over 70 years of age, and the third most common in males (lung cancer is no. 1; colon-rectum no. 2), accounting for about 17,000 deaths each year.

Autopsy studies in men over 50 years of age reveal histological prostatic cancer in 20%. This means that there are 5,000,000,000 men in the United States with unsuspected prostatic cancer. Obviously, most of these prostatic cancers remain only as histological tumors and do not progress to become clinically significant.

This tumor primarily involves older men, rarely occurring before the age of 40, with increasing incidence each succeeding decade to a peak incidence at ages 65 to 75 (Table I).

Pathology

Carcinoma may originate from any area of the prostate where there is glandular tissue, but it most commonly arises from the *peripheral portion*-—posterior lobe and outer portion of the lateral lobes (Fig. 10).

The focus of carcinoma cells induces a fibrous tissue response and this hardens the carcinoma, making it palpable as a firm nodule. It extends very early to the perineural spaces, and it tends to grow in a cephalocaudad direction, eventually extending to the seminal vesicle and bladder base and often obstructing one or both ureters. The rectum is *not usually involved*, for Denonvilliers' fascia between the prostate and rectum acts as an effective barrier to cancer cells, probably because it lacks lymphatics. Metastases occur via the lymphatics and blood vessels with earliest sites

TABLE I
Clinical Prostatic Cancer (Flocks—4,000 cases)

Age	Incidence	
yrs	%	
<50	1	
50–60	9	
60–69	32 ⎫	90% are discovered
70–79	43 ⎬	in men over 60
80	15 ⎭	years of age.

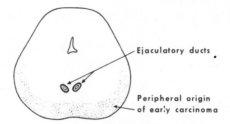

Fig. 10. Drawing of the prostate showing the peripheral origin of most early carcinomas.

being iliac and para-aortic lymph nodes and lumbosacral spine and pelvis. Bone metastases are most commonly osteoblastic but may be osteolytic or a mixture of both. The pathway for these bone metastases is the vertebral venous system. This valveless system of veins communicates with systemic veins at each segmental level. When the intra-abdominal pressure is suddenly increased as with coughing or straining to void, blood from the intracavitary veins (caval system) is diverted to the extracavitary veins (vertebral veins) permitting embolic tumor cells to reach the bones.

The incidence of both nodular hyperplasia (BPH) and carcinoma increases progressively with age, so that though separate lesions, they are often found together in the same prostate. The following system is in general use for classification of prostatic cancer.

Stage A—Clinically *latent;* identified in tissue removed at surgery or at autopsy.

Stage B—Clinically *early;* palpable nodule apparently confined within capsule; no clinical, laboratory or x-ray evidence of local extension or metastases.

Stage C—Clinically *locally extensive;* area of abnormal induration extends locally beyond the capsule of the prostate; no evidence of distant metastases.

Stage D—Clinically *metastatic*, evidence of distant metastases.

Grade I—Well differentiated.

Grade II—Intermediate.

Grade III—Poorly differentiated.

Prostatic cancer has a *very variable natural history*, and it may remain latent (stage A) for many years.

Clinical Findings

Since carcinoma of the prostate is so common in men over 50 years of age and usually arises in the periphery of the prostate, the portion most accessible to the examining finger, one would anticipate a high early detection and cure rate. The sad fact is that *less than 10% of patients with prostatic cancer are discovered early enough to be cured* (Table II).

What are the reasons for this low cure rate?

1. When potentially curable, prostatic cancer *produces no symptoms.*

A. This is due to the peripheral origin of the cancer far from the urethra. (Fig. 11). By the time the tumor has grown from its site of origin to the periurethral region producing obstructive symptoms, it has usually grown through the capsule and become incurable.

2. Some prostatic cancers are not detectable early.

A. They may arise in a nonpalpable area of the prostate.

B. They may be soft with consistency similar to normal prostate. These tumors are usually very cellular and anaplastic, carrying a poor prognosis.

3. Infrequent rectal examinations in men over 50 years of age.

A. When yearly rectal examinations were performed on Army personnel, 50% of the tumors were detected when still potentially curable as contrasted with the nationwide figure of 5 to 10%.

4. A lack of aggressive attack on this particular cancer by many physicians.

A. Since this tumor is discovered in older men (90% over 60 years of age), other significant medical problems often coexist.

B. The majority of patients with prostatic cancer do not die as a result of this tumor.

C. A few may live 10 to 15 years without any treatment.

Despite these reasons, it should be emphasized that 70% of patients are dead within 3 years of diagnosis of prostatic cancer.

Physical Examination

Prostatic Nodule

Carcinomatous nodules are usually firm to hard in consistency and may be detected in any area of the prostate. All hard nodules are not cancer! Half of them are one of the following.

1. Isolated adenoma of BPH—smooth, movable nodule with adjacent prostate having normal rubbery consistency.

TABLE II
Prostatic Cancer

Percentage	Clinical Presentation	Stage
5–10	Routine rectal examination	B
60–70	Symptoms of prostatic obstruction	C
10–20	Metastatic bone pain	D
10	Detected after prostatectomy for apparent BPH	A, B

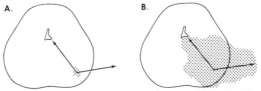

Fig. 11. Drawing showing the usual local growth spread for a peripheral carcinoma.

2. Calculus—very hard, may detect crepitation on gentle palpation, visible on x-ray.

3. Granulomatous prostatitis—irregularity often involves most of the surface of the gland.

4. Phleboliths—tiny, BB-sized, hard movable nodules in vessels adjacent to the prostate.

In the most common form of presentation (stage C), the prostate is hard and irregular, and there is extension beyond the prostate, most frequently to the seminal vesicles and bladder base.

Laboratory Studies

Acid Phosphatase

This enzyme is present in small amounts in the lysosomes of many body tissues, but its richest source is the *normal prostate gland*. The acid phosphatases from the different tissues have the same functional activity but slightly different molecular structures, and this permits identification of the source of the enzyme by special physiochemical methods. Men and women have a similarly low serum acid phosphatase (SAP), since prostatic acid phosphatase does not enter the circulation. This enzyme does not appear in great quantity in the prostate until after puberty. Gutman's report of the quantities of acid phosphatase in relation to age is shown in Table III.

After puberty, acid phosphatase is secreted normally in the prostatic fluid and appears in high concentration in the ejaculate. Carcinomatous prostatic tissue retains the ability to form acid phosphatase, and lacking any duct system, the enzyme is picked up by the general circulation with resultant elevation of SAP. Prostatic cancer tissue produces less acid phosphatase than noncancerous prostate. The production of this enzyme is a function of the maturity of the cell, so that the high grade, anaplastic tumors may secrete little or no enzyme with resultant normal SAP. When the carcinoma is still confined to the prostate (stage A or B), the SAP is usually normal, so that this test *does not detect potentially curable prostatic cancer*. With locally invasive lesions (stage C), the SAP is elevated in 40 to 50% of cases, and when there are metastases (stage D), it is elevated in 70 to 80%. With osteoblastic bone metastases, the involved bone

TABLE III
Acid Phosphatase in Prostatic Tissue in Relation to Age

Age	Acid Phosphatase
yrs	*units/g fresh tissue*
4	1.5
13	73
Adult	525–2,300

produces increased amounts of both acid and alkaline phosphatase with resultant increased serum levels. With acid phosphatase, it is the *extent* of the metastases rather than the site that determines the amount of enzyme in the blood. With alkaline phosphatase, it is the *extent and rapidity of development* of the osteoblastic metastases that determines the blood level (Table IV).

Transitory slight elevations of the SAP may occur with the following.

1. Palpation or surgical manipulation of the prostate.
2. Prostatic infarct.

Slight-to-moderate elevations of SAP are occasionally seen in the following.

1. Paget's disease.
2. Multiple myeloma.
3. Metastatic bone disease.
4. Primary hyperparathyroidism.
5. Gaucher's disease.
6. Benign and malignant bone tumors.

Clinical Usefulness of Acid Phosphatase Determinations

1. *High* levels are virtually diagnostic of metastatic carcinoma of the prostate.
2. If elevated initially, it is a useful indicator of the patient's clinical response to endocrine therapy.

A. If the tumor is androgen-dependent and responds to endocrine manipulation, the SAP rapidly returns to normal levels, and when the tumor eventually relapses, it again becomes elevated.

3. This determination can also be performed on *bone marrow aspirate*, and Lattimer and his group believe this may be the most sensitive indicator of bone metastasis—better than serum acid phosphatase, bone x-rays, or bone scans.

X-Ray Studies

The intravenous urogram may show evidence of ureteral obstruction as the prostatic cancer encroaches on the base of the bladder. Bone metastases, both osteoblastic and osteolytic, should be searched for in the

TABLE IV
Phosphatase Levels from Gutman

	Acid Phosphatase	Alkaline Phosphatase
	units/g	*units/g*
Normal adult prostate	525–2,300	0.4–1.5
Carcinomatous prostate	0–100	
Normal bone	0.9	3.3
Osteoblastic bone metastases	19	39.4

lumbosacral spine and pelvis, their most frequent sites. Addition of a bone scan will increase the detection rate of bone metastases.

Special Studies

Cystoendoscopy

The prostatic urethra may be rigid, and multiple nodules of varying size may project into the prostatic urethra. With invasion of the bladder neck area, a mosaic, cobblestone appearance may be evident as the tumor extends submucosally.

Diagnosis

Palpation of the prostate gland is the key to making the diagnosis! Any firm areas should be considered carcinoma until proved otherwise. Tissue biopsy of the prostate is the *only certain way* to establish the diagnosis. This may be accomplished by open perineal biopsy or by needle biopsy via perineum or rectum. Elevated SAP levels or presence of osteoblastic bone metastases to the pelvis suggest the diagnosis of metastatic carcinoma of the prostate, but *do not embark on a program of treatment without tissue confirmation of carcinoma.*

The majority of patients with both BPH and prostatic carcinoma consult their physicians because of voiding problems, and although their symptoms may be the same, their clinical histories are often quite different. Patients with BPH usually give a history of voiding difficulties over a number of years with frequent variation in the severity of symptoms from time to time. In contrast, the patient with prostatic cancer often has a relatively short history of voiding difficulties, frequently 6 months or less, and once initiated, the symptoms usually progress inexorably. By the time obstructive symptoms appear, the carcinoma is usually extensive, involving a major portion of the prostate and the firm, unyielding nature of the tumor, and continued growth account for the short, progressive history.

Treatment

There are three modes of treatment which have some impact on prostatic cancer—surgery, endocrine therapy, and irradiation—and the choice and timing of these treatments is still hotly debated.

The natural history of the tumor and of the host must be considered in each case (Tables V and VI).

The natural history of stage A and B tumors is not definitely known, but it is estimated that it takes about 20 years for a stage A lesion to become stage B.

Surgery

Surgical excision is the *only known cure* for prostatic cancer! This is feasible only when the tumor is confined to the prostate gland, stage A and B, and unfortunately less than 20% of cases fall into this group.

TABLE V
Life Expectancy of Males

Age Group	Life Expectancy
yrs	*yrs*
50–55	23
55–60	19
60–65	16
65–70	13
70–75	10
75–80	8
Over 80	5

TABLE VI
Natural History of Untreated Carcinoma of Prostate Stages C and D

Stage	Diagnosis to Death, No Treatment
	yrs
C (local invasion)	2–3
D (metastases)	1–2

In stage A tumors, the tiny tumor foci may have been completely removed at the time of "prostatectomy" so that no further treatment may be necessary. If the area involved is more extensive, it should be classified as stage B.

In stage B tumors, the prostatic nodule should be biopsied, and if it is cancer, a *total prostatectomy* is performed with removal of the seminal vesicles.

In stage C and D tumors, bladder outlet obstruction may necessitate a transurethral resection of the prostate.

Endocrine Therapy

Rationale

Prior to puberty, the prostatic cell is small and does not secrete, but when sufficient testosterone becomes available, the cell enlarges and secretes. Withdrawal of testosterone causes the cell to shrink but not die. Prostatic cancer cells often retain their androgen dependence, but unlike normal cells, they *die* when deprived of androgen.

Seventy percent of all prostatic cancers are androgen-dependent and will respond for an *unpredictable* period of time to androgen deprivation. It is not known why the remaining 30% are not androgen-dependent, but many of these tumors are poorly differentiated. The tumor may remain androgen-dependent for several months to many years, but *most tumors escape from androgen control after 2 to 3 years*. When this occurs, further endocrine manipulations are usually futile and most patients die in 1 to 2 years.

Endocrine therapy is usually reserved for stage C and D lesions, which make up 90% of all diagnosed prostatic cancers. Androgen deprivation is most commonly achieved by bilateral orchiectomy or estrogen therapy. Estrogens are believed to work primarily by inhibiting pituitary production of gonadotrophins with resultant testicular atrophy and loss of androgen production (chemical castration). There is a difference of opinion regarding the timing of endocrine therapy. Whitmore[34] noted no difference in survival time of patients with stage C (local invasion) prostatic cancer between those treated *initially* versus those treated when metastases developed.

$$\text{Stage C} \quad \xrightarrow[\text{treatment}]{\text{Endocrine}} \quad \text{Death—average 48 months}$$

$$\text{Stage C} \longrightarrow \text{Metastases} \quad \xrightarrow[\text{treatment}]{\text{Endocrine}} \text{Death—average 48 months}$$

Today, many urologists delay hormonal therapy until bone pain or urinary obstruction develops. Their reasons for this approach are the following.
1. Side effects of orchiectomy or estrogen therapy are postponed.
   A. Orchiectomy—psychological trauma, hot flashes.
   B. Estrogens—swelling of breasts, nausea, fluid retention.
   C. *Sexual potency is retained.*
2. Cardiovascular complications secondary to estrogens are avoided.
   A. Recent study indicated that patients receiving 5 mg of stilbestrol daily for prolonged periods had increased incidence of cardiovascular complications.
3. There is no clear-cut evidence that early hormone treatment produces a longer survival time.

The response to orchiectomy is almost instantaneous, whereas the response to estrogen therapy takes 1 to 2 weeks. It is not unusual for severe bone pain secondary to osteoblastic bone metastases to disappear *within 24 hours after orchiectomy.* If the acid phosphatase is elevated, it will return to normal levels in 2 to 3 days.

Androgen control is palliative and does not cure prostate cancer, but in the 70% of patients with androgen-dependent tumors, it probably extends their life 1 to 2 years.

Irradiation

Irradiation of the prostate has been employed on a limited scale to date, but it seems to offer promise chiefly for stage C lesions. High energy source external irradiation is the usual method of treatment, but Flocks[7] has effectively employed interstitial irradiation with radioactive gold, and

Whitmore[35] has similarly employed radioactive iodine. Proctitis often accompanies treatment but is usually transient and not debilitating.

Irradiation is useful in two other clinical situations.

1. Spot irradiation to pain-producing bone metastases relieves pain about 50% of the time.

2. Irradiation of both male breasts *prior* to estrogen therapy prevents gynecomastia.

Advantages of Irradiation

1. Two out of three patients treated with irradiation retain their sexual potency.

2. The side effects of endocrine therapy are avoided.

3. If the patient does not respond to irradiation—or having responded, relapses—he may still be treated with endocrine therapy.

A summary of the above treatments is shown in Table VII.

INFECTIONS OF THE PROSTATE GLAND

Bacterial infections of the prostate gland are uncommon. Many urinary infections are called "prostatitis," but careful studies, as recommended by Stamey, show that many of these are urethral. To locate the source of lower urinary tract infection, he suggested the following procedure.

1. After careful cleansing of the glans penis, three 10-ml samples of urine are obtained and bacterial colony counts performed.

VB_1—initial 5 to 10 ml is voided into first culture tube.

VB_2—without stopping, the patient continues to void, and when about 150 ml have been voided, another 10 ml are caught in a second culture tube.

VB_3—patient stops voiding, his prostate gland is massaged, and the first 10 ml voided afterwards are caught in a third culture tube (valid test if this fluid is more cloudy than VB_1 and VB_2, indicating presence of prostate secretion).

2. Findings in primary urethral and primary prostate infection (Table VIII).

TABLE VII
Summary of Results of Treatment of Prostatic Cancer

	Treatment	Survival Time		
		5 years	10 years	15 years
		%	%	%
Expected survivorship, age 65		80	60	40
Stage B (prostatic nodule)	Surgery	75	50	35
Stage C (locally invasive)	Irradiation	50		
	Endocrine	50	20	
Stage D (metastases)	Endocrine	25	0	

TABLE VIII
Determination of Site of Infection Based on Bacterial Count

	Urethra	Prostate
Suprapubic aspiration of bladder	0	0
VB_1	++++	++
VB_2	+	+
VB_3	++	++++

A. In both urethral and prostatic infections, bladder urine is sterile.

B. The midstream urine, VB_2, shows the least number of bacteria.

C. In primary urethral infections, VB_1 has the most bacteria, whereas in primary prostatic infections, VB_3 has the most.

Clinical

Acute Prostatitis

Often very explosive in onset, this infection is usually accompanied by severe dysuria, frequency, urgency, and general malaise. Patients may complain of perineal discomfort and difficult voiding.

The prostate is usually swollen and exquisitely tender and should be palpated very gently, *never massaged*. Treatment includes appropriate antimicrobials and hot sitz baths. Catheterization should be avoided, if possible.

Rarely, prostatitis may progress to an abscess and this may be suspected if the patient has severe perineal pain, chills, and fever. Fluctuation, if present, is diagnostic. Drainage is most effectively accomplished by open perineal incision. Additional treatment includes hot sitz baths and high doses of appropriate antibiotics. Urinary diversion via suprapubic cystostomy is often advisable.

Chronic Prostatitis

This label is often applied to a group of men with soft, mushy prostates who give a history of intermittent perineal and low back ache sometimes accompanied by urinary symptoms. Symptoms are probably due to stasis of secretions in the prostate and seminal vesicles, for urine cultures usually disclose no bacterial infection. The most effective treatment is hot sitz baths. Prostatic massage may be helpful in selected cases.

True chronic *bacterial* prostatitis infrequently occurs and is best managed by long-term antimicrobial therapy, such as nitrofurantoin, 50 mg b.i.d.

REFERENCES AND SUGGESTED FURTHER READING

Benign Prostatic Hyperplasia

1. Blandy, J. P. Benign prostatic enlargement. Br. Med. J. 1:31, 1971.
2. Dowd, J. B. and Emmett, E. E. Silent prostatism (unrecognized bladder neck obstruction). J.A.M.A. 178:296, 1961.

3. Randall, A. *Surgical Pathology of Prostatic Obstructions*. Williams & Wilkins, Baltimore, 1931.
4. Scott, F. B., Cardies, D., Quesada, E. M., and Rites, T. Uroflometry before and after prostatectomy. South. Med. J. 60:948, 1967.
5. Semple, J. E. Surgical capsule of the benign enlargement of the prostate—its development and action. Br. Med. J. 1:1640, 1963.

Carcinoma—General

1. Arnheim, F. K. Carcinoma of the prostate gland: study of postmortem findings in 176 cases. J. Urol. 60:599, 1948.
2. Batson, O. V. The function of the vertebral veins and their role in the spread of metastases. Am. Surg. 112:138, 1940.
3. Batson, O. V. The vertebral system of veins as a means for cancer dissemination. In *Progress in Clinical Cancer*, Vol. III, edited by I. M. Ariel. Grune & Stratton, New York, 1967.
4. Bumpus, H. C., Jr. Carcinoma of the prostate: clinical study of 1,000 cases. Surg. Gynecol. Obstet. 43:150, 1926.
5. Connolly, J. G., Thomson, A., Jewett, M. A. S., Hartman, N., and Webber, M. Intraprostatic lymphatics. Invest. Urol. 5:371, 1968.
6. Cowan, D. R. and DeLong, R. P. The role of the vertebral venous system in the metastasis of cancer to the spinal column. Cancer 4:610,1951.
7. Flocks, R. H. Clinical cancer of the prostate: a study of 4,000 cases. J.A.M.A. 193:559, 1965.
8. Greene, L. F. and Simon, H. B. Occult carcinoma of the prostate. J.A.M.A. 158:1494, 1955.
9. Gutman, A. B., The development of the acid phosphatase test for prostate carcinoma. Bull. N. Y. Acad. Med. 44:63, 1968.
10. Hudson, P. B., Finkle, A. L., Hopkins, J. A., Sproul, E. E., and Stout, A. D. Prostatic cancer. XI. Early prostatic cancer diagnosed by arbitrary open perineal biopsy among 300 unselected patients. Cancer 7:690, 1954.
11. Huggins, C. and Hodges, C. V. Studies on prostatic cancer: effect of correlation of estrogen and androgen injection on serum phosphatase in metastatic carcinoma of the prostate. Cancer Res. 1:293, 1941.
12. Jewett, H. J. Prostatic cancer (editorial). J. Urol. 108:829, 1972.
13. Jorgens, J. The radiographic characterization of carcinoma of the prostate. Surg. Clin. North Am. 45:1427, 1965.
14. Kahler, J. E. Carcinoma of the prostate gland—a pathologic study. J. Urol. 41:557, 1939.
15. McNeal, J. Origin and development of carcinoma in the prostate. Cancer 23:24, 1969.
16. Melicow, M. M. The prostatic nodule—a challenge and a problem. J. Am. Geriatr. Soc. 16:631, 1968.
17. Olsen, B. S. and Carlisle, R. W. Adenocarcinoma of the prostate simulating primary rectal malignancy. Cancer 25:219, 1970.
18. Rodin, A. E., Larson, D. L., and Roberts, D. K. Nature of the perineural space invaded by prostatic carcinoma. Cancer 20:1772, 1967.
19. Rosenberg, S. E. Is carcinoma of the prostate less serious in older men? J. Am. Geriatr. Soc. 13:791, 1965.
20. Scott, R., Jr. Needle biopsy in carcinoma of the prostate. J.A.M.A. 201:958, 1967.
21. Scott, R., Jr., Mutchnik, D. L., Laskowski, T. Z., and Schmalhorst, W. R. Carcinoma of the prostate in elderly men: incidence, growth characteristics and clinical significance. J. Urol. 101:602, 1969.
22. Woodard, H. O. The clinical significance of serum acid phosphatase. Am. J. Med. 27:902, 1959.

Carcinoma—Treatment

23. Bagshaw, M. A. Cancer of the urogenital tract—prostatic cancer: definitive radiotherapy in carcinoma of the prostate. J.A.M.A. 210:326, 1969.
24. Barnes, R. W. and Minan, C. A. Carcinoma of the prostate—biopsy and conservative therapy. J. Urol. 108:897, 1972.
25. Brendler, H. Cancer of the urogenital tract—prostatic cancer: therapy with orchiectomy or estrogens or both. J.A.M.A. 210:1074, 1969.

26. Dykhuizen, R. F., Sargent, C. R., George, F. W., III, and Kurahara, S. S. Use of cobalt-60 teletherapy in treatment of prostatic carcinoma. J. Urol. 100:333, 1968.
27. Emmett, J. L., Greene, L. F., and Papantoniou, A. Endocrine therapy in carcinoma of the prostate gland—10-year survival studies. J. Urol. 83:471, 1960.
28. Jewett, H. J., Bridge, R. W., Gray, G. F., Jr., and Shelley, W. M. The palpable nodule of prostatic cancer—results 15 years after radical excision. J.A.M.A. 203:403, 1968.
29. McCollough, D. L. and Leadbetter, W. F. Radical pelvis surgery for locally extensive carcinoma of the prostate. J. Urol. 108:939, 1972.
30. Ray, G. R., Cassady, J. R., and Bagshaw, M. A. Definitive radiation therapy of carcinoma of the prostate—a report on 15 years of experience. Radiology 106:407, 1973.
31. Scott, W. W. and Boyd, H. L. Combined hormone control therapy and radical prostatectomy in the treatment of selective cases of advanced carcinoma of the prostate—a retrospective study based upon 25 years of experience. J. Urol. 101:86, 1969.
32. Veterans Administration Cooperative Urological Research Group. Factors in the prognosis of carcinoma of the prostate. J. Urol. 100:59, 1968.
33. Veterans Administration Cooperative Urological Research Group. Treatment and survival of patients with cancer of the prostate. Surg. Gynecol. Obstet. 124:1011, 1967.
34. Whitmore, W. F., Jr. Rationale and results of ablative surgery for prostatic cancer. Cancer 16:1119, 1963.
35. Whitmore, W. F., Jr., Hilaris, B., and Grabstald, H. Retropubic implantation of iodine[125] in the treatment of prostatic cancer. J. Urol. 108:918, 1972.

17

Disorders of the Penis and Urethra

ARTHUR W. WYKER, JR.

ANATOMY OF THE PENIS AND MALE URETHRA

1. The penis is made up of three cylinders of spongy, erectile tissue—the paired dorsal corpora cavernosa and the single ventral corpus spongiosum.

A. Most of the erectile tissue is contributed by the solid corpora cavernosa.

B. The smaller corpus spongiosum acts primarily as a wall for the urethra. It is expanded proximally to form the bulb and distally to form the glans penis.

1) The hollowed out glans fits like a cap over the distal end of the corpora cavernosa. They are firmly fused together, and the vessels and nerves from the corpora cavernosa continue into the glans.

2. The deep fascia of the penis is a tough membrane which encases all three corpora.

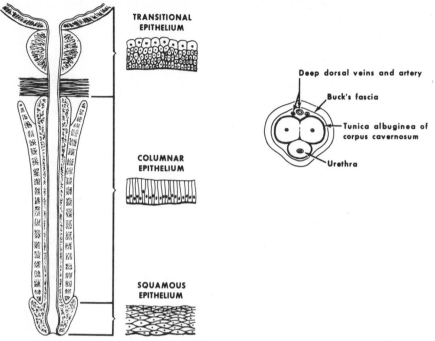

TRANSITIONAL
EPITHELIUM

Deep dorsal veins and artery

Buck's fascia

Tunica albuginea of
corpus cavernosum

COLUMNAR
EPITHELIUM

Urethra

SQUAMOUS
EPITHELIUM

Fig. 1. Transverse and cross-section of the male urethra and penis.

A. A transverse septum divides the penis into a dorsal compartment containing the two corpora cavernosa and a ventral compartment containing the
corpus spongiosum.

1) This cleavage plane allows easy separation of the two compartments.
3. The urethral mucosa is not uniform in type.

A. At the bladder end of the urethra, transitional cell epithelium continues
down to the urogenital diaphragm lining both the prostatic and membranous
portions.

B. At the outer end of the urethra, stratified squamous epithelium extends back into the urethra a short distance, lining the urethra within the
glans penis.

C. The major remaining portion of the urethra is lined by *pseudostratified
columnar epithelium.*

ERECTION

An erection occurs when the corpora of the penis become distended with
blood.

1. Initiation. The increased blood flow is due to dilation of the penile
arteries induced by stimulation of the parasympathetic pelvic nerves
(vasodilators) or by inhibition of the thoracolumbar sympathetics (vasocon-
strictors). There are two types of erection—reflex and psychogenic.

2. Reflex erection.

A. The parasympathetic erection reflex may be activated by tactile stimulation of the external genitalia or by a distended bladder.

3. Psychogenic erection.

A. The brain is bombarded by various sex-arousing stimuli—sights, sounds, smells, thoughts, and images.

B. These impulses from the brain are probably mediated via the thoracolumbar sympathetics, since this form of erection occurs even when the erection reflex arc has been destroyed.

Conte in 1952 found that the amount of blood entering and leaving the penis was determined by *autonomically controlled* muscular pillars in the walls of the blood vessels.

In the normal flaccid state, these muscular gates constrict the arterioles but leave the venules and A-V shunts open. The results of the restriction of inflow are small amount of blood in the corpora, low penile blood pressure, and low flow rate.

In the erect state, the opposite occurs with constriction of the venules and A-V shunts and open arterioles. The results of this restriction of outflow are distension of all three corpora with blood, penile blood pressure approximating that in the aorta, and high flow rate.

4. Experimental. Newman induced erections in normal human volunteers by perfusion of the corpora cavernosa. To obtain a typical erection, it was necessary to perfuse at the rate of 20 to 50 ml/min, but once erection was achieved, it could be maintained at a lower rate, 12 ml/min.

5. Maintenance of erection. Erection is sustained by compression occlusion of the deep veins between the distended, high pressure cavernous spaces and the surrounding, unyielding tunica albuginea and Buck's fascia.

6. Subsidence of erection. When the stimulus which evoked the erection is no longer present, vasoconstriction of the penile arteries occurs, reducing blood flow to the penis with resultant lowering of penile blood pressure, release of compressed veins, and resumption of the normal flaccid state.

PRIAPISM

Priapism may be defined as a prolonged, painful erection *not associated with sexual desire*. It is a serious disorder which often leaves the patient impotent and sometimes kills him. There are a number of significant differences between erection and priapism (Table I).

1. Physiopathology. The usual mechanism responsible for prolonged distension of the corpora cavernosa is obstruction to the venous outflow from the penis. Fitzpatrick recently studied the venous drainage in priapism by performing spongiosograms and cavernosograms. A summary of his findings follows.

A. Corpus spongiosum and glans penis are not involved in idiopathic priapism because they drain to the superficial dorsal veins of the penis outside Buck's fascia.

1) These veins remain patent during idiopathic priapism.

TABLE I
Differences between Erection and Priapism

	Erection	Priapism
Portion of penis involved	Corpora cavernosa + corpus spongiosum and glans (3)	Corpora cavernosa (2)
Cause	Vasodilation of penile arteries	Obstruction of venous outflow
Sexual desire	Present	Absent
Pain	Absent	Present
Duration	Minutes–hours	Hours–days

B. Cavernosograms in priapism outlined the distended corpora cavernosa, but there was no runoff to the deep dorsal veins below Buck's fascia.

C. Cavernosum-spongiosum shunt was successful in relieving priapism because the stagnated blood in the corpora cavernosa was drained off through the corpus spongiosum and the superficial dorsal veins of the penis. If venous obstruction is unrelieved, the following sequence of events takes place.

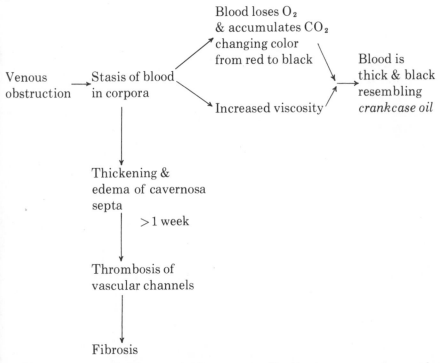

2. If no treatment is given, priapism eventually disappears spontaneously, but the extensive fibrosis of the corpora cavernosa prevents future erections, and the patient is permanently impotent.

3. To reduce the priapism yet retain potency, treatment must be successfully accomplished before the vascular channels become thrombosed.

4. Etiology

   A. Idiopathic.

   1) The majority of patients have no known cause for their priapism although in some it follows prolonged, vigorous intercourse.

   B. Hematological.

   1) Sickle cell disease.

   2) Leukemia.

   C. Malignant tumors.

   1) Primary lymphoma of the penis.

   2) Metastases to corpora cavernosa.

   D. Neurogenic lesions involving the spinal cord.

   1) Multiple sclerosis.

   2) Trauma to spinal cord.

   3) Neurogenic lesions produce an atypical form of priapism.

      a. All three corpora may be involved.

      b. Erection is not as marked as in the idiopathic form, and the patient usually experiences no pain.

5. Diagnosis. This may usually be made on the basis of the history and a brief physical examination. The penis is erect and somewhat tender to palpation and manipulation. The dorsal corpora cavernosa are turgid and tense, in marked contrast to the soft and yielding ventral corpus spongiosum and glans penis. Appropriate studies should be performed to rule out the known causes of priapism.

6. Treatment.

   A. Time is important, for the sooner treatment is instituted, the greater the chance of resolving the priapism and retaining potency.

   B. Medical measures generally have been unsuccessful.

   C. Needle aspiration combined with irrigation and massage of the corpora is occasionally successful in early cases.

   1) To evacuate completely the thick, black oily blood from the corpora, massage them until you see bright red blood.   ·

   D. Most patients are best managed by a prompt bypass surgical procedure.

   1) Cavernosum-spongiosum shunt.

      a. This procedure is feasible because the corpus spongiosum is *uninvolved* in priapism.

      b. When these two bodies are joined, venous runoff takes place via the corpus spongiosum and the superficial dorsal veins.

   2) Cavernosum-saphenous shunt.

      a. This procedure is feasible because the nearby saphenous vein can be detached distally and connected to the corpus cavernosum.

      b. Venous runoff takes place via the saphenous vein, femoral vein, and the vena cava.

   E. Whatever treatment is employed, it is helpful to minimize stimuli to the external genitalia.

1) Voiding difficulty is common and this should be managed with a cysto-cath, not a urethral catheter.

2) Give the patient adequate doses of analgesics and sedatives to keep him pain-free and calm.

F. Anticoagulants should be used in selected patients with priapism.

PHIMOSIS

Phimosis exists when an abnormally small opening in the prepuce prevents its retraction over the glans penis. If the urethral meatus and preputial opening are not accurately superimposed during voiding, a difficult task at best, some urine will splash into the preputial pouch causing inflammation of the glans penis and prepuce. If the preputial opening is smaller than the urethral meatal orifice, it obstructs the urinary stream and causes back-pressure changes on the entire urinary tract. The treatment for phimosis is circumcision.

PARAPHIMOSIS

Paraphimosis exists when the prepuce, once retracted, cannot be returned to its normal position. The tight opening in the prepuce constricts the venous return of the glans penis causing edema.

Manual reduction should be performed as soon as possible. The penis is grasped so that both thumbs compress and push the glans, while at the same time the fingers gently but steadily pull the prepuce over the corona and glans penis. If this cannot be accomplished, the constricting fibrous band may be divided under local anesthesia and a circumcision performed later when all inflammation has subsided (Fig. 2).

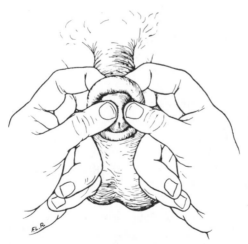

A method for the manual reduction of a para-phimosis

Fig. 2. (Reproduced with permission from *Textbook of Urology*, Victor F. Marshall, 2nd Ed., Hoeber Medical Division, Harper & Row Publishers, New York, 1969).

PEYRONIE'S DISEASE

Peyronie's disease, or fibrous induration of the penis, is an uncommon disorder seen most often in men over 35. The etiology is unknown! One or more fibrous plaques develop in the corpora cavernosa, but for unknown reasons the corpus spongiosum is not involved, so there is no interference with urination. These plaques do, however, restrict the expansion of the involved corpus during erection causing the penis to bend toward the plaque. This bending is usually accompanied by some local discomfort, and sexual intercourse may be inhibited. The plaques histologically resemble ordinary scar tissue and may involve the tunica albuginea and the underlying corpus cavernosum. Occasionally they become calcified or ossified.

1. Clinical. There are two symptoms which induce the patient to seek medical advice.

A. A hard lump or lumps on the penis.

1) He often fears that the lump is a carcinoma.

B. Erection deformity. The plaques are located on the dorsal and lateral surface of the corpora cavernosa, more commonly near the base of the penis. The plaques are slightly elevated and smooth, usually with well demarcated margins. Since they develop deep to Buck's fascia, they have no attachment to the overlying skin.

Metastases to the corpora cavernosa may sometimes mimic Peyronie's disease, but they usually are *very rare* and usually are late manifestations of previously diagnosed, far advanced genitourinary or rectal carcinoma.

2. Treatment. There is no specific form of therapy which is uniformly successful in the treatment of Peyronie's disease. Fortunately in the majority of the patients, the plaques remain stationary or spontaneously improve so that treatment is unnecessary. Once reassured that the hard lump in the penis is benign, patients usually adjust to their relatively mild symptoms. When the disease progresses to the point where the painful curvature of the penis prevents sexual intercourse, one of the following treatments may be tried.

A. Oral administration of potassium aminobenzoate (Potaba), 12 g/day.

1) This drug has an antifibrosis effect, and the plaques may soften after 1 to 3 months of treatment.

B. Local injection of steroids into and around the plaque.

1) This often reduces penile discomfort, but it is less successful in reversing the curvature of the penis.

C. Surgical excision of the plaque.

1) Devine and Horton reported good results using dermal grafts to replace the excised plaque.

CARCINOMA

1. Etiology and incidence. Penile carcinoma is uncommon in the U.S., accounting for less than 1% of all deaths from cancer in men. It occurs most

commonly in middle-aged men with 70% of patients being over 50. Two factors play a role in the etiology of this tumor—circumcision and local hygiene.

   A. Most cases occur in *uncircumcised* males.

   B. The timing of circumcision is significant.

     1) When performed as a newborn, the chances that he will develop carcinoma of the penis are almost zero.

     2) When performed at age 5 to 10, there is very low incidence.

     3) When performed at age over 10, there is low incidence.

   C. Poor hygiene was noted in most cases.

2. Pathology. Penile carcinoma usually begins on the prepuce or glans penis, so it is a squamous cell carcinoma. It looks and behaves like skin cancers elsewhere, but the presence of the preputial pouch encourages secondary infection which may mask the presence of the underlying tumor. It is a slow growing tumor staying localized for long periods of time, but eventually this tumor spreads by direct extension down the shaft of the penis and by metastases to the inguinal and pelvic lymph nodes. It infrequently penetrates the tough fascial envelope around the corpora, so hemic dissemination is uncommon.

There are five penile lesions which are considered precancerous, and except for one, they show varying degrees of hyperplasia of the squamous cell layers, but in all, *the basement membrane remains intact.*

PRECANCEROUS LESIONS

1. Leukoplakia—white or grayish white plaques.

2. Erythroplasia of Queyrat—shiny red, papular lesion confined to the glans penis.

3. Carcinoma-in-situ (Bowen's disease)—reddish papule, sometimes ulcerated.

4. Condyloma acuminata (venereal warts)—warty growths which may appear anywhere on the genitalia.

   A. These lesions are caused by a virus.

   B. The larger ones may resemble carcinoma.

5. Balanitis xerotica obliterans—perimeatal whitening of the skin which may obstruct the urethral meatus.

   A. Unlike the previous four lesions, the epithelium is thin and atrophic.

3. Clinical findings.

   A. Symptoms. The most common complaint is a *penile sore which fails to heal.* This is seen chiefly in patients with a retractable prepuce. When the prepuce is nonretractable, the patient may note a lump, foul discharge or bleeding, itching, edema, or pain. One would anticipate that the majority of penile carcinomas would be detected early, since the penis is at least casually inspected and handled 4 to 5 times each day. This is not the case, however, for the lesion usually has been present for at least 6 months before the patient sees his physician. What are the reasons for this surprising delay?

1) Lesions are usually painless.
2) Lesions are often invisible.
   a. The presence of the prepuce may hide the lesion.
3) Misinterpretation of findings.
   a. The patient may attribute the changes in his penis to local infection or venereal disease.
4) Fear of losing his penis.

4. Physical and laboratory findings. Most patients present with a hard lump, dirty ulcer, or a fungating mass near the end of their penis. Approximately 60% have enlarged, often tender inguinal lymph nodes, only half of which turn out to be metastases.

In the usual case, laboratory findings are normal. If the tumor results in an infection in the preputial pouch, the urinalysis will show evidence of infection and the urine culture will be positive.

5. Diagnosis. This is established by *biopsy* under local anesthesia, excising a small piece of viable tissue from the growing edge of the lesion. This is important for chancroid or large condyloma acuminata may occasionally mimic carcinoma.

6. Treatment.

A. A partial or total penectomy is done in most cases removing at least a 2-cm margin proximal to the tumor.

B. Small superficial lesions may sometimes be managed by circumcision or irradiation.

C. Bilateral inguinal lymphadenectomy is performed when there are metastases in the groin.

1) Experts differ as to the advisability of node dissection when these nodes are not enlarged—some do it, some don't.

URETHRA

Urethral Stricture

A urethral stricture is a pathological narrowing of the urethral lumen due to fibrous tissue replacement of the corpus spongiosum and urethra. It is caused by infection or trauma.

1. Infection-induced strictures.

A. The gonococcus is the usual culprit, and, because it attacks only columnar epithelium, strictures develop only in the anterior urethra.

1) Urethritis must be severe and persist for many days to cause stricture formation, so that most patients with gonococcal urethritis *do not* form strictures.

B. They are often multiple.

2. Traumatic strictures.

A. Unlike infection-induced strictures, those resulting from trauma are characteristically single.

B. The location of the stricture varies with the injury.

1) Fractured pelvis—membranous urethra.

2) Straddle injury—bulbous urethra.

3) Instrumentation with sounds, catheters, or resectoscope—any portion of the urethra.

3. Pathophysiology. When a urethral stricture obstructs urine flow, it causes back-pressure effects on the proximal urethra, bladder, ureters, and kidneys. The bladder muscle contracts more vigorously to force urine by the narrow area, and for a variable period of time, this compensatory hypertrophy enables the bladder to empty itself. The forceful bladder contraction raises the pressure inside the bladder and may force the mucosa between the thickened, spread apart muscle fibers producing cellules and diverticula. These anatomical changes in the bladder wall often cause dysfunction of the ureterovesical junction with resultant obstruction or, less commonly, reflux. Eventually the overworked bladder muscle becomes fatigued and is unable to empty the bladder. This residual urine makes the urinary tract more vulnerable to infection. The resting pressure inside the bladder is now higher than normal, disturbing the ureter-bladder pressure gradient and making it more difficult for urine to reach the bladder. Back-pressure produces hydroureter and hydronephrosis, with resultant loss of renal function.

4. Clinical findings.

A. Symptoms. The primary complaint is a *weak urinary stream*. Other symptoms which may be present—prolonged voiding time, dribbling at end of urination, two-stage voiding, and painful urination.

B. Physical examination.

1) Watch the patient void!

a. Since the urinary flow rate varies with the amount of urine in the bladder (the higher the volume, the greater the flow rate), be sure that the patient's bladder is comfortably full.

b. The presence of a weak urinary stream voided with obvious straining is strong evidence of infravesical obstruction.

2) Palpate the urethra.

a. Strictures may be detected as localized areas of induration or tenderness.

3) Look for complications of long standing urethral obstruction and infection—urethrocutaneous fistulas, diverticula, and periurethral abscesses.

C. Laboratory findings. Urinalysis may reveal bacteriuria and pyuria if infection is present.

D. Diagnosis. Strictures may be diagnosed by *urethrograms* or by *calibration of the urethra* with graduated bougies, sounds or catheters, or by *panendoscopy*.

1) Urethrograms. This easily performed, relatively painless x-ray study has some distinct advantages over instrumental evaluation.

a. It detects multiple strictures often not appreciated by passage of a catheter or sound.

b. It pinpoints the location of the stricture or strictures and also defines their length—important considerations if surgery is contemplated.

c. It may identify additional pathology in the urethra such as stone, diverticulum, false passage, or fistula.

d. It provides a permanent objective record of the findings.

e. It is atraumatic and carries virtually no morbidity when performed on the noninfected individual.

2) Calibration of the urethra.

a. A significant stricture narrows the urethral lumen so that normal sized catheters or instruments pass up to but not through the stricture. The caliber of this stricture may be determined by finding what size catheter can be passed through the stricture.

3) Panendoscopy.

a. This instrument permits one to both visualize and calibrate the stricture.

b. It also allows one to assess the effects of urethral obstruction on the proximal urethra and bladder.

E. Treatment.

1) Urethral dilation. When a stricture is first identified, the urethra should be progressively dilated up to normal size using graduated instruments—filiforms and followers, sounds, or soft catheters.

a. Unfortunately, the effects of this dilation are *not permanent*, and in time the stricture contracts down again, and the patient notes a gradual weakening of his urinary stream.

b. Patients who void freely between dilations done every 4 to 6 months may continue to be managed in this fashion.

2) Surgery. Surgery should be considered when one of the following situations exist.

a. The stricture cannot be adequately dilated.

b. Voiding difficulties remain even after maximal urethral dilation.

c. The beneficial effects of urethral dilation last only 1 to 2 months necessitating too frequent treatments.

d. Significant complications develop—fistulas, sepsis, stone, or tumor.

The following surgical procedures have been employed.

a. Internal urethrotomy—the stricture is incised from inside the urethra using special instruments, and a large size catheter is left as a splint for 6 weeks.

b. Excision—small, localized accessible strictures may be totally excised and an end-to-end anastomosis accomplished after mobilization of the proximal and distal urethral segments.

c. External urethrotomy—the stricture is incised longitudinally, opening into normal urethra at both ends, and the resultant urethral defect may be closed primarily with a free skin graft or by two-stage techniques using scrotal skin.

Tumors of the Male Urethra

There are three significant tumors of the male urethra—the benign tumors, condyloma acuminata and papilloma, and carcinoma.

1. Condyloma acuminata (venereal warts). These are ordinary warts which tend to grow more exuberantly on the genitalia because of local moisture and warmth.

A. They are caused by a virus which may be transmitted by sexual intercourse.

B. They may appear anywhere on the genitalia, but the only portion of the urethra involved is the meatus.

C. Presenting complaints.

    1) Irritation or itching sensation at the urethral meatus.

    2) Spraying of the urinary stream.

    3) Initial hematuria or just a bloody discharge.

    4) The patient may have noted the lesion by examining his meatus.

D. Treatment. They may be eradicated with local application of Podophyllin, by electrodissection, or by surgical excision.

2. Papilloma.

A. These tumors resemble bladder papillomas and may occur anywhere along the urethra.

    1) Lesions at the urethral meatus are hard to differentiate from condyloma acuminata, but papillomas tend to be softer and more friable.

B. The primary complaint usually is urethral bleeding.

    1) Lesions at the meatus may cause local irritation and spraying of the urinary stream.

C. Diagnosis is made by visualization of the tumor with the panendoscope.

D. These tumors usually can be safely and completely excised transurethrally.

3. Carcinoma.

A. It is fortunate that these tumors are rare, for they have a bad prognosis.

B. They develop most commonly in middle-aged men with long standing urethral strictures.

    1) Chronic or recurrent irritation of the columnar epithelium lining the major portion of the urethra causes squamous metaplasia which occasionally progresses to squamous cell (epidermoid) carcinoma.

    2) These stricture-associated carcinomas usually are diagnosed late, since symptoms due to the tumor are initially attributed to the stricture.

C. Prostatic urethral carcinomas usually are transitional cell.

1) They behave like bladder tumors and should be managed in similar fashion.

a. Superficial, low grade tumors are treated by transurethral resection, whereas the deeply infiltrative ones may require radical surgery or irradiation.

2) They may invade the prostate and be detected as a hard lump on rectal examination.

a. Unlike adenocarcinoma of the prostate, these tumors are unaffected by endocrine therapy.

D. Signs and symptoms.

1) The earliest sign may be a change in the behavior of the urethral stricture.

a. It may become difficult or impossible to dilate.

2) Complications of urethral obstruction and infection may appear.

a. Urethral cutaneous fistulas.

b. Periurethral abscess.

3) A mass or lump along the urethra may be noted by the patient or his physician.

4) Urethral obstruction or bleeding may occur.

E. Diagnosis.

1) All suspicious areas in the urethra or perineum must be biopsied, sometimes repeatedly, to establish the diagnosis.

F. Treatment.

1) Radical surgery offers the only hope of cure, and it is infrequently successful.

Tumors of the Female Urethra

There are two significant tumors of the female urethra—the benign caruncle and carcinoma.

1. Caruncle.

A. These soft, red tumors occur at the urethral meatus, most commonly on the posterior lip.

B. They usually are quite vascular, often bleeding after slight trauma.

C. Usual symptoms.

1) The patient may note blood in the urine or on the toilet paper after voiding.

2) Sometimes the bright red tumor is seen by the patient.

3) Local irritation and itching may be present.

D. Treatment.

1) Small tumors may be treated with silver nitrate stick. The larger ones should be totally excised.

2) If there is any suspicion of malignancy, the tumor should be totally excised and sent for pathological examination.

2. Carcinoma.

A. Urethral carcinoma occurs more commonly in women than in men, with a ratio of 5:1.

1) This is surprising considering the disparity in length of the male and female urethra and the fact that most urinary tract tumors occur more commonly in men.

B. The most common histological type is epidermoid carcinoma.

C. Middle-aged women are the usual victims, 90% of patients being over 50 years of age.

D. Signs and symptoms.

1) Virtually all patients have blood in their urine or have a bloody vaginal discharge.

2) Other common urinary symptoms—painful urination, urinary frequency, and urgency.

3) Other gynecological symptoms—vaginal discharge, itching, and dyspareunia.

4) Some patients are aware of a mass at the vaginal introitus.

E. Physical findings.

1) The most common site is the urethral meatus, and the tumor may present as an ulcer, nodule, or mass.

2) Sometimes it spreads along the entire urethra, so that the urethra feels like a rigid pipe.

3) Inguinal and pelvic lymph node metastases occur in about one-third of patients.

F. Diagnosis.

1) Since urethral carcinoma may masquerade as a caruncle, polyp, or prolapse, all urethral lesions should be evaluated carefully and suspicious lesions should be biopsied.

G. Treatment.

1) Lesions of the distal urethra usually can be managed by a partial urethrectomy.

2) Lesions of the entire urethra are best treated with a combination of irradiation and radical surgery.

a. Despite this aggressive therapy, the prognosis is poor, and less than 10% of patients are cured.

Urethral Diverticulum

Although occasionally congenital in origin, most diverticula of the female urethra are secondary to lower urinary tract infections. There are numerous suburethral glands which drain into the floor of the urethra, and when their duct becomes obstructed by inflammatory edema, an abscess may form. When this abscess eventually ruptures into the urethra, it leaves a thick walled, poorly draining pouch—a diverticulum. These diverticula retain urine, so that infection is common and stone formation occurs in about 10%.

1. Signs and symptoms.

A. The large majority of patients are married women, 30 to 50 years of age, with a long standing history of urinary infections.

1) Their infections often recur at frequent intervals and are difficult to eradicate.

B. The most common sympton is *painful urination*.

C. Other symptoms.

1) Frequency and urgency of urination.

2) Dribbling after urination.

3) Dyspareunia.

4) Awareness of a mass in the vagina.

2. Physical findings. A mass usually is seen in the anterior vaginal wall which on palpation results in a gush of cloudy urine from the urethral meatus. The mass usually is tender and about 10% of these masses contain stones.

3. Diagnosis. All women with a history of frequent urinary infections should have a careful examination of the urethra to determine if a diverticulum is present.

A. If a characteristic, expressible tender mass is palpable in the anterior vaginal wall, the diagnosis is established.

B. Inspection of the urethra with the panendoscope is confirmatory and allows inspection of the ostium, usually in the midposterior urethral wall.

C. Radiographic demonstration of the diverticulum may be accomplished but not without some difficulty.

1) Intravenous urogram—it may be seen on the pre- or postvoiding film.

2) Urethrogram—special catheters often are necessary to distend adquately the urethra to outline the diverticulum.

4. Treatment. After a 2-week course of appropriate antibiotics, the urethral diverticulum should be excised and the urethra repaired.

Prolapse of the Urethra

Eversion of the mucosa at the urethral meatus, a mild form of prolapse, is common in older women and is of no clinical significance. Occasionally this process progresses to prolapse, at which time a 2- to 4-cm long portion of the urethra projects from the urethral meatus. The resultant mass usually partially obstructs the urethra causing voiding difficulty. Blood may be noted in the urine or on the toilet paper. The mass involves the entire circumference of the urethra, and it is commonly purplish because of venous obstruction. There is a well demarcated line between the normal pink urethra and the bulging, soft gangrenous portion.

1. Treatment. Most prolapses can be managed in the following simple fashion.

A. Insert a No. 24 Foley catheter through the prolapsed and normal urethra into the bladder and distend the balloon.

B. Place a heavy silk suture around the entire urethra and its catheter, and tie it down securely at the junction of the normal and gangrenous portions.

1) The gangrenous, prolapsed urethra usually sloughs in several days, and the patient subsequently voids normally with continence. The gangrenous portion of the urethra may also be excised surgically, and this should be done if there is any suspicion of tumor.

REFERENCES AND SUGGESTED FURTHER READING

Penis

1. Conti, G. L'érection du penis humain et ses bases morphologicovasculaires. Acta Anat. 14:217, 1952.
2. Daseler, E. H., Anson, B. J., and Relmann, A. F. Radical excision of the inguinal and iliac lymph glands—a study based upon 450 anatomical dissections and upon clinical observations. Surg. Gynecol. Obstet. 87:679, 1948.
3. deKernion, J. B., Tynberg, P., Persky, L., and Fegen, J. P. Carcinoma of the penis. Proc. of the National Conference on Urologic Cancer, p. 1256, Washington, D.C., March, 1973.
4. Devine, C. J., Jr., and Horton, C. E. Surgical treatment of Peyronie's disease with dermal graft. J. Urol. 111:44, 1974.
5. Ekstrom, T. and Edsmyr, R. Cancer of the penis: a clinical study of 229 cases. Acta. Chir. Scand. 115:25, 1958.
6. Fitzpatrick, T. J. Spongiosograms and cavernosograms: a study of their value in priapism. J. Urol. 109:843, 1973.
7. Garrett, R. A. and Rhamy, D. E. Priapism management with corpus-saphenous shunt. J. Urol. 95:65, 1966.
8. Grace, D. A. and Winter, C. C. Priapism: appraisal of the management of 23 patients. J. Urol. 99:301, 1968.
9. Grayhack, J. T., McCullough, W., O'Conor, V. J., Jr., and Trippel, O. Venous bypass to control priapism. Invest. Urol. 1:509, 1964.
10. Hardner, G. J., Bhanalaph, T., Murphy, G. P., Albert, D. J., and Moore, R. H. Carcinoma of the penis—analysis of therapy in 100 consecutive cases. J. Urol. 108:428, 1972.
11. Henderson, V. E. and Roepke, M. H. On mechanism of erection. Am. J. Physiol. 106:441, 1933.
12. Hinman, F., Jr. Priapism—reasons for failure of therapy. J. Urol. 83:420, 1960.
13. Jackson, S. M. The treatment of carcinoma of the penis. Br. J. Surg. 53:33, 1966.
14. Johnson, D. E., Fuerst, D. E., and Ayala, A. G. Carcinoma of the penis—experience with 153 cases. Urology 1:404, 1973.
15. Kossow, J. H., Hotchkiss, R. S., and Morales, P. A. Carcinoma of the penis treated surgically—analysis of 100 cases. Urology 2:169, 1973.
16. Smith, B. H. Peyronie's disease. Am. J. Clin. Pathol. 45:670, 1966.

Urethra

1. Beard, D. E. and Goodyear, W. E. Urethral stricture—a pathological study. J. Urol. 59:619, 1948.
2. Engel, R. M. E., Wise, A. A., and Whitaker, R. H. Otis internal urethrotomy with longterm urethral intubation—a comparison of latex and silastic catheters. South. Med. J. 65:55, 1972.
3. Grabstald, H. Tumors of the urethra in men and women. Cancer 32:1236, 1973.
4. Weaver, R. G. and Schulte, J. W. Clinical aspects of urethral regeneration. J. Urol. 93:247, 1965.
5. Yelderman, J. J. and Weaver, R. G. The behavior and treatment of urethral strictures. J. Urol. 97:1040, 1967.
6. Zeigerman, J. H. and Gordon, S. F. Cancer of the female urethra—a curable disease. Obstet. Gynecol. 36:785, 1970.

18

Disorders of the Scrotum and Testes

JAY Y. GILLENWATER

CYSTIC LESIONS OF THE SCROTUM

Cystic lesions of the scrotal wall and its contents are common.

1. Sebaceous cysts. These cysts of the scrotum resulting from overproduction of secretions or obstruction to the sebaceous glands are common. Occasionally they become infected. Treatment is not required for small cysts. Multiple or large cysts require surgical excision.

2. Hydrocele. A hydrocele is an accumulation of a straw-colored fluid between the two layers of the tunica vaginalis. Hydroceles are common and may be seen as frequently as 1% in older men.

A. Etiology. The etiology is either overproduction of fluid by some irritative process of the tunica or a defect in the absorption of the fluid through the lymphatics. Acute hydroceles are seen after trauma, inflammations, or tumors.

B. Diagnosis. Diagnosis of hydrocele in an adult is usually easy. The patients present with a history of a slowly developing cystic mass in the scrotum. Transillumination with a bright light shows transmission of the light. A hernia can usually be differentiated by palpation at the external inguinal ring showing no inguinal impulse or mass on coughing. A hematocele (bloody fluid) or *chylocele* (lymphatic fluid) usually does not transmit light. A *spermatocele* contains sperm and usually consists of distinct cystic masses separate from the testes and located behind the testes with an attachment in the region of the upper pole of the epididymis.

C. Hydroceles of childhood. Hydroceles of childhood are usually due to a small communicating hernia which allows peritoneal fluid to enter and accumulate within the tunica vaginalis. Most of these will be cured spontaneously by 1 year of age.

D. Treatment. Operative intervention is not indicated in small children unless there is an accompanying herniation of the intestines. In older children, operative treatment may be necessary. In the adult, small hydroceles require no treatment. For larger hydroceles, surgical excision of the tunica vaginalis is necessary. Aspiration is usually contraindicated because of the risk of introducing infection and can be expected to recur fairly rapidly.

3. Hematocele. A hematocele is a collection of blood in the tunica vaginalis

most often occurring after trauma or needling. Hematoceles do not transilluminate. Treatment is usually nonsurgical, consisting of scrotal elevation and bedrest.

4. Spermatocele. This is a cystic lesion which transmits light, is separate from the testis, and may give the impression of an additional testis. The etiology is partial obstruction of part of the sperm-carrying system. Spermatoceles are most often asymptomatic and require no treatment unless they become very large.

5. Varicocele. This is an abnormal dilation of the pampiniform venous plexus in the scrotum. Venous drainage of the testes is from the internal spermatic vein which drains into the renal vein on the left and vena cava on the right, from the external spermatic vein which drains into the epigastric vein, and the veins of the vas deferens which drain into the internal iliac veins. All three groups of veins anastomose in the scrotum.

A. Etiology. Varicoceles result from reverse flow of blood due to defective valves in the internal spermatic vein and most of the time are on the left side (99%).

B. Symptoms. Symptoms are usually a dull scrotal pain that disappears on lying down.

C. Diagnosis. Diagnosis is made by examining the patient in the upright position and feeling the distended veins ("bag of worms"). Varicoceles should disappear when the patient lies down. Secondary varicoceles are due to intra-abdominal venous obstruction and will not disappear on lying down. These patients need to be studied to determine the cause of the venous obstruction.

D. Relationship to infertility. Varicoceles have been of interest recently as a cause of infertility. Why varicoceles cause low sperm counts is not known. Postulated mechanisms have been that the varicoceles elevate scrotal temperature or bring high concentrations of adrenal steroids (since one of the left adrenal veins empties into the renal vein opposite the point where the internal spermatic vein drains) to the testis, inhibiting spermatogenesis.

E. Treatment. Treatment is indicated for infertility or for patients with marked pain. The surgical procedure consists of ligation of the internal spermatic veins near the internal inguinal ring through a herniorrhaphy type of incision (Fig. 1).

UNDESCENDED TESTIS

1. Embryology. The genital or gonadal ridge first appears in the 4-week embryo on each side between the mesonephros and the dorsal mesentary. Germ cells migrate to the testis from the dorsal mesentary of the hindgut during the 6th week. Under the stimulus of a Y chromosome, the medulla of the indifferent gonad develops into the testis from the 6th to the 8th week of development. The testis descends to the inguinal ring which is 10 segments

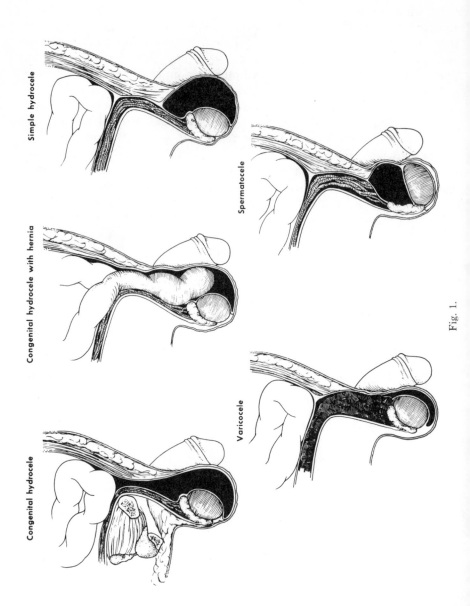

Simple hydrocele

Spermatocele

Congenital hydrocele with hernia

Varicocele

Congenital hydrocele

Fig. 1.

below its origin from the 3rd to the 5th month. The testis descends into the inguinal canal after the 7th month and into the scrotum by the 9th month.

2. Incidence. Failure of normal descent is reported to be about 5%, and if one excludes retractile testis, the incidence is 2.7%. The adult incidence of cryptorchidism is reported to be 2 to 8%.

3. Harmful effects. Failure of normal descent is believed to be harmful for several reasons.

A. Increased temperature of the body, as compared to the lower (by 2 to 3°) temperature of the scrotum causes the testis to remain infantile and become fibrotic. The testicular changes are thought to become irreversible at between 5 and 10 years of age.

B. There usually will be no spermatogenesis and perhaps lower testosterone production from the fibrotic changes.

C. The undescended testes has an increased chance of malignancy whether or not it is brought down.

D. An increased risk for trauma to the testis in the inguinal canal is reported.

E. An undescended testis may cause psychological problems.

4. Classification. Undescended testes may be separated into 5 categories for management purposes.

A. The retractile testis. This is the largest group and is caused by an active cremasteric reflex which draws the testis out of the scrotum when the child is frightened or examined by a physician with cold fingers. These testes are normal histologically and will most often spontaneously descend by puberty, so surgery is not necessary.

B. Anatomic abnormalities. This group involves anatomic abnormalities of the inguinal canal, gubernaculum, shortness of vascular supply, or the vas deferens. These cases require surgical correction to bring the testis into the scrotum.

C. Dysgenetic testis. The dysgenetic testis is histologically abnormal and usually requires surgical treatment.

D. Endocrine abnormalities. The primary endocrine abnormalities are most often lack of pituitary gonadotrophin hormones. These will usually respond to hormone therapy.

E. Ectopic testis. This is usually a normal testis histologically which lies out of the scrotum, in the region near the external inguinal ring, perineum, or penis. Surgery is required in most cases to bring these testes into the scrotum (Fig. 2).

5. Therapy.

A. Surgery. Operation before the age of 10 is believed to lead to acceptable fertility rates (60 to 80%). There is little information on surgery after the age of 10. Changes appear to become irreversible after 13 years of age.

Surgical correction for the mechanically obstructed or ectopic testis is

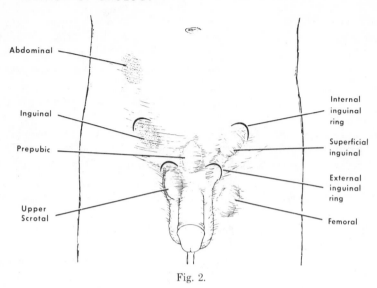

Fig. 2.

done by making an inguinal incision and locating the testis to bring it down into the scrotum without tension. Added length can be obtained by freeing up the internal spermatic artery and vas deferens retroperitoneally, transplanting the cord to the medial portion of the canal, or occasionally by cutting the internal spermatic artery and relying on the external spermatic artery and artery to the vas deferens to provide the necessary blood supply. The optimal age for this procedure is before age 13; many surgeons operate at about age 5 before the child begins school. If an associated inguinal hernia is present, the operation should be performed, regardless of age.

Cancer is reported to occur 30 to 50 times more frequently in the undescended testis whether or not it is operated upon. This probably does not apply to the retractile and ectopic testis. Thus, when operating on undescended testes, most surgeons prefer to place the testis in the scrotum where it can be palpated, or remove it.

B. Hormones. Chorionic gonadotropin can be administered in a short course (3,300 units every other day × 3) or a long course (500 units, 3 × each week to a total of 10,000 units). Results are reported to be 33% successful in bilateral undescended testes, 16% successful in unilateral (where presumably there was enough natural hormone to bring down the testis on the other side), with a total success rate of 23%. This method brought the best results in patients 2 to 5 years old. Hormonal therapy should be tried in undescended testes due to primary endocrine dysfunction; however, these may be indistinguishable from the testes that are dysgenetic or mechanically obstructed, and a course of gonadotropin therapy may be tried empirically. Too much hormone therapy can produce precocity and closing of the epiphyses.

TORSION OF THE SPERMATIC CORD

Torsion of the spermatic cord with resultant infarction of the testis occurs most frequently during the 1st year of life or around puberty. The main etiology factor is believed to be abnormal motility of the spermatic cord and testes.

1. Types. Two types of lesions are usually described, extravaginal and intravaginal.

A. Extravaginal torsion is commonly seen in children because of the loose attachment of the tunica vaginalis to the scrotal lining. In this type, the spermatic cord undergoes rotation above the testes.

B. Intravaginal torsion occurs when there is an abnormality of the visceral layer of the tunica vaginalis giving rise to the so-called bell-clapper deformity.

2. Etiology. Normally, the tunica vaginalis is attached to the epididymis and spermatic cord. Motility of the testes is prevented by attachment of the lower end of the spermatic cord and epididymis to the scrotum by the scrotal ligament. Attachment of the tunica vaginalis higher up on the spermatic cord with the tunica completely surrounding the testis and epididymis allows more freedom of motion by preventing attachment to the scrotum. The immediate cause of torsion may be a forceful contraction of the cremasteric muscle.

3. Diagnosis. Diagnosis of torsion of the spermatic cord should be suspected in any boy who has scrotal pain or swelling. Classically, torsion causes excruciating testicular pain, vomiting, and collapse. More often, the onset of pain is gradual and may initially be in the abdomen or groin. Soon there will be local tenderness of the testis with edema and hyperemia of the overlying skin. An experienced observer may diagnose torsion by noting the horizontal position of the affected or opposite testis. In addition, elevation of the testis usually increases the pain, where in epididymitis, elevation of the scrotum usually provides pain relief (Prehn's sign).

4. Differential diagnosis. Differential diagnosis in patients with torsion of the spermatic cord is usually between torsion of the appendix testis or appendix epididymis, epididymo-orchitis, trauma, idiopathic scrotal edema, or incarcerated or strangulated inguinal hernia. Torsion of the appendix testis or epididymis causes much less tenderness and swelling, and if seen early enough, point tenderness may be palpated in the cephalad portion of the testis or epididymis. Orchitis is rare in children, and patients with epididymitis usually will have pyuria.

5. Therapy. Treatment is operative exploration with fixation of the testis to the scrotum by two or more sutures if it is viable. Since the anatomic defect is most often bilateral, it is important also to do an orchiopexy on the other side. Immediate surgery, less than 24 hours after onset, is necessary to save the testis. *The most frequent cause for delay is failure of the primary physician to suspect torsion of the spermatic cord.*

INFECTIONS OF THE SPERMATIC CORD

Inflammation restricted to the vas deferens (deferentitis) and inflammations of the tissues except the cord (funiculitis) are uncommon unless associated with infections of the epididymis or prostate. Infection spreads to the structures of the spermatic cord through the lumen or by the lymphatics. Gonococcal infections and tuberculosis were the most commonly reported specific infections. The symptoms are pain in the area of the cord. Physical examination shows swelling, induration, and nodularity of the cord. Treatment is the administration of the appropriate antibacterial agent.

ORCHITIS

An acute infection involving solely the testis is uncommon. Occasionally, infections are seen with most bacteria, and there may be an epididymo-orchitis. Orchitis secondary to mumps occurs in approximately 18% of cases. Mumps orchitis rarely occurs prior to puberty. The mumps orchitis usually is unilateral and may result in testicular atrophy in 50% of cases. Onset of the orchitis is usually seen 4 to 6 days after the parotitis and subsides in 7 to 10 days. There is no specific treatment or means of preventing its occurrence.

EPIDIDYMITIS

Epididymitis is a common infection constituting as high as 25% of urological admissions in military hospitals. Epididymitis causes significant morbidity in civilian and military populations and also in animals.

1. Etiology. In California, 25 to 35% of rams have epididymitis caused by a specific organism, *Brucella ovis*. Unfortunately, the etiological factors in human epididymitis are not as clear. Two major theories for the causation of acute epididymitis have been advanced.

A. Retrograde passage of urine during stress to the epididymis through the vas deferens causing a chemical epididymitis.

B. Bacterial infection secondary to infection of the genitourinary tract or blood borne from a distant site.

There is more than just an academic interest in carefully defining the etiology of acute epididymitis, since if it can be caused by retrograde passage of urine to the epididymis by heavy straining, then it is compensatory by industry.

During the last decade, Miley B. Wesson championed the fight to show that epididymitis was not caused by retrograde reflux of urine into the vas deferens, stating that no one has demonstrated this in *normal* patients. To my knowledge, no one has yet demonstrated reflux of dye into a normal vas deferens. Wesson also stated that urine can normally be injected retrograde through the vas deferens only under considerable pressure, and then the urine only goes into the distal portion (tail) of the epididymis. The reports of demonstration of retrograde flow have been in patients with benign prostatic hypertrophy or urethral stricture by demonstrating a silver solution introduced into the bladder seen in the vas deferens the following day when a segment was removed; or passage of some urine through a vasostomy in a few patients with benign prostatic hypertrophy while they were urinating. The advocates of retrograde passage of urine to the epididymis say that when straining with a full bladder, urine is forced through the bladder neck into the prostatic urethra where it is held by the external urinary sphincter, and passage of some urine into the prostatic and ejaculatory ducts may occur. Graves and Engel in 1950 did show that injection of sterile urine into a dog's vas deferens caused an inflammatory reaction which was usually confined to the epididymis.

In the last 10 years, several large series of patients with epididymitis have been studied. Epididymitis in some has been found to be associated with lower urinary tract infection and upper respiratory infection. However, in most patients, no etiological factor could be found, as shown by the percentage with no etiology in the following series: Gartman, 55%; Ross, 95%; Mittemeyer, 55%. Nilsson in 1968 performed direct aspiration of the testes of patients with epididymitis and found only 4 of 11 who had positive cultures. In 1971, Wolin reported on 28 patients with epididymitis who all had negative bacterial and viral cultures from aspirations of the epididymis and prostate. Thus, it seems safe to say that we do not know what the etiological factor is in most cases of epididymitis.

2. Diagnosis. The symptoms and signs of acute epididymitis are pain, tenderness, and swelling of the epididymis. There may be an accompanying acute hydrocele. Edema and erythema of the overlying scrotal skin are common. Unless the epididymis can be palpated, it is difficult to distinguish between orchitis, epididymitis, or epididymo-orchitis. It is also important and sometimes difficult to make a clinical distinction between epididymitis and torsion of the spermatic cord or tumors of the testis. The presence of pyuria and fever is helpful in diagnosing epididymitis. Also in many cases of epididymitis, the pain will be relieved by scrotal elevation.

3. Therapy. Treatment of epididymitis may be both medical and surgical. Scrotal support and application of cold initially with later use of heat will relieve the pain. Specific antibiotic therapy should be used with isolation of the bacteria usually being done by culturing urine or prostatic secretions. Temporary relief of pain has been reported by injecting the spermatic cord with local anesthetic agents. The use of anti-inflammatory and proteolytic enzymes has not been shown to be helpful. In the elderly patient who develops epididymitis after prostatectomy, removal of the epididymis under local anesthesia will provide prompt improvement, prevent complications, and shorten the hospital stay. Vasectomy prior to prostatectomy in patients with uninfected urine and prior to instrumentation may prevent epididymitis.

TESTIS TUMORS

1. Incidence. The incidence of testicular tumors in the United States is 2.1

per 100,000 males per year. Testicular tumors account for 0.64% of all male cancer deaths. There is evidence that the incidence of testicular tumors is increasing, with a doubling in certain countries (U.S., New Zealand, Denmark). Testicular tumors are relatively rare in the black population.

2. Etiology. The etiology of testicular tumors is unknown. An increased incidence of 10 to 20 times the normal number of testicular tumors has been reported in patients with undescended testes. This figure is derived from the fact that 3 to 14% of testicular tumors are reported in undescended testes, while only about 0.25% of the total adult male population has cryptorchidism. Successful correction of the undescended testis before age 6 may provide some prophylaxis against subsequent tumor formation. Orchiopexy after the age of 6 seems to afford no protection against subsequent development of tumor in the undescended testis. Tibbs reviewed the recorded cases of malignant testicular tumors in the north of England. He found 10% of the malignancies occurred in undescended testes, or 90 testicular tumors over a period of 50 years in the 6,000 men with undescended testes (0.2% of 3,000,000). Thus, the individual had 90/6,000 (or $1/67 = 1.5\%$) chance of developing a malignancy in his undescended testis during an adult life span of 50 years. The male population with normally descended testes was calculated to have 1/3,654 (0.027%) chance of developing a testicular tumor during the same 50 years. Mostofi quotes other authors as stating that 1/80 inguinal testes and 1/20 abdominal testes will become malignant. It has also been shown that if both testes are abdominal and one develops a testicular tumor, there is a 1/4 chance that the other testis will also have a tumor.

Although over 10% of patients with testicular tumor give a history of trauma, there is no convincing evidence that the trauma was responsible for the development of the tumor. Trauma is considered a factor in experimental testicular tumors. A possible endocrine role has been postulated because of several observations.

A. A number of patients with testicular tumor show a persistent elevation of pituitary gonadotropins even after removal of all the tumor.

B. Testicular tumors in man usually occur during high androgen activity.

C. Experimental induction of teratomas in the fowl by injection of zinc salts occur only during pituitary gonadotropin secretion.

D. Androsterone accelerates growth of certain testicular tumors in tissue culture.

E. Gonadotropin and/or estrogens are produced by a number of testicular tumors. Genetic factors have been postulated to play a role, since there is a higher than normal incidence of testicular tumor in the families of these cases (16%). There is a higher than normal incidence of a testicular tumor developing in the other testis of these patients.

There are two theories on the development of testicular teratomas. The

American theory is that these tumors arise from a primordia of the germ cell. This has been substantiated in strains of mice that have a 14% incidence of testicular tumor. The English theory is that these tumors develop from undifferentiated cells that have escaped influence.

3. Pathology. Primary testicular tumors are usually classified into two types: germ cell tumors (seminoma, embryonal carcinoma, teratoma, and choriocarcinoma) which constitute over 94%; and tumors of gonadal stroma (Leydig cell, Sertoli cell, granulosa cell, and the carcinoma cell tumors). Sixty percent of germ cell tumors show a single cell pattern and 40% are mixed.

A. Germ cell tumors.

1) Seminoma. Seminoma comprises 40 to 50% of testicular tumors and is composed of clear, uniform cells that resemble primordial germ cells. These tumors have not been reported in children and peak incidence is in the 4th and 5th decades. Seminomas are usually very sensitive to radiation and first metastasize via the lymphatics to the retroperitoneal lymph nodes near the renal pedicle. A histologically similar tumor occurs in the ovary and is called dysgerminoma.

2) Embryonal carcinoma. Embryonal carcinoma comprises about 20% of testicular tumors. Histologically, these tumor cells have an embryonic and anaplastic epithelial cell appearance and a variable pattern of acinar, tubular, papillary, solid, and/or reticular appearance. Embryonal testicular tumors are highly malignant and also usually metastasize to the retroperitoneal lymph nodes. They are moderately radiosensitive.

3) Teratomas. Teratoma of the testis shows elements that are derived from more than one germ layer:

a. Ectoderm represented by squamous epithelium and neural tissue.

b. Endoderm represented by gastrointestinal, respiratory, and urinary tract tissue.

c. Mesoderm represented by bone, cartilage, muscle, and lymphoid tissue.

Teratomas of the testis should not be considered benign tumors in the adult since 29% metastasize, usually via the lymphatics. The cut surface of these tumors shows cysts of various sizes.

4) Choriocarcinoma. This is a highly malignant testicular tumor that comprises less than 1% of testis tumors. Histologically, this tumor has synctiotrophoblastic and cytotrophoblastic cells present. Chorionic gonadotropin titers are always elevated. Choriocarcinoma of the testis metastasizes by both hematogenous and lymphatic routes. Hemorrhage is usually seen in the histological specimens.

B. Tumors of the gonadal stroma. These comprise less than 6% of testicular tumors.

1) Leydig cell (interstitial cell) tumors represent about 3% of testicular tumors. These tumors cause masculinization in children and feminization,

or no symptoms, in the adult. Twenty-five percent of the adult patients with Leydig cell tumors have gynecomastia. Ten percent of these tumors metastasize. Histologically, these tumors consist of uniform cells with granular or clear cytoplasm.

2) Sertoli cell tumors have an histologically easy to recognize columnar cell with a large nucleus and distinct nuclear membrane surrounding a fine chromatin network. About 10% of the Sertoli cell tumors are malignant. These tumors may produce endocrine abnormalities that are not well defined.

C. Secondary testicular tumors. Secondary testicular tumors are most frequently lymphomas. Histologically, most of these tumors are reticulum cell sarcoma. Hodgkin's disease has not been reported as occurring primarily in the testis. In contrast to germ cell tumors, lymphomas of the testis occur in the older age group and, in fact, are the most common type of testicular tumor after age 60. If these tumors present as a manifestation of disseminated lymphoma, the prognosis is poor. The prognosis is relatively favorable after orchiectomy and radiation therapy to the regional lymph nodes. "Primary" lymphoma of the testis tends to involve skin and the nasopharynx when dissemination occurs.

4. Diagnosis. A painless swelling is the most common symptom of testicular tumor and occurs in 65% of cases. Less frequently (9%), the patient may have pain or a heavy sensation in the testis. Unfortunately, about 10% have back pain as a consequence of retroperitoneal node involvement or a neck mass due to supraclavicular lymph node metastasis. Gynecomastia is not unusual and may occur with any type of testicular tumor.

Examination of the testes should be done with both hands, carefully examining for all the scrotal contents, vas deferens, epididymis, and testes. Any palpable mass should be transilluminated in a dark room to determine if it is solid or fluid-filled. Usually a testicular tumor will be a painless mass in the testis with no discoloration or fixation of the overlying skin. With seminoma, the entire testis may be replaced with a dense, heavy rubbery mass. Embryonal carcinoma or teratocarcinoma may replace part of the testis distorting the capsular surface as a lump. Epididymo-orchitis, hydrocele, varicocele, spermatocele, hematocele, and torsion have to be differentiated and these have been discussed earlier in this chapter. If testicular tumor is suspected, the physician should note the presence or absence of retroperitoneal and supraclavicular lymph nodes as well as gynecomastia.

5. Preoperative studies. Preoperative diagnostic studies should include chest x-ray, intravenous urograms, baseline titers of chorionic gonado-tropins to determine if these decrease to normal, postoperatively. Biopsy of the testis by needle or open biopsy through the scrotum should never be done because of the rapid spread of the tumor to the scrotum once the tough tunica albuginea is violated. The lymphatic metastases of the testicular

tumor from the scrotal extension would then also include inguinal lymph nodes. If the patient has had prior inguinal or scrotal injury, the lymphatic spread also may be to the inguinal nodes. Lymphatic spread to the inguinal region is bad because excision of these nodes by a groin dissection carries considerably more morbidity than a retroperitoneal node dissection.

6. Staging. Staging of testicular tumors is important from the standpoints of prognosis and of treatment. The terminology has not been uniformly agreed upon, but the two systems most widely used are presented below.

    A. Stage A or IA—tumor confined to the testis.

    Stage IB—same as IA plus histological evidence of lymphatic, spread to iliac or para-aortic lymph nodes.

    B. Stage B or II—tumor spread to retroperitoneal lymph nodes, but not beyond.

    C. Stage C or III—tumor spread to a site other than retroperitoneal lymph nodes.

7. Treatment. Treatment depends upon the pathological type and stage of the testicular tumor. Surgery, irradiation, and chemotherapy all are important in the management of these tumors.

    A. Orchiectomy. Orchiectomy through an inguinal incision with separation ligation of the vas deferens and spermatic vessels is the accepted initial treatment. In doubtful cases, the vas deferens and spermatic vessels are clamped with a rubber shod clamp, the testis delivered from the scrotum through the inguinal incision, examined, and if any question of tumor exists, the testis should be removed. Local scrotal recurrences after this type of orchiectomy are almost never seen. Cure after orchiectomy alone averages around 50% in seminomas and 20 to 30% in embryonal and teratocarcinomas.

    B. Staging. Further staging studies such as lymphangiograms. Gallium scans, and vena cavograms (if the testis tumor is on the right) can be done. If there is a clinical suggestion of metastasis to the retroperitoneal nodes, a left supraclavicular node biopsy should be done and will be positive in 15% of cases.

    C. Treatment of seminoma. With a pathological diagnosis of seminoma and a stage A(I) clinically, prophylactic irradiation of the retroperitoneal nodes in doses ranging from 2,000 to 3,500 rads over a 2- to 4-week period is usually given. Whether these patients with stage A(I) should also receive irradiation to the mediastinum or neck, or chemotherapy with an alkylating agent has not been answered. The cure rate with seminoma, stage A(I), is over 95%. In seminoma patients with stage B(II), irradiation to both the retroperitoneal area, mediastinum, and left supraclavicular area is usually given with a cure rate of over 75%. In stage C(III) seminoma patients, a combination of irradiation and chemotherapy is employed with a cure rate of 10 to 20%. The overall cure rate for all patients with seminoma of the testis averages about 90%.

D. Treatment of embryonal and teratocarcinoma. For patients with nonseminoma, germinal cell testicular tumor, there is some disagreement about the role of surgical excision of the retroperitoneal nodes and use of irradiation to the retroperitoneal lymph nodes as well as irradiation to the mediastinum and left supraclavicular node areas. Many questions are unanswered because of the lack of carefully controlled clinical series, lack of accurate pathological staging in the radiation treatment series, and use of actual survival in most surgical series, while actuarial or projected survival by life tables (Berkson-Gage) is used by most radiation series. In addition, the various authors writing on the subject have tended to use series or even interpret the same series differently toward their own bias. Thus, the student should interpret the following paragraph in the knowledge that it is written by a surgeon who believes that one sure way of curing cancer is to cut it all out!

The results of the various series in relation to surgical excision of the retroperitoneal lymph nodes versus radiotherapy will be discussed.

1) Retroperitoneal node dissection. In embryonal testicular tumor, Staubitz had an 86% 5-year cure rate (20/23) in stage A(I) and 83% (10/12) in stage B(II) using only surgical excision of the retroperitoneal lymph nodes. Whitmore, using surgery with and without postoperative irradiation, had 86% (18/21) stage A(I) survival and 50% (12/24) stage B(II). Skinner and Leadbetter, using surgery with and without irradiation, reported a 66% (4/6) stage A(I) and 66% (10/15) stage B(II) survival.

2) Radiotherapy to retroperitoneal nodes. Caldwell summarized all major series and reports a survival of 60% (254/421) (stages I, II, III) in nonseminoma germinal cell tumor treated by radiotherapy. Skinner and Leadbetter, reviewing many of these same series, report a survival of 30.6% (204/666) (stages I, II, III) in nonseminoma germinal cell tumor with radiotherapy.

3) Chemotherapy. Chemotherapy is effective treatment in a small percentage of metastatic nonseminoma germinal cell tumors of the testis. The Memorial Hospital reported a complete remission (this is not the same as survival since the tumor may reappear and later kill the patient) with actinomycin D alone of 23% (5/22). Mithramycin was reported (manufacturer's brochure (305 patients)) to have an 11% complete response and 26% partial response. The National Cancer Institute reported 29% (5/17) complete remission with a combination of drugs (S-fluorouracil, cyclophosphamide, Methotrexate, and vincristine).

Certain information is clear from the above studies. Examination of retroperitoneal lymph node specimens shows a 30 to 60% chance of having nodal metastasis in the nonseminoma testicular tumors. If the retroperitoneal nodes are histologically negative for tumors, 10 to 20% will have metastasis to the mediastinum and supraclavicular node areas. The studies of Ray and Whitmore of excised retroperitoneal lymph nodes showed 13% of right-sided testicular tumors metastasized to contralateral aortic nodes and 20% of left-sided testicular tumors metastasized to the contralateral nodes. The lymphangiographic studies (which may not reproduce physiological flows since the contrast is injected in the feet) show more frequent crossing of retroperitoneal lymphatics from the right to the left.

4) Management at the University of Virginia Medical Center. Management of nonseminomal germinal cell testicular tumors at our institution has usually consisted of bilateral retroperitoneal lymph node dissection through a vertical midline incision. If the excised nodes are negative, no further treatment is given. If the nodes have only microscopic tumor involvement, chemotherapy (actinomycin) is given for 2 years. If the retroperitoneal nodes have more extensive involvement, then irradiation and chemotherapy are used. Solitary chest metastases are surgically excised if no more lesions appear after chemotherapy and irradiation to the lungs. Some authors advise prophylactic chemotherapy if the retroperitoneal lymph nodes are negative to treat the 10 to 20% of patients who might be expected to have lung metastases.

5) Effects of irradiation on renal and testicular function. Renal function has usually not been impaired after irradiation to the retroperitoneal lymph nodes. It has been calculated that the shielded (by a lead cup) remaining testis receives 50 to 70 rads with retroperitoneal irradiation and 90 to 110 rads if the inguinal region is also irradiated. The unshielded (without lead cup) testis receives 150 rads with retroperitoneal irradiation and 250 rads if the inguinal area is also irradiated. No teratogenic effects of the irradiation have been noted in the patients. After the irradiation, the patients are subfertile for 1 to 4 years and should not have children for at least 1 year. Testicular irradiation with a 600-rad single dose causes permanent sterility, 250 rads cause sterility for 12 months, and 35 rads cause temporary oligospermia for 18 months.

6) Sexual function after retroperitoneal node dissection. After bilateral retroperitoneal lymph node dissection, many patients are infertile because of lack of emission of sperm. These patients have normal libido, erection, and orgasm. The lack of seminal emission is due to loss of sympathetic nerve stimulation of emission, and in some cases, retrograde ejaculation into the bladder from loss of sympathetic control of the internal sphincter (bladder neck). Erection is due to vasodilation of the penile arteries and partial occlusion of the penile veins. The pudendal nerve carries the afferent, and sacral nerves (n. erigentes) carry the efferent fibers for erection. Emission of sperm is from afferent fibers in the sacral nerves (n. erigentes) and efferent fibers which come from the T12-L4 sympathetic ganglia, with the L2 sympathetic ganglia being the most important.

7) Extragonadal testicular tumors. Extragonadal testicular tumors have been reported most frequently in the mediastinum and retroperitoneum. However, primary occurrence of testicular tumors has been reported

in the pineal gland, bladder, prostate, stomach, ovary, omentum, and thymus gland. These tumors are postulated to arise from remnants of the urogenital ridge or from primitive rests of the totipotiental germ cells. Most of these tumors have had the histological appearance of seminoma, but the other cell types have also been reported. The question always arises as to whether or not these tumors are really metastatic from small or healed tumors in the testes. Autopsy studies have shown normal testes in a few of the patients and a few have had microscopic changes that were interpreted as autorejected tumor sites. In my opinion, if the testes feel normal, bilateral orchiectomy should not be done in these extragonadal testicular tumors.

8. Testicular tumors in childhood. Testicular tumors are also seen in children, but with a lower incidence than in the adult (2 to 5% of testicular tumors are in children). Seminoma has not been reported in children and the teratoma has not been reported to metastasize in children. The embryonal testicular tumor in children should be treated by retroperitoneal node dissection and/or irradiation to the retroperitoneal lymph nodes. The prognosis is better for the children than for the adults.

REFERENCES AND SUGGESTED FURTHER READING

1. Boatman, D. L., Culp, D. A., and Wilson, V. B. Testicular neoplasms in children. J. Urol. 109:315, 1973.
2. Caldwell, W. L. Why retroperitoneal lymphadenectomy for testicular tumors? South. Med. J. 62:1232, 1969.
3. Ehrlich, R. M., Dougherty, L. J., Tomashefsky, P., and Lattimer, J. K. Effect of gonadotropin in cryptorchism. J. Urol. 102:793, 1969.
4. Houser, R., Izant, R., and Persky, L. Testicular tumors in children. Am. J. Surg. 110:876, 1965.
5. Kelly, J. M., Massey, B. D., Harrison, E. G., and Utz, D. C. Lymphoma of the testis. Cancer 26:847, 1970.
6. Leape, L. L. Torsion of the testis. J.A.M.A. 200:669, 1967.
7. Levin, A. and Sherman, J. O. The undescended testis. Surg. Gynecol. Obstet. 136:473, 1973.
8. Maier, J. G. and Sulak, M. H. Radiation therapy in malignant testis tumors. Cancer 32:1212, 1973.
9. Skinner, D. G. and Leadbetter, W. F. The surgical management of testis tumors. J. Urol. 106:84, 1971.
10. Staubitz, W. J., Early, K., Magoss, I. V., and Murphy, G. P. Surgical treatment of non-seminomatous germinal testes tumors. Cancer 32:1206, 1973.
11. Tibbs, D. J. Unilateral absence of the testis (appendix). Br. J. Surg. 48:607, 1961.
12. Tsuji, I., Nakajima, F., Nishida, T., Nakanoya, Y., and Inoue, K. Testicular tumors in children. J. Urol. 110:127, 1973.
13. Utz, D. C. and Buscemi, M. F. Extragonadal testicular tumors. J. Urol. 105:271, 1971.
14. Wolin, L. H. On the etiology of epididymitis. J.Urol. 105:531, 1971.

Texts

1. *Paediatric Urology*, edited by D. I. Williams. Appleton-Century-Crofts, London, 1969.
2. *Urology*, edited by M. F. Campbell and J. H. Harrison, Chap. 16 and 30. W. B. Saunders & Co., Philadelphia, 1970.

19

Disorders of the Adrenal

ARTHUR W. WYKER, JR.

The adrenal is really two distinct glands—cortex and medulla—which just happen to be anatomically confined within a common capsule. They differ in many ways.

1. Embryology.

A. The cortex is derived from mesoderm.

B. The medulla is derived from neuroectoderm and can be considered modified nervous tissue.

2. Physiology.

A. The cortex responds to *humoral* stimuli secreting a wide variety of steroid hormones.

B. The medulla responds to *nerve* stimuli secreting the catecholamines: epinephrine and norepinephrine.

3. Is it vital?

A. The cortex, not the medulla, is the life-maintaining portion of the adrenal.

ANATOMY

The adrenal glands are small (5 to 7 g each), yellow, flat caplike structures sitting on top of each kidney within Gerota's fascia. They have an unusual blood supply. They do not have a main or single adrenal artery but instead, numerous small arterial branches from the inferior phrenic, renal artery, and aorta enter the gland from all sides. There is, however, a single adrenal vein on each side—the right one draining into the adjacent vena cava, the left one into the left renal vein. The nerve supply is rich with many sympathetic nerve fibers reaching the gland to connect *exclusively* with the medulla.

ADRENAL CORTEX

This metabolic factory produces a wide variety of steroids with the most important ones, physiologically, being cortisol and aldosterone. The other hormones normally have only a small biological effect and become significant only when produced in excess.

Cholesterol is the starting block for all adrenal steroids, and it is converted to cortisol, aldosterone, or androgens by a number of steps, each one requiring the presence of a specific enzyme.

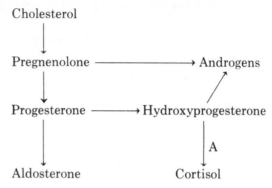

Formation of Adrenal Cortical Hormones

If an enzyme is deficient or absent, the block in the steroid pathway results in an increased secretion of those steroids proximal to the block and decreased secretion of those steroids distal to the block. For example, if there is an enzymatic block at A, less cortisol is formed and there is an increased secretion of hydroxyprogesterone and androgens.

There are three zones in the adrenal cortex—the outer zona glomerulosa, the middle zona fasciculata, and the inner zona reticularis. The zona glomerulosa produces aldosterone and is not adrenocorticotropic hormone-dependent, its chief stimulus being the renin-angiotensin system. The zona fasciculata and reticularis are a *functional unit* producing both cortisol and androgens when stimulated by adrenocorticotropic hormone (ACTH).

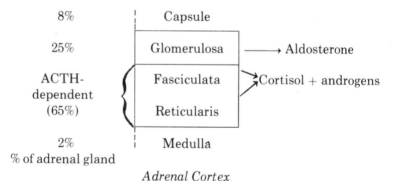

Adrenal Cortex

ADRENOCORTICOTROPIC HORMONE

ACTH is produced *only* by selected cells of the anterior pituitary gland—basophils and some large chromophobe cells. They secrete ACTH only when the hypothalamus permits it, via its ACTH-releasing hormone. This hypothalamic-pituitary-adrenal axis is affected by three factors.
1. The blood level of free cortisol.

A. The amount of ACTH secreted is *inversely related* to the cortisol level.

    1) A rising free cortisol level leads to decreased ACTH production.

    2) A falling free cortisol level leads to increased ACTH production.

B. Servoregulation via circulating levels of cortisol is primarily hypothalamic.

2. Stress.

    A. Many, but not all, types of stress result in an increased production of ACTH.

    B. Stressful stimuli reaching the cerebral cortex excite the hypothalamus with resultant secretion of ACTH-releasing hormone.

3. Sleep-wake habit.

    A. ACTH secretion rises during sleep and falls during waking hours, so that blood levels of ACTH are highest in the early morning, lowest in the late evening.

Melanocyte-stimulating hormone (MSH) is produced by the anterior pituitary in conjunction with ACTH, and this sister hormone causes hyperpigmentation of the skin and mucous membranes. Whenever hypocortisolism is present, as in adrenocortical insufficiency, both ACTH and MSH blood levels will be high, and the patient will be hyperpigmented.

1. Stress, sleep-wake pattern, and circulating levels of free cortisol all initiate ACTH release by their effect on the central nervous system (CNS) and the hypothalamus (Fig. 1).

    A. The anterior pituitary may also respond to cortisol.

2. The hypothalamus is the control center for ACTH production and release.

HYPOTHALAMIC - PITUITARY - ADRENAL AXIS

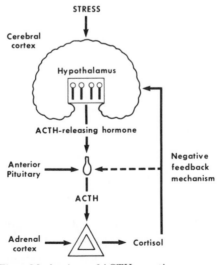

Fig. 1. Mechanisms of ACTH secretion.

A. Its *secretory neurons* secrete ACTH-releasing hormone into the blood vessels going to the anterior pituitary, and when this hormone reaches the anterior pituitary, ACTH is released and a few minutes later, cortisol is secreted by the adrenal cortex.

CORTISOL

This is the only adrenal cortical hormone which is *essential for life*. Its major effects are as follows:

1. Carbohydrate-protein metabolism.

A. The conversion of protein to carbohydrate is affected by the amount of cortisol present.

  1) Protein $\xrightleftharpoons{\text{cortisol}}$ carbohydrate——normal

  2) Protein $\overrightarrow{}$ $\rightleftarrows$ carbohydrate——hypercortisolism

  3) Protein $\rightleftarrows$ _____ carbohydrate——hypocortisolism

B. With excess cortisol, as in Cushing's syndrome, this reaction is pushed to the right, with resultant *protein depletion in tissues*.

  1) Loss of protein from the skin → striae

                            bones → osteoporosis

                            muscles → weakness

                            blood vessels → increased fragility.

C. With insufficient cortisol, as in adrenocortical insufficiency (ACI) the reaction is pushed to the left, with resultant *depletion of carbohydrate*.

  1) This decreased carbohydrate formation results in hypoglycemia, low tissue glycogen levels, and poor tolerance to fasting.

2. Resistance to stress.

A. Cortisol helps the body blunt the effects of stress.

  1) When insufficient cortisol is present (ACI and some forms of the adrenogenital syndrome), there is an increased susceptibility to the harmful effects of heat, cold, infection, operation, or injury.

3. Immunological and inflammatory response.

A. When there is excess cortisol present (hypercortisolism), the normal responses are suppressed.

  1) Wound healing is impaired and the spread of infection is enhanced.

4. Suppresses pituitary production of ACTH.

A. This brake mechanism probably works via the hypothalamus rather than by direct action on the anterior pituitary (see Fig. 1).

ALDOSTERONE

Aldosterone is an electrolyte-regulating hormone affecting the kidney, salivary and sweat glands, and the gastrointestinal (GI) tract.

1. Kidney.

A. Its primary action is on the distal renal tubule where it causes retention of sodium and water while enhancing the excretion of potassium and hydrogen ions.

1) The sodium ion-retaining effect is *transient* because of "renal escape."

2) The potassium ion-losing effect is persistent.

B. The magnitude of this sodium ion-potassium ion exchange is directly related to the number of sodium ions reaching the tubule.

1) Aldosterone increases urinary potassium ion *only* if sodium ions are available!

a. In animals on sodium ion-free diets, aldosterone has no effect on the kidney and urine potassium ion is not increased.

2) A low salt diet limits the sodium ion-potassium ion exchange, whereas a high salt diet permits it to operate maximally.

C. Renal escape.

1) After 2 to 3 days of aldosterone administration, the kidneys escape from the sodium ion-retaining effect, urinary sodium ion excretion returns to normal levels, and the patient *does not become edematous.*

2) Before renal escape occurs, the extracellular fluid (ECF) compartment is expanded by the retention of sodium ions and water, and the patient usually gains 2 to 3 kg.

3) Urinary sodium ion returns to normal, not because aldosterone loses its sodium ion-retaining effect on the distal tubule, but because a volume sensitive, salt-losing hormone (third factor) causes *decreased sodium ion reabsorption by the proximal tubule.*

a. This decreased sodium ion reabsorption throws an added load on the distal tubule, balancing out the enhanced sodium ion reabsorption due to aldosterone. This trade-off returns urinary sodium ion excretion to normal.

2. Salivary and sweat glands, and GI tract.

A. Aldosterone has a similar but less important effect here, reducing sodium ion concentration and increasing potassium ion concentration.

1) The finding of reduced sodium ion concentration in the sweat was the evidence of excess aldosterone activity used by Dr. J. W. Conn in 1954 when he introduced a new clinical syndrome—primary aldosteronism (PA).

There are three *direct* stimuli to aldosterone production—ACTH, angiotensin II, and potassium ion.

1. ACTH.

A. This pituitary hormone is of minor importance in the day-to-day aldosterone output, since it stimulates aldosterone release only in emergency or acute situations and for only a short period of time.

2. Angiotensin II.

A. The renin-angiotensin system (R-A) is the chief regulator of aldosterone secretion, and it accomplishes this via a negative feedback loop.

B. The R-A system is activated by a *reduction in effective blood volume* which may be the result of hemorrhage, dehydration, low salt diet, or loss of body fluids.

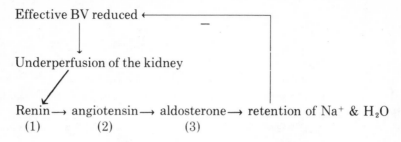

Effective BV reduced ←

Underperfusion of the kidney

Renin→ angiotensin→ aldosterone→ retention of Na⁺ & H₂O
(1)   (2)   (3)

1) When the effective blood volume is reduced, the R-A system increases aldosterone production and the resultant retention of sodium ions and water returns the blood volume towards normal, thereby shutting off the R-A system (negative feedback).

2) In this system, the levels of renin, angiotensin, and aldosterone *move together* so that a low salt diet would cause a rise in blood levels of all three.

3. Potassium ion.

A. Potassium ion levels play a dominant roll in regulation of aldosterone secretion only when the R-A system is absent (*e.g.*, after bilateral nephrectomy) or loses its responsiveness (*e.g.*, primary aldosteronism).

B. Hyperkalemia causes increased aldosterone production, which enhances the urinary excretion of potassium ion, returning plasma potassium ion levels to normal, thereby removing the stimulus.

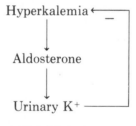

Hyperkalemia ←

Aldosterone

Urinary K⁺

ANDROGENS

Adrenal androgens are biologically weak! Much less potent than testosterone, they cannot prevent the clinical picture of hypogonadism seen after loss of testicular androgens in young males. They promote anabolism of protein in both sexes, but their most identifiable effect is the production of pubic and axillary hair in girls at puberty.

ADRENAL CORTICAL INSUFFICIENCY

The normal adrenal cortex has such a large functional reserve that signs and symptoms of hypofunction do not develop unless approximately 90% of the cortical tissue is nonproductive (Table I).

Hypofunction may result from atrophy or destruction of adrenocortical tissue (primary) or from ACTH deficiency due to hypopituitarism (secondary).

TABLE I

% Normal Adrenocortical Function	Signs and Symptoms of ACI
> 25 (25–100)	Absent
10–25	Present only after stress
< 10	Present

1. Primary.

   A. Since the pathological process affects all zones of the cortex to an equal degree, there is a reduction in output of *all* adrenal cortical hormones with low or absent levels of cortisol, aldosterone, and adrenal androgens.

   B. Since the amount of ACTH secreted by the pituitary varies inversely with the blood cortisol level, hypocortisolism results in an elevated blood level of both ACTH and its sister hormone, melanocyte-stimulating hormone (MSH).

   1) *Hyperpigmentation* due to increased levels of MSH is the most common physical finding of primary ACI or Addison's disease.

   C. Etiology.

   1) Atrophy—50%.

   a. Destruction is probably the result of an autoimmune reaction.

   2) Tuberculosis—35%.

   3) Carcinoma, primary or metastatic—10%.

   4) Miscellaneous—5%.

2. Secondary.

   A. Hypopituitarism may be due to atrophy or destruction of the pituitary or to pituitary suppression.

   1) The most common form of ACI is *iatrogenic* caused by pituitary adrenal suppression from prior administration of cortisone.

   B. The presence of ACTH deficiency reduces the levels of the ACTH-dependent hormones—cortisol and adrenal androgens—but *does not* reduce the level of aldosterone.

   C. Since ACTH and MSH levels are low, hyperpigmentation does not occur.

ADDISON'S DISEASE

Clinical Picture

Hyperpigmentation is the hallmark of Addison's disease and is the most useful diagnostic clue! High MSH levels cause a brownish pigmentation of exposed areas of skin and a purplish brown pigmentation of the buccal mucosa.

The signs and symptoms shown in Table II result from the inadequate amounts of normal adrenocortical hormones—aldosterone, cortisol, and androgens.

TABLE II

Incidence of Common Signs and Symptoms

Sign or Symptom	Incidence
	%
1. Weakness, easy fatigability	100
2. Weight loss	100
3. Hyperpigmentation	95
4. Hypotension	90
5. GI symptoms	85
6. Early morning hypoglycemia	70

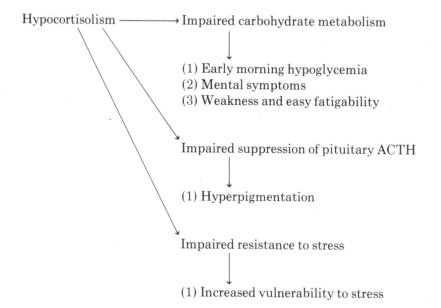

Hypoaldosteronism ⟶ Loss of salt and water

      ↓

   (1) Hypotension
   (2) Weight loss
   (3) Dizziness and syncopal attacks

Hypocortisolism ⟶ Impaired carbohydrate metabolism

      ↓

   (1) Early morning hypoglycemia
   (2) Mental symptoms
   (3) Weakness and easy fatigability

   Impaired suppression of pituitary ACTH

      ↓

   (1) Hyperpigmentation

   Impaired resistance to stress

      ↓

   (1) Increased vulnerability to stress

Hypoadrenal androgens ⟶ Reduced androgenic activity

      ↓

   (1) Reduction in axillary & pubic hair, primarily in women

Diagnosis

In the usual case of Addison's disease, plasma and urinary levels of cortisol, aldosterone, and adrenal androgens are *low*. The finding of a low plasma cortisol level in the face of a high plasma ACTH level should confirm the diagnosis of ACI, but there are two drawbacks to this approach.
1. Plasma ACTH levels are difficult to measure.
2. Basal plasma cortisol levels in mild ACI may overlap the normal range. The best test for ACI is the determination of plasma cortisol after ACTH stimulation.

ACTH Stimulation Test

1. In ACI, plasma cortisol already low, does not respond to exogenous ACTH, because the adrenal cortex is already being maximally stimulated by endogenous ACTH.
2. Method of performing test.
  A. A single intramuscular injection of 25 units of aqueous ACTH is used to stimulate the adrenal glands.
    1) Plasma cortisol is determined prior to and 1 hour after the injection.
    2) Urinary cortisol is determined prior to and 1 to 2 hours after the injection.
3. In Addison's disease, baseline plasma and urinary levels of cortisol are low, and they do not change significantly after ACTH stimulation.

Treatment

Replacement therapy in patients lacking significant adrenocortical function requires 25 to 37.5 mg of cortisone to correct hypocortisolism and 0.1 to 0.2 mg of Florinef to correct hypoaldosteronism. In some patients, it may be advisable to place them on a high salt, high carbohydrate diet.

PRIMARY ALDOSTERONISM

This syndrome, first identified by Conn in 1954, has as its chief manifestations hypertension and weakness.

Etiology and Pathology

A small adenoma of the adrenal cortex accounts for around 75% of the reported cases, the remaining 25% being due to adrenocortical hyperplasia. The adenoma is unilateral in 95% of cases and is bright yellow in color. It is small because aldosterone is an unusually potent hormone. Each day, only 0.1 mg is produced by the normal adrenal cortex and chronic production of as little as 0.2 mg/day, only two times the usual output, can cause symptomatic primary aldosteronism. This amount can be produced by an adenoma less than 2 mm in size. It is not surprising, then, that of the reported adenomas, 85% have been less than 10 g in size; 75% have been less than 3 cm in diameter.

Clinical Findings

Hypertension and hypokalemia are the key findings in primary aldosteronism.

1. Hypertension.

A. This is usually long standing and benign with diastolic pressures usually less than 130 mm Hg.

B. The mechanism of hypertension is thought to be retention of sodium ion and water, with expansion of the ECF volume, making this a form of *steroid hypertension*.

C. In the early phase of PA before hypokalemia develops, this may be the only abnormality, the patient being asymptomatic or complaining only of nocturia.

2. Hypokalemia.

A. This is present in all the full blown cases, but it is absent in the early phase.

B. It is responsible for *most* of the signs and symptoms.

1) Muscle weakness.

2) Nocturia secondary to polyuria and polydipsia.

3) Paresthesias and tetany due to reduction in the level of ionized calcium secondary to hypokalemic alkalosis.

4) Impaired carbohydrate tolerance.

5) Abnormal electrocardiogram (EKG).

PA occurs most commonly in the 30 to 50 age group (70%) and the ratio of female to male patients is 2 to 3:1.

Differential Diagnosis

The diagnosis of PA must be considered in any patient with hypertension, but particularly so if it is associated with hypokalemia and weakness.

1. Urinalysis—possible early clue.

A. Urine is *persistently dilute, relatively alkaline, or alkaline.*

1) Urine specific gravity is usually around 1,010 (1,005 to 1,015).

2) Urine pH is usually around 7.0 (6.5 to 7.5).

B. Do serial A.M. urines for pH and specific gravity.

1) The early A.M. urine specimen normally is the most concentrated and most acid one excreted each day.

2) Rule out other possible causes of alkaline urine such as drugs and urea-splitting urinary tract infection.

2. Screening test.

A. Plasma potassium concentration is determined after the patient has been off all medications and on a high salt, moderate potassium diet for 2 weeks.

1) Plasma potassium greater than 3.5 mEq/liter—the patient *does not* have aldosteronism.

2) Plasma potassium less than 3.5 mEq/liter—the patient *may* have aldosteronism.

B. The high salt diet is used for two reasons.

1) In normal people, a high salt diet expands the ECF volume, thereby suppressing the R-A mechanism and decreasing the secretion of aldosterone.

    a. With low secretion rates of aldosterone, urinary potassium ion levels are low and plasma potassium remains unchanged.

2) In patients with PA, the autonomous production of aldosterone is *not suppressed* by the high salt diet, and the availability of plenty of sodium ions permits the aldosterone present to exert its maximal effects.

    a. With the potassium ion-sodium ion exchange operating maximally, the resultant high urinary excretion of potassium ion causes hypokalemia.

3. The first step in making the definitive diagnosis of PA is to establish that the patient is *overproducing aldosterone*.

A. The amount of aldosterone secreted and excreted each day is markedly affected by the quantity of salt ingested, so any determination of aldosterone production must be correlated with the urinary sodium level (Table III).

B. To widen the gap between normal patients and those with PA, aldosterone determinations are performed while the patient is on a high salt diet.

1) Abnormally high levels of aldosterone in plasma or urine establish the diagnosis of aldosteronism.

4. Overproduction of aldosterone (aldosteronism) may be primary or secondary.

A. Primary.

 → ↑ Aldosterone → ↑ Circulating BV → ↓*Renin*

1) The primary pathology is in the adrenal cortex and the expansion of the blood volume induced by the excess aldosterone removes the stimulus to renin production, so *renin levels are very low*.

TABLE III
Relationship of Salt Intake to Aldosterone Secretion

Normal	Aldosterone Secretion
	μg/day
Average salt intake	100–200
Low salt intake	Up to 3,000
High salt intake	Down to 0

B. Secondary.

 Underperfusion of the kidneys → ↑ *Renin* → ↑ Aldosterone

1) The primary pathology is in the kidneys with functional renal hemodynamic changes stimulating the R-A mechanism with resultant overproduction of aldosterone.

2) In contrast to PA, *renin levels are consistently high*, for the induced aldosteronism is unable to shut off the renin mechanism.

C. To widen the gap between normal and PA, the plasma renin is performed while the patient is on a low salt diet and after 3 to 4 hours in the upright position.

1) Upright posture doubles the plasma renin in a normal individual.

2) Low salt diet (10 mEq/day) triples the plasma renin in a normal individual.

5. Primary aldosteronism may be due to a functioning adenoma or to adrenal hyperplasia, and every effort should be made to identify correctly the pathological lesion present, since the adenoma is managed surgically, hyperplasia medically.

A. Since the majority of the adenomas are small and relatively hypovascular, they are not detectable by the usual techniques—intravenous urogram (IVP), nephrotomography, arteriography, or retroperitoneal pneumography.

B. Selective adrenal venography successfully outlines the adenoma in around 80% of cases.

1) The adenoma displaces the adrenal venules but does not cause a tumor blush.

C. Adrenal venous blood is sampled at the time of venography.

1) If you detect high levels of aldosterone on the side of the lesion (via venography) with close to peripheral levels on the unaffected side, the probability of a functioning adenoma being present approaches 100%.

2) In hyperplasia, both sides will have high, approximately equal, levels of aldosterone.

D. Isotopic adrenal scanning.

1) 19-iodocholesterol labeled with radioactive iodine-131 is used.

2) The adenoma shows up as a "hot spot."

3) Adrenal hyperplasia shows diffuse uptake of radioactivity or bilateral small "hot spots."

E. Patients with bilateral hyperplasia tend to have less severe hypokalemia and lower aldosterone secretion than do those with a functioning adenoma.

Management

1. Adenoma.

A. Hypokalemia is corrected prior to surgery either by administration of spironolactone, an aldosterone blocker, or by giving a low salt, high potassium diet.

1) This is important, for hypokalemia increases cardiac irritability, predisposing to arrhythmias, and weakens the respiratory muscles, predisposing to respiratory insufficiency.

B. A total unilateral adrenalectomy is performed.

1) Over 90% of functioning adenomas are unilateral.

C. The electrolyte abnormalities return to normal in 5 to 10 days, but the blood pressure may take many months to descend to normal levels.

2. Adrenal hyperplasia.

A. The treatment of choice is spironolactone, an aldosterone blocker.

1) This brings the blood pressure down to the normal range and corrects the hypokalemia.

B. When aldosteronism is part of the adrenogenital syndrome, it is successfully treated with dexamethasone.

C. Surgery is *not advised* because, although it usually corrects the hypokalemia, it usually does not correct the hypertension.

CUSHING'S SYNDROME

Cushing's syndrome refers to the clinical picture resulting from excess cortisol, *regardless of the underlying cause.* Cushing's disease is a less inclusive term denoting only those patients with Cushing's syndrome due to overproduction of ACTH by the pituitary gland. Spontaneous Cushing's syndrome is rare!

Classification of Cushing's Syndrome

1. Primary hypercortisolism—due to primary disorder of the adrenal cortex.

A. Adrenal tumor—25%.

1) Adenoma.

2) Carcinoma.

3) Bilateral adenomas or microadenomatosis.

2. Secondary hypercortisolism—normal adrenal cortex is *overstimulated* by ACTH.

A. Adrenal hyperplasia—75%.

1) Excess pituitary ACTH (Cushing's disease).

2) Ectopic ACTH syndrome.

3. Iatrogenic hypercortisolism—cortisol-like drugs are taken exogenously.

Clinical Picture

This disease primarily affects young adults 20 to 40 years old, but it has been reported in all age groups; 80% of the reported cases have been women. The signs and symptoms are due to the physiological effects of excess cortisol.

1. Metabolism.

A. Protein $\xrightarrow{\text{cortisol}}$ carbohydrate.

1) This reaction is pushed to the right, causing protein depletion in *all* tissues.

    a. Skin—striae.

    b. Bones—osteoporosis.

    c. Muscles—weakness and fatigue.

    d. Blood vessels—marked fragility.

B. Fat.

1) There is an increased amount of fat deposited in facial, shoulder, and abdominal regions but *not in the extremities.*

2. Normal immunological and inflammatory response is *suppressed.*

A. Wound healing is impaired so there is a constant threat of wound dehiscence following surgery.

B. Spread of infection is enhanced.

1) There is a decreased resistance to *all* types of infection—bacterial, viral, fungal, and parasitic.

3. Gonadal function is *suppressed.*

  A. Men tend to be impotent.

B. Women tend to have oligomenorrhea or amenorrhea.

4. Chief threats to life.

A. Hypertension with cardiovascular complications.

B. Abnormal mental reactions.

C. Likelihood of poor wound healing or of unusual infections.

Diagnosis

1. The physical appearance of the patient is often diagnostic.

A. Central obesity is the hallmark of Cushing's syndrome.

1) Most but not all patients have gained weight, but there is a redistribution of fat to the facial and truncal areas in all patients.

2) The relatively thinner extremities stand out in marked contrast to the rest of the body.

B. Face is round, plethoric, and hairy.

C. Skin is thin, transparent, and fragile.

1) Blue striae over the lower abdomen are characteristic.

2) Ecchymoses, acne, and fungal lesions are common.

3) Mottled cyanosis of the hands and feet may be present.

2. Screening tests for Cushing's syndrome.

A. Urinary free cortisol.

1) The urinary excretion of cortisol is a better indication of hypercortisolism than the excretion of 17-hydroxycorticosterone (17-OHCS) because it is a function of the unbound cortisol of plasma, the physiologically active portion.

2) In the past, considerable confusion arose when obese women with

mild hypertension and hirsutism were found to have increased urinary 17-OHCS, *but urinary cortisol levels are not elevated in obese people.*

    3) Level: 60 to 350 μg/24 hours—normal.

          > 350 μg/24 hours—probable Cushing's syndrome.

  B. Overnight dexamethasone suppression test.

    1) Test—1 mg of dexamethasone is given orally between 11:00 P.M. and 12:00 midnight, and at 8:00 A.M. the following morning, plasma cortisol is determined.

    2) Level: < 10 μg/100 ml—normal.

          > 10 μg/100 ml—probable Cushing's syndrome.

  C. Both of these tests can be performed on an outpatient basis with minimal inconvenience and high diagnostic accuracy.

    1) Five to 10% of Cushing's syndrome suspects have positive screening tests, and these people are admitted for the more exacting tests by the endocrinologists designed to determine the underlying pathology.

3. High dose dexamethasone test—8 mg/day for 2 days—separates patients with Cushing's disease (pituitary-induced adrenal hyperplasia) from those with adrenal tumors or with ectopic ACTH syndrome due to a nonendocrine tumor.

  A. Urinary levels of cortisol or 17-OHCS are *lowered* only in Cushing's disease.

    1) The servomechanism is set at a higher level, like setting one's heat thermostat at 75° instead of 70°. The furnace can be turned off but it takes more heat to do it.

3. Adrenal function tests helpful in determining the underlying cause of Cushing's syndrome (Table IV).

  A. Determination of urinary 17-ketosteroid (17-KS) may aid in differentiating adrenal adenoma from carcinoma.

    1) Adenoma—17-KS usually normal.

    2) Carcinoma—17-KS markedly elevated.

TABLE IV
Adrenal Function Test

	Plasma ACTH	Response of Urinary 17-OHCS or Cortisol to:		
		8 mg Dexamethasone	ACTH	Metyrapone
Adrenal hyperplasia due to pituitary ACTH	↑	↓	↑	↑
Adrenal adenoma	↓	0	0	0
Adrenal carcinoma	↓	0	0	0
ACTH-producing nonendocrine tumor	↑↑	0	0	0
Nodular hyperplasia of the adrenal glands	↓	0	0	0

↑ = increased ↑↑ = markedly increased ↓ = decreased 0 = no change

4. X-ray studies.

A. Intravenous urogram with tomography.

1) This will detect the majority of the carcinomas and the large adenomas.

B. Skull films.

1) If a pituitary tumor is present and is of sufficient size, there may be widening or erosion of the sella turcica.

C. Lumbosacral spine films.

1) Osteoporosis is best demonstrated here.

D. Chest x-rays.

1) This may detect a tumor which produces ACTH.

a. Bronchogenic carcinomas (small cell) and thymic tumors are the two most common causes of ectopic ACTH syndrome, accounting for two-thirds of the total.

2) Metastases from the adrenal or other primary tumors may be evident.

E. Arteriography and venography.

1) These studies are useful in selected cases.

Management

1. Adenoma.

A. Surgical excision of the involved adrenal usually results in complete resolution of the Cushing's syndrome.

2. Carcinoma.

A. Many of these are large and have involved vital structures or have metastasized so that complete surgical excision is not always possible.

B. Incurable cancers may be treated with a drug called ortho-P-DDD, an agent which inhibits cortisol synthesis and sometimes causes shrinkage of the primary tumor and its metastases.

3. Bilateral adrenal hyperplasia.

A. This pituitary-induced form of Cushing's syndrome may be treated by bilateral adrenalectomy or by irradiation or surgery to the pituitary.

B. Irradiation alone or combined with unilateral adrenalectomy will produce a clinical remission in about 50% of patients with the *less severe forms of the disease.*

1) Advantages.

a. Patients usually do not require any replacement therapy.

b. Hyperpigmentation which is frequently seen after bilateral adrenalectomy is avoided.

2) Disadvantages.

a. It takes 3 to 6 months before remission occurs.

b. 50% of patients treated do not respond and will require additional treatment.

C. Bilateral adrenalectomy is recommended for all patients with moderate to severe forms of the disease.

1) Advantages.

a. This immediately eliminates the most lethal threat to the patient—vascular complications secondary to hypertension.

b. 100% of patients gain a clinical remission.

2) Disadvantages.

a. Patients are required to take replacement therapy for the rest of their lives.

b. The continuing high levels of ACTH and MSH often cause unpleasant hyperpigmentation.

4. ACTH-producing nonendocrine tumors.

A. The primary tumor should be surgically excised if possible.

All patients undergoing unilateral or bilateral adrenalectomies receive hydrocortisone before, during, and after surgery. After unilateral adrenalectomy, replacement therapy is usually not necessary after 1 week. After bilateral adrenalectomy, replacement therapy is gradually tapered down to long range maintenance by the end of 1 week. Most patients require 25 to 37.5 mg of cortisone and 0.1 mg of Florinef daily.

ADRENOGENITAL SYNDROME

This virilizing syndrome is due to overproduction of androgens by the adrenal glands. The usual cause is congenital adrenal hyperplasia secondary to an intra-adrenal enzyme deficiency.

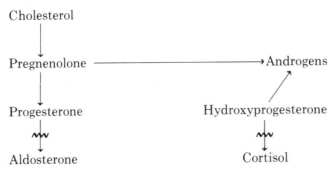

1. Deficiency of the enzyme 21-hydroxylase shown above (⋁⋁) is the most common cause of the adrenogenital (AG) syndrome.

A. This partial steroid block results in an increased secretion of steroids proximal to the block—hydroxyprogesterone and androgens—and decreased secretion of those steroids distal to the block—aldosterone and cortisol.

B. With deficient production of cortisol, there is a compensatory increase in ACTH production by the pituitary gland with resultant adrenal cortical hyperplasia.

1) This overstimulation of the adrenal glands further increases the output of androgens, but since the blockage usually is only partial there is also some increased production of cortisol.

a. This increase in cortisol secretion may be enough to avert any symptoms of cortisol deficiency.

2. Other enzyme deficiencies affecting different portions of the steroid pathway may similarly cause the AG syndrome. An adenoma or carcinoma of the adrenal cortex is a relatively rare cause of the AG syndrome. The clinical picture will be discussed in the chapter on intersex.

ADRENAL CANCER

This rare carcinoma, accounting for only 2% of all cancer deaths, occurs with equal frequency in both men and women, most commonly between the ages of 30 and 50.

Clinical Picture

These tumors may or may not produce adrenal cortical steroids.
1. Functional tumors—80%.
   A. Cushing's syndrome—most common—50% of total.
   B. Virilization—30%.
   C. Both above—10%.
   D. Feminization in men—rare.
   E. Hypoglycemia—rare.
2. Nonfunctional tumors—20%.
   A. Signs and symptoms.
      1) Fever—100%.
      2) Abdominal or chest pain—65%.
      3) Fatigue syndrome—50%.
      4) Abdominal mass—30%.
      5) Metastases in lung or liver.
3. Adrenal carcinomas are usually large when first detected, and so the prognosis generally is poor.
   A. Tumors are *hormonally silent* when small.
      1) They either form no steroids at all (nonfunctional) or they are inefficient synthesizers of steroids (functional).
   B. Tumors are *symptomatically silent* when small.
      1) The hidden location of the adrenal glands make them nonpalpable unless they become very large.
      2) The mobility of adjacent structures prevents dysfunction or pain from compression by an adrenal tumor.
4. Clinical findings suggesting adrenal carcinoma.
   A. Mixed clinical picture, usually Cushing's syndrome with virilization.
   B. Pronounced virilization often associated with marked elevation of the urinary 17-KS, usually over 50 mg/day.
   C. Abrupt onset with rapid progression of symptoms.
   D. Cushing's syndrome in a *child*.
   E. Demonstration of large vascular adrenal tumor.

1) Most adrenal carcinomas are larger than 100 g, whereas benign adenomas are usually less than 50 g.

F. Tumor is usually autonomous with negative dexamethasone suppression and ACTH stimulation tests. The treatment of adrenal carcinoma is discussed in the previous section on Cushing's syndrome.

ADRENAL MEDULLA

The adrenal medulla, originating from the neural crest, has two types of cells—chromaffin cell and the ganglion cell. The chromaffin cell produces the hormones, epinephrine (E) and norepinephrine (NE) in a 4:1 ratio; and tumors derived from these cells are called pheochromocytomas. Ganglion cells produce no hormones, and tumors derived from these cells are called ganglioneuromas (benign) or neuroblastomas (malignant) depending on the degree of differentiation.

PHEOCHROMOCYTOMA

This tumor is the best defined cause of curable hypertension today, accounting for about 5% of all cases of hypertension. At the present time, we have the capability of diagnosing *100%* of these tumors with relatively simple, safe, inexpensive *biochemical tests*; but despite this, an estimated 1,000 persons die each year in the United States from complications of unrecognized pheochromocytoma.

Location of Tumor

Pheochromocytomas may occur wherever chromaffin tissue is found. The largest collection of chromaffin tissue is in the adrenal medulla, but there are discrete collections in association with sympathetic plexuses in the abdomen, pelvis, thorax, and neck (Table V).

1. Multiple tumors are more apt to occur in children and in familial pheochromocytoma with reported incidence of 20 to 50%.

2. About 5% of pheochromocytomas are malignant.

TABLE V
Location of Reported Cases of Pheochromocytoma

	Abdomen—97%	
	Thorax—2-3%	
	Neck— <1%	

	Adults	Children
	%	%
One adrenal	80	50
Both adrenals	10	20
Multiple tumors	10	30
Extra-adrenal	10	20

3. The bladder is an occasional site for extra-adrenal pheochromocytoma.

A. Patients often complain of headache during or after voiding.

B. 50% have hematuria.

C. Tumors are usually identifiable in the bladder wall on cystoscopy, although the overlying mucosa appears uninvolved.

Pathophysiology

These tumors produce catecholamines, and it is the pharmacological effects of these drugs that determine the clinical findings in a given case. There are two points to keep in mind.

1. E and NE have different pharmacological actions.

2. Tumors produce both E and NE, or NE only, but *not E only*.

There are two types of receptor sites in the tissues—alpha and beta—so the net pharmacological effect depends upon how much each of these sites is stimulated (Table VI).

Actions of E and NE

1. NE acts predominantly on alpha-receptors, whereas E acts predominately on beta-receptors but both stimulate the beta-receptors of the heart (Table VII).

2. Mechanism of hypertension.

A. Pressure = cardiac output × total peripheral resistance.

B. NE raises the pressure because it causes widespread arteriolar constriction with resultant *increase in peripheral resistance*.

C. E raises the pressure by its direct effect on the heart, increasing the rate and force of contraction with resultant *increase in cardiac output*.

3. The effect of E and NE on the heart rate is not what you would anticipate.

A. E ⟶ tachycardia.

B. NE ⟶ bradycardia.

C. E + NE ⟶ normal rate.

D. The difference in action of these two drugs on the heart rate is due to a *physiological reflex*.

TABLE VI

Cardiovascular Receptors

Organ	Receptor	Response to stimulation	
Blood vessels	Alpha	Arteriolar constriction (NE)	
	Beta	Arteriolar dilatation (E)	
Heart	Beta only	↑ Rate of contraction	NE
		↑ Force of contraction	+
		Arrhythmias	E

TABLE VII

Drug	Cardiac Stimulation	Mean Pressure ↑	Vagal Stimulation	Net
NE	+	↑↑20%	+ + +	Pulse ↓
E	+ +	↑10%	+	Pulse ↑

1) Both drugs increase the heart rate by their direct effect on the heart, and both drugs decrease the heart rate by evoking vagal stimulation secondary to the mean pressure effect on the baroreceptors.

2) NE causes bradycardia because the vagal effect outweighs the cardiac effect.

3) E causes tachycardia because the cardiac effect outweighs the vagal effect.

4) In the isolated heart, or if the vagal reflex is knocked out by atropine, E and NE have the same action on the heart—increasing heart rate and increasing the strength of contractions.

4. E is responsible for virtually all the symptoms experienced by patients with pheochromocytomas.

A. Patients with tumors producing only NE—50% of the total—may have no symptoms whatever, the only finding being hypertension.

Clinical Picture

1. Hypertension.

A. The majority of patients have a sustained, usually fluctuating, hypertension with only a small number experiencing true paroxysmal hypertension.

2. Sudden attacks or spells are the *hallmark of pheochromocytoma*.

A. Most patients have intermittent rather than persistent symptoms.

B. Attacks appear *suddenly* and are *relatively brief*, usually lasting less than 1 hour, often for only 15 to 30 min.

C. Usually two or more symptoms are experienced together, and each attack tends to be a carbon copy of the previous one.

D. The most common symptoms are the following.

1) Headache—80%.
2) Perspiration—70%.
3) Palpitation—65%.
4) Pallor—40%.
5) Nausea and vomiting—40%.
6) Nervousness and anxiety—35%.

E. The frequency of these attacks is quite variable, but about one-fourth of the patients will have one or more each day, and about two-thirds will have one or more each week.

3. Patients tend to be *thin*.

A. Chronic outpouring of catecholamines causes a hypermetabolic state so that 60% of patients are underweight.

B. Only 10% of these patients are overweight in marked contrast to the majority of patients with essential hypertension who are overweight.

4. Familial occurrence.

A. Pheochromocytomas are frequently familial.

5. Associated disorders.

A. Pheochromocytomas may occur in association with other tumors of neuroectodermal origin such as thyroid or parathyroid or with certain neurocutaneous diseases such as neurofibromatosis, probably because of their common embryological origin from the neural crest.

Diagnosis

1. The diagnosis of pheochromocytoma hinges on *biochemical confirmation* of the overproduction of catecholamines.

Urinary Excretion of Catecholamines and Their Metabolites

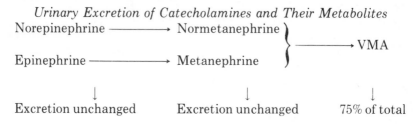

A. Urine normally contains small quantities of the free catecholamines and their metabolites—the metanephrines and vanillylmandelic acid (VMA).

B. The excretion of *all three* of these compounds is persistently high in almost every patient with pheochromocytoma, even those with paroxysmal hypertension.

1) There are no reported cases with negative tests for all three determinations.

C. Urinary total metanephrines.

1) 95% accurate.

2) Widely used because the test is simple and reliable.

3) False positive values may occur if patients are taking a monoamine oxidase inhibitor.

D. Urinary VMA.

1) 90% accurate.

2) Chief end product of catecholamine metabolism.

3) Good screening test because it is a relatively simple test.

4) Drugs have no significant effect on determination.

E. Urinary free catechols.

1) 99% accurate.

2) Technically demanding test so less often used for screening.

3) False values may occur if patient is taking one of the following drugs.

a. Vasopressor drugs—bronchodilators or nasal decongestant sprays.

b. Methyldopa.

c. Fluorescent drugs—tetracycline, chloropromazine, quinidine.

4) *This test aids in localizing the site of the pheochromocytoma.*

a. If the urine contains increased amounts of epinephrine as well as norepinephrine, 90% of the tumors will be found in the adrenal gland, 10% in the organs of Zukerkandl near the origin of the inferior mesenteric artery.

b. However, if the urine contains increased amounts of norepinephrine only, 60 to 70% will be found in the adrenal gland.

2. Pharmacological tests are *not recommended* because they are more hazardous, more expensive, and less accurate than urinary assays.

A. Up to 25% of patients with proven pheochromocytomas may have negative pharmacological tests.

Localization of the Tumor

Once the diagnosis of pheochromocytoma is established by chemical means, do not make a special effort to localize the site of the tumor.

1. There are two reasons for this approach.

A. At surgery, one *always* examines both adrenal glands and the para-aortic and pelvic regions, the usual sites for intra-abdominal tumors.

B. All efforts should be directed at avoiding stimulation of the tumor with catecholamine release.

1) Diagnostic procedures such as arteriography and retroperitoneal gas insufflation often stimulate the tumor and have caused some deaths.

2. X-ray studies.

A. Chest x-rays are performed to rule out the 1 to 2% intrathoracic tumors.

B. A double dose intravenous urogram with tomography is performed, looking for depression and flattening of the upper pole of the kidney.

C. Arteriography and venography are performed only in special cases.

1) If these studies are performed, put the patient on protective pharmacological blockade with alpha-blocker phenoxybenzamine (Dibenzyline) and have an infusion in place with both alpha- and beta-blockers available in the x-ray suite.

3. Urinary free catechol determinations indicate the probability of finding the tumor in the adrenal glands.

4. Plasma catechol determinations via vena cava sampling at different levels are reserved for those patients requiring a *second* surgical exploration for pheochromocytoma—either for a recurrent tumor or for a previously missed tumor.

Management

1. Preoperative.

A. The primary aim of the preoperative preparation and the anesthetic management is to minimize stimuli to the pheochromocytoma to prevent sudden and dangerous alterations in heart rate, rhythm, and arterial pressure.

B. The key point of this preparation is partial alpha-adrenergic blockade with long acting phenoxybenzamine (Dibenzyline).

1) Blood pressure is lowered to normal or near normal levels.

2) Symptoms are lessened.

3) Surgical course is smoother and less hazardous.

4) Plasma volume is expanded with resultant drop in hematocrit of 5 to 10%.

C. Beta-adrenergic blockade is used *only in selected cases*.

1) Persistent tachycardia or arrhythmia despite adequate adrenergic blockade.

2. Surgery.

A. Continous monitoring of blood pressure, central venous pressure, and cardiac activity is established *prior to induction*.

1) Induction is almost as tumor-stimulating as manipulation of the tumor itself during surgery.

B. Every effort is made to minimize or avoid the following stimuli known to cause the tumor to release catecholamines.

1) Positioning of the patient or intubation.

2) Muscle twitching.

3) Hypercarbia or hypoxia.

4) Drugs—curare, cyclopropane.

C. Halothane is the anesthetic agent of choice.

1) It elicits no sympathoadrenal activity, and it blunts the peripheral vascular response to norepinephrine.

D. Surgery.

1) A subcostal transabdominal incision is used, permitting careful examination of both adrenal glands, the para-aortic region, and the pelvis.

2) Removal of the tumor usually causes a significant fall in blood pressure which is readily corrected by volume replacement.

a. If arterial pressure does not drop, or if after a short period of hypotension, it bounces back up to supernormal levels, look around for a second tumor.

b. 10% of patients have more than one tumor, and if the patient is a child or has familial pheochromocytoma, the probability of a second tumor increases to 20 to 50%.

3. Cardiovascular problems during surgery.

A. Hypertension due to stimulation or manipulation of the tumor.

1) This usually is easily controlled with a short acting alpha-adrenergic blocker, phentolamine, given by IV drip.

2) Sodium nitroprusside may be used if the phentolamine drip is ineffectual.

a. It lowers arterial pressure by direct action on smooth muscle, allowing one to titrate the pressure down to the desired level.

B. Hypotension after removal of the tumor.

1) With adequate preoperative alpha-adrenergic blockade, this is usually not a problem.

2) In most cases, volume expansion with albumin and Ringer's lactate corrects the hypotension.

C. Cardiac arrhythmias.

1) Many of these can be controlled by reducing the concentration of halothane and giving IV lidocaine.

2) If arrhythmia does not respond promptly, give 1 to 2 mg of the beta-blocker, propranolol.

ADRENAL CYSTS

Adrenal cysts are relatively rare! They may be classified as follows.

1. Parasitic and epithelial account for 15%.

2. Endothelial and pseudocyst account for 85%.

Endothelial cysts usually arise from lymphangiomatous tissue, are generally small, and are *clinically insignificant*. The most common type of adrenal cyst seen clinically is the pseudocyst, due to hemorrhage into a normal adrenal gland or into an adrenal tumor. One interesting form of this is *calcified adrenal hemorrhage in a newborn*.

1. These newborns are found to have a mass above one or both kidneys, often outlined by a rim of calcification.

2. Usually there is no evidence of adrenal insufficiency or excessive blood loss.

3. The etiology is thought to be *trauma*, since most of these babies are the product of a difficult breech delivery.

4. If the diagnosis is secure, surgery is not necessary.

NEUROBLASTOMA

This malignant adrenal medullary tumor occurs primarily in children, and it will be discussed in conjunction with kidney masses in children in the chapter on the kidney.

REFERENCES AND SUGGESTED FURTHER READING

General

1. Bennett, A. H., Harrison, J. H., and Thorn, G. W. Neoplasms of the adrenal gland. J. Urol. 106:607, 1971.
2. Colapinto, R. F. and Steed, B. L. Arteriography of adrenal tumors. Radiology 100:343, 1971.
3. Dunlop, D. Eighty-six cases of Addison's disease. Br. Med. J. 2:887, 1963.
4. Eisenstein, A. B. Addison's disease: etiology and relationship to other endocrine disorders. Med. Clin. North Am. 52:327, 1968.
5. Hartman, G. W., Witten, D. M., and Weeks, R. E. The role of nephrotomography in the diagnosis of adrenal tumors. Radiology 86:1,030, 1966.

6. Liddle, G. W. Regulation of adrenocortical function in man. In *The Human Adrenal Cortex*. Chap. 2, Harper & Row, New York, 1971.
7. McAlister, W. H. and Koehler, P. R. Diseases of the adrenal. Radiol. Clin. North Am. 5:205, 1967.

Primary Aldosteronism

1. Biglieri, E. G., Stockigt, J. R., and Schambilan, M. Adrenal mineralocorticoids causing hypertension. Am. J. Med. 52:623, 1972.
2. Cain, J. P., Tuck, M. L., Williams, G. H. Dluhy, R. G., and Rosenoff, S. H. The regulation of aldosterone secretion in primary aldosteronism. Am. J. Med. 53:627, 1972.
3. Conn, J. W. Primary aldosteronism. A new clinical syndrome. J. Lab. Clin. Med. 45:3, 1955.
4. Conn, J. W. The evolution of primary aldosteronism. 1954–1967 Harvey Lectures 62:257, 1968.
5. Conn, J. W., Knopf, R. F., and Nesbit, R. M. Clinical characteristics of primary aldosteronism from an analysis of 145 cases. Am. J. Surg. 107:159, 1964.
6. Conn, J. W., Morita, R., Cohen, E. L., Beierwaltes, W. H., McDonald, W. J., and Herwig, K. R. Primary aldosteronism; photoscanning of tumors after administration of [131]I-19-Iodocholesterol. Arch. Intern. Med. 129:417, 1972.
7. Dustan, H. P., Corcoran, A. C., and Page, I. H. Renal function in primary aldosteronism. J. Clin. Invest. 35:1,357, 1956.
8. Horton, R. and Finck, E. Diagnosis and localization in primary aldosteronism. Ann. Intern. Med. 76:885, 1972.
9. Laragh, J. H. Renal and adrenal factors in hypertension: diagnostic approaches. Bull. N. Y. Acad. Med. 45:859, 1969.
10. Melby, J. C., Spark, R. F., Dale, S. L., Egdahl, R. H., and Kahn, P. C. Diagnosis and localization of aldosterone-producing adenomas by adrenal-vein catheterization. N. Engl. J. Med. 277:1,050, 1967.
11. Rovner, O. R., Conn, J. W., Knopf, R. F., Cohen, E. L., and Hsueh, MT-Y. Nature of renal escape from the sodium-retaining effect of aldosterone in primary aldosteronism and in normal subjects. J. Clin. Endocrinol. Metab. 25:53, 1965.
12. Scoggins, B. A., Oddie, C. J., Hare, W. S. C., and Coughlan, J. P. Preoperative lateralization of aldosterone-producing tumors in primary aldosteronism. Ann. Intern. Med. 76:891, 1972.
13. Silen, W., Biglieri, E. G., Slaton, P., and Gilante, P. Management of primary aldosteronism: evaluation of potassium and sodium balance, technic of adrenalectomy and operative results in 24 cases. Ann. Surg. 164:600, 1966.

Cushing's Syndrome
Classic Article

Cushing, H. The basophilic adenomas of the pituitary body and their clinical manifestations. Bull. Johns Hopkins Hosp. 50:137, 1932.

1. Glenn, F., Horwith, H., Peterson, R. E., and Mannix, H. Total adrenalectomy for Cushing's disease. Trans. South. Surg. 73:352, 1971.
2. Liddle, G. W. Tests of pituitary-adrenal suppressibility in the diagnosis of Cushing's syndrome. J. Clin. Endocrinol. Metab. 20:1,539, 1960.
3. Liddle, G. W. The ectopic ACTH syndrome. Cancer Res. 25:1,057, 1965.
4. Nichols, T., Nugent, C. A., and Tyler, F. H. Steroid laboratory tests in the diagnosis of Cushing's syndrome. Am. J. Med. 45:116, 1968.
5. O'Neal, L. W. Correlation between clinical pattern and pathological findings in Cushing's syndrome. Med. Clin. North Am. 52:313, 1968.
6. Rovit, R. L. and Berry, R. Cushing's syndrome and the hypophysis—a re-evaluation of pituitary tumors and hyperadrenalism. J. Neurosurg. 23:270, 1965.
7. Seidenstecker, J. F., Folk, R. L., Wieland, R. G., and Hamwi, G. J. Screening tests for Cushing's syndrome with plasma 11-hydroxycorticosteroids. J.A.M.A. 202:87, 1967.

Adrenogenital Syndrome

1. Eberlein, W. R. and Bongiovanni, A. M. Pathophysiology of congenital adrenal hyperplasia. Metabolism 9:326, 1960.

Adrenal Cancer

1. Hutter, A. M., Jr. and Kayhoe, D. E. Adrenal cortical carcinoma—clinical features of 138 patients. Am. J. Med. 41:572, 1966.
2. Lipsett, M. B., Hertz, R., and Ross, G. T. Clinical and pathophysiologic aspects of adrenocortical carcinoma. Am. J. Med. 35:374, 1963.
3. Schteingart, D. E., Obermann, H. A., Friedman, B. A., and Conn, J. W. Adrenal cortical neoplasms producing Cushing's syndrome—a clinicopathologic study. Cancer 22:1,005, 1968.
4. Wood, K. F., Lees, F., and Rosenthal, F. D. Carcinoma of the adrenal cortex without endocrine effects. Br. J. Surg. 45:41, 1957.
5. Georgetown Tumor Board Conference. Adrenocortical Carcinoma. Am. J. Surg. 109:242, 1965.

Pheochromocytoma

Reviews

1. Hume, D. M. Pheochromocytoma in the adult and in the child. Am. J. Surg. 99:458, 1960.
2. Page, L. B. and Copeland, R. B. Pheochromocytoma. Disease of the Month. Jan. 1968.
3. Stackpole, R. H., Melicow, M. M., and Uson, A. C. Pheochromocytoma in children. Report of 9 cases and review of the first 100 published cases with follow-up studies. J. Pediatr. 63:315, 1963.
4. Thomas, J. E., Rooke, E. D., and Kvale, W. F. The neurologist's experience with pheochromocytoma—a review of 100 cases. J.A.M.A. 197:754, 1966.

Catecholamines

1. Ahlquist, R. P. A study of the adrenotropic receptors. Am. J. Physiol. 153:586, 1948.
2. Crout, J. R. and Sjoerdsma, A. Catecholamines in the localization of pheochromocytoma. Circulation 22:516, 1960.
3. Goldenberg, M., Pines, K. L., Baldwin, E., Greene, D. G., and Roh, C. E. Hemodynamic response of man to norepinephrine and epinephrine and its relation to the problem of hypertension. Am. J. Med. 5:792, 1948.

Diagnosis and Treatment

1. Berry, K. W., Jr., and Scott, E. V. Z. Pheochromocytoma of the bladder. J. Urol. 85:156, 1961.
2. Brown, W. G., Owens, J. B., Berson, A. W., and Henry, S. R. Vanillylmandelic acid screening test for pheochromocytoma and neuroblastoma. Am. J. Clin. Pathol. 46:599, 1966.
3. Crout, J. R. and Brown, B. R., Jr. Anesthetic management of pheochromocytoma—the value of phenoxybenzamine and methoxyflurane. Anesthesiology 30:29, 1969.
4. Engelman, K. Principles in the diagnosis of pheochromocytoma. Bull. N. Y. Acad. Med. 45:851, 1969.
5. Engelman, K. and Sjoerdsma, A. Chronic medical therapy for pheochromocytoma. Ann. Intern. Med. 61:229, 1964.
6. Freis, J. G. and Chamberlin, J. A. Extra-adrenal pheochromocytomas—literature review and report of a cervical pheochromocytoma. Surgery 63:268, 1968.
7. Pertsemlidis, D., Gitlow, S. E., and Kark, A. E. Pheochromocytoma: advances in diagnosis and treatment. Surg. Annu. 4:345, 1972.
8. Rosenberg, J. C. and Varco, R. L. Physiologic and pharmacologic considerations in the management of pheochromocytoma. Surg. Clin. North Am. 47:1,453, 1967.
9. Rossi, P., Young, T. S., and Panke, W. F. Techniques, usefulness and hazards of arteriography of pheochromocytoma. Review of 99 cases. J.A.M.A. 205:547, 1968.

20
Intersexuality

JAY Y. GILLENWATER

Genital anomalies that require plastic surgical procedures frequently are associated with or are the result of one of the intersex disorders. It is very important to recognize the disorders of abnormal sexual development early because some are life-threatening (congenital adrenogenital syndrome); in some, the sex of rearing will need to be changed to preserve fertility (female pseudohermaphroditism resulting from adrenogenital syndrome); and in some, there is a high incidence of malignancy of the gonad (testicular feminization). It is also important to assign the appropriate sex early to avoid psychological problems.

1. Criteria of sex. In evaluating patients with a question of intersexuality, it is helpful to define the five morphological criteria of sex.

    1) Chromosomal sex.

    2) Gonadal structure.

    3) Morphology of internal genitalia.

    4) External genital appearance.

    5) Hormonal status.

The two psychological criteria of sex are:

    1) Sex of rearing.

    2) Psychological gender role.

Intersexuality usually is defined as one or more contradictions in the five morphological criteria of sex. The terms "male" or "female pseudohermaphrodite" are assigned according to whether the gonads are testes or ovaries, and "true hermaphroditism" defines the individual having both gonadal structures.

2. Chromosomal sex.

A. Karyotyping. The chromosomal sex can be evaluated by karyotyping (the basic process by which chromosomes are identified and studied) or by studying the nuclear chromatin pattern (Barr bodies). The first accurate count of human chromosomes was made by J. H. Tijo and Albert Levan in 1956.[10] In the succeeding 14 years, much information has been gathered

---

* The material in this chapter first appeared in *Plastic and Reconstructive Surgery of the Genital Area*, edited by Charles E. Horton, Chap. 5, Little Brown & Co., Boston, 1973, and an article by J. Y. Gillenwater, A. W. Wyker, Jr., M. Birdsong, and W. N. Thornton, J. Urol. 103:500, 1970.

concerning the chromosomal structure in the various intersex disorders. Karyotyping is done by culturing human cells, usually lymphocytes, and by arresting the division in metaphase using a substance such as colchicine. In metaphase, the chromosomes are discrete and easily visible; when placed in a hypotonic solution, the cell swells, spreading the chromosomes apart. The preparation is fixed, stained, and photographed, and the photograph is cut so that the chromosomes can be arranged in a standardized order. Humans have 46 chromosomes, of which 44 are autosomes and two are sex chromosomes. The normal female has 44 autosomes and 2 X sex chromosomes (46/XX). The normal male has 44 autosomes and an X and Y sex chromosome (46/XY). Chromosomal mosaicism exists when different cell lines have varying numbers or types of chromosomes in the same individual. Structural abnormalities of individual chromosomes have been described that are caused by translocation or the formation of an isochromosome by an error in meiosis.

B. Barr body. In 1949 Barr and Betram[1] noted that it was possible to identify the sex of an individual by a clump of chromatin that is visible in the nuclei of female cells and absent from those of males. The nuclear chromatin, or Barr body, is found in most tissue of the female with the exception of the primary oocyte. It usually is found in 20% or more of the nuclei of cells examined from the normal female, and in less than 1 to 2% of cells from the normal male. An individual with no chromatin bodies is said to be "chromatin-negative"; one having 5% or more chromatin bodies is said to be "chromatin-positive."

C. Sex chromosome. The Y chromosome is believed to be the male organizer that leads to the differentiation of a testis. The testis, through the inducer substance and testosterone secretion, leads to male genital differentiation. There are no true Y-linked disorders. However, there are more than 75 X-linked disorders. The 47/XXX has a decreased IQ, and the 48/XXXX has an even greater reduction in IQ.

3. Gonadal sex. Of the various criteria of sex, probably the most important and most difficult to obtain is the microscopic identity of the gonad. It is important that the gonadal structure be identified by microscopic examination, since the gross appearance may be deceptive. The identity of the gonad is necessary to classify the true hermaphrodite and to confirm the diagnosis of male or female pseudohermaphroditism.

4. Morphology of internal genitalia. The morphology of the internal genitalia may be extremely variable, since every normal embryo has both wolffian and mullerian ducts. The development into male internal genitalia with inhibition of female structures is dependent on the male gonadal inducer substance. The identity of the internal genitalia may influence the choice of sex of rearing, as in the female with adrenogenital syndrome, since fertility may be possible when the individual is reared as a female. The morphology of the internal genitalia may be identified by using appropriate x-ray studies or by laparotomy.

5. External genital appearance. The appearance of the external genitalia is the most readily identifiable criterion for sex differentiation, but it is the least reliable. The assignment of sex usually is based on the appearance of the external genitalia; however, ambiguity of external genitalia is often the first suggestion that an intersex problem exists. The external genital development will influence the assignment of sex; if an individual cannot function sexually as a male, the female sex gender will most often be assigned. It is much easier surgically to create a functioning vagina than a functioning phallus.

6. Hormonal sex. The hormonal environment is important in determining the appearance of the external genitalia and is responsible for the secondary sex characteristics. The hormonal state frequently may not correlate with the gonadal tissue, as in cases of testicular feminization or congenital adrenal hyperplasia. The knowledge of hormonal secretions is important in defining and treating intersexuality.

7. Psychological criteria of sex. The sex of rearing usually is assigned to the patient by the physician and parents. It has been shown by Money et al.[7] that sexual orientation depends upon assignment of sex and rearing rather than upon genetic determination. Unless there is some contradiction in the five morphological criteria of sex, there is, by definition, no intersexuality. Thus the individual who sees himself in a contradictory gender role (e.g., a transvestite) does not belong to any of the various hermaphroditic classifications per se. However, the gender role of the individual is an extremely important consideration when deciding the sex of rearing because of the psychological problems that may be caused or prevented by the correct assignment of sex.

8. Normal sexual development.

A. Undifferentiated gonad. The undifferentiated gonad appears in the fetus about the 4th week as a genital ridge medial to the mesonephros, and it develops into either an ovary or a testis. The genetic sex is believed to determine gonodal sex by inhibiting one part of the gonad.

B. Internal genitalia. The further differentiation of the internal genitalia is delayed until the 25- to 30-mm (8th to 9th week) stage. According to the work of Jost,[5] this differentiation is dependent upon whether a normally functioning testis is present. In a series of experiments on rabbits (Fig. 1), Jost[5] found that if the gonad was removed (either testis or ovary) prior to this stage of differentiation of the internal genitalia, the wolffian duct system was inhibited, and the internal and external genitalia developed toward female organogenesis. If the testis was removed from one side, then only that side developed along female lines with inhibition of that wolffian duct. If a testis was transplanted to one side, that side developed along male lines with development of the wolffian duct and inhibition of the mullerian duct system. He found that no available synthetic androgen could cause these local changes of the fetal internal genitalia; thus, he postulated that

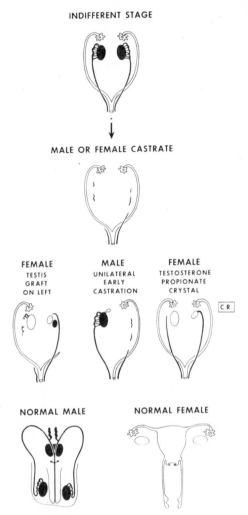

INDIFFERENT STAGE

MALE OR FEMALE CASTRATE

FEMALE
TESTIS
GRAFT
ON LEFT

MALE
UNILATERAL
EARLY
CASTRATION

FEMALE
TESTOSTERONE
PROPIONATE
CRYSTAL

NORMAL MALE

NORMAL FEMALE

Fig. 1. Schematic representation of the development of the internal and external genitalia as proposed by Jost.

the fetal testes have some other masculinizing hormone that causes the local effects of stimulating the wolffian duct and inhibiting the mullerian duct in the fetus. When a crystal of testosterone propionate was implanted unilaterally, there was persistence of the complete wolffian duct system and no inhibition of the mullerian duct. The external genitalia would become masculinized. Jost found that the stage of development at which the testis was removed or implanted was critical. If differentiation was already proceeding along male lines, then the later removal of the testis (or later malfunction of the testis) would produce a wide variety of abnormalities of the mullerian and wolffian duct systems. Thus, any abnormality of the internal duct systems could be explained by the presence or absence of the male inducer substance at various stages of development.

C. Summary of normal sexual development. In summary, Jost's classic work shows that the normal testis possesses a locally acting male inducer substance that inhibits the mullerian duct system and stimulates the wolffian duct system. In the absence of this inducer substance, the mullerian structures persist and the wolffian duct structures disappear. If not virilized, the external genitalia also will progress along female lines.

D. External genitalia. The external genitalia remain in an undifferentiated state until the 12th fetal week.

E. Adrenal development. The human adrenal primordium appears during the 16th fetal week and reaches its maximal relative size in the 3rd and 4th fetal months. This is the same period in which androgen stimulus is necessary to masculinize the external genitalia and urogenital sinus in the female fetus to produce a female pseudohermaphrodite.

9. Effect of androgen in fetal sexual development. The age of the fetus is a critical factor in the response of the sex primordia to androgens, since the capacity to stimulate the external genitalia, urogenital sinus, and development of the wolffian duct is limited to a specific period of life. For the development of a complete phallic urethra in the female fetus, the androgenic stimulus must occur before the 11th fetal week. This concept is supported both by experimental work and by observations in humans. Androgens have been found to be readily transmitted across the placental barrier in humans. They can modify female fetal development of the external genitalia, urogenital sinus and, rarely, the wolffian duct. Overzier[8] stated that the differentiation of the genital ducts is almost complete at the time the fetal adrenal cortex begins to produce androgens, but seminal vesicles and prostatic glands have been found in female patients with noticeable virilism. It is of interest that four cases of masculinization of the female infant have been reported after the mother had received stilbestrol during pregnancy. It was postulated that perhaps this effect was due to adrenal hyperplasia consequent to the administration of estrogens. Conversely, feminization of the male fetus leading to a severe hypospadias has been reported after maternal administration of estrogens and progesterones.

A. Classification of masculinization of the urogenital sinus. Prader[9] has divided the different degrees of masculinization of the urogenital sinus into five types (Fig. 2):

Type 1. Androgen administration after the 20th week of fetal life. The vulva has been formed and only clitoral hypertrophy results.

Type 2. Androgen administration after the 19th week of fetal life. The vulva gapes but is funnel-shaped and the clitoris is enlarged. The vagina and urethra open separately.

Type 3. Effect of androgens at about the 14th to 15th fetal week. The

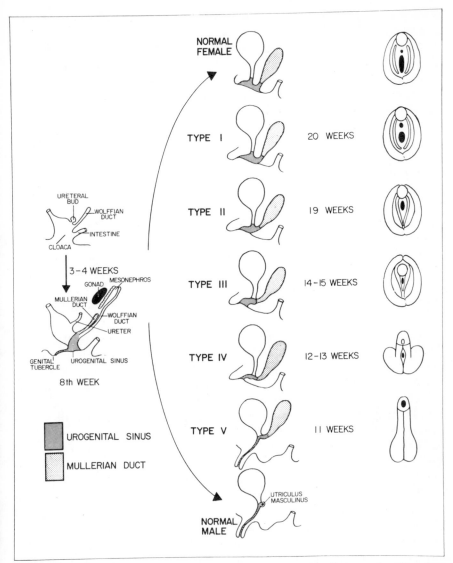

Fig. 2. Effect of androgenic hormones on the development of mullerian and wolffian ducts (adapted from original description by Prader[10]).

vagina and urethra open into a common urogenital sinus. The clitoris is larger and penis-like.

Type 4. Effects of androgens at about the 12th to 13th fetal week. The perineum is thrust forward, the narrow urogenital sinus is formed, and the labia form a bifid scrotum. The urogenital sinus opens at the base of the penis corresponding to a hypospadial penis.

Type 5. Effect of androgens at about the 11th week of fetal life. The external genitalia have a male appearance except for the absence of testes in the scrotum.

10. Klinefelter's syndrome. In 1942, Klinefelter, Reifenstein, and Albright[6] described nine men who had small testes, azoospermia, elevated urinary gonadotropins, normal external genitalia, and gynecomastia.

A. Gonad. Testicular biopsies revealed hypoplastic, sclerotic, and hyalinized tubules. The Leydig cells were clumped in some patients and even appeared hyperplastic.

B. Genitalia. In Klinefelter's syndrome, the internal and external genitalia are as those of the normal male. Gynecomastia is present in some but not all of these patients.

C. Hormone. The patients with Klinefelter's syndrome have been shown to have a decrease in plasma testosterone.

D. Karyotype. The contradiction in the morphological criteria of sex results from the karyotype abnormality of an extra X chromosome (47/XXY). Thus, these individuals also would be chromatin-positive. Other karyotypes of 48/XXXY, 49/XXXXY, 49/XXXYY, and 46/XX have been described. Eighty percent of patients with Klinefelter's syndrome are chromatin-positive. The incidence is reported to be 1 in 400 live births and 1 in 100 male mental defectives.

The patients with Klinefelter's syndrome usually are seen by the physician because of gynecomastia or infertility. The diagnosis can be established by obtaining a sperm count, chromatin pattern, or testicular biopsy specimen. The patients usually have a normal male phenotype, but the testes are small and firm. In the patients with small testes resulting from trauma or postinflammatory disease, the testes ordinarily are not as firm as those of the Klinefelter patients.

11. Turner's syndrome (gonadal dysgenesis). Turner's syndrome is a term used synonymously with gonadal dysgenesis. The syndrome includes females of short stature who have congenital anomalies, hypoestrinism, streak gonads, and increased urinary gonadotropins. Other abnormalities encountered in females who have Turner's syndrome include sexual infantilism, primary amenorrhea, webbing of the neck, shield chest, pigmented moles, lymphedema, mental retardation, coarctation of the aorta, deafness, cubitus valgus, retardation of growth, and low set ears. In the newborn female, the syndrome may present as webbing of the neck and nonpitting edema of hands and feet due to large, dilated vascular spaces. A negative chromatin pattern would verify the gonadal dysgenesis. However, 20 to 40% of such individuals have positive buccal smears.

A. Karyotype. In gonadal dysgenesis, it is postulated that there is a defect in the second sex chromosome in some of the patient's cells. The predominant group is 45/XO and chromatin-negative. Some patients are mosaics, with the most common combination being XO/XX. Some patients have been reported with 46/XX and are believed to have a structural abnormality of the second X.

B. Genitalia. The internal and external genitalia are those of an immature female.

C. Gonad. The gonads usually are described as "streak gonads."

D. Hormone. The hormone studies show hypoestrinism with increased urinary gonadotropins.

Turner's syndrome is believed to represent the human counterpart of the cases in Jost's studies involving rabbits in which the absence of a gonad leads to female differentiation of the internal and external genitalia. The failure of the primitive germ cells to reach the gonad has been postulated as one of the causes of streak gonads.

12. Mixed gonadal dysgenesis. Recently a syndrome of intersexuality has been described which may bridge the gap between Turner's syndrome and male pseudohermaphroditism.

A. Gonad. The gonadal structures have included the following manifestations:

1) An immature inguinal testis on one side and a streak gonad on the other.

2) A streak gonad on one side and gonadal tumor on the other.

3) Unilateral gonadal agenesis.

B. Genitalia. The internal genitalia have usually been symmetrical Fallopian tubes, uterus, and upper vagina. The external genitalia have a wide spectrum including normal and hypospadiac penis, females with clitormegaly, Turner's phenotype, and normal female. Most have been reared as females.

C. Karyotype. All reported cases have been chromatin-negative.

13. True hermaphrodites. The true hermaphrodite is an individual who has both ovarian and testicular tissue. Hermaphrodites usually have been classified according to location and lateralization of the conflicting gonads.

A. Gonad. The gonads may be combined, such as ovotestes, or there may be an ovary and a testis or an ovary or testis with or without an ovotestis.

B. Genitalia. The internal and external genital differentiation can vary widely from almost normal female to male with some degree of hypospadias. Most hermaphrodites have been raised as males (70%), most develop gynecomastia (75%), and half of them menstruate.

C. Karyotype. The predominant karyotype is 46/XX, and the nuclear chromatin test is positive.

D. Hormone. The hormonal status has been variable. The diagnosis of true hermaphroditism can be made only by microscopic confirmation of the presence of both gonadal and testicular tissue.

The following case history (U.V.H. #57 42 20) has been reported: An infant was born at the University of Virginia Hospital on 2-23-67 with ambiguous external genitalia. The mother's pregnancy had been normal. No medications had been taken. Examination of the genitalia showed a 3.5-cm phallus with a bifid scrotum and perineal hypospadias as well as cryptorchidism. The karyotyping showed 46/XX chromosomes, and the urinary steroid excretion was normal. The parents were told that the child had an intersex problem and that laparotomy and endoscopy should be performed when the child was older. It was suggested that the child be reared as a female. At 4 months of age, the child was readmitted and ketosteroids were found to be less than 2 mg/24 hours, which is normal for that age. Endoscopy showed a female type of urogenital sinus leading to a normal bladder and vagina, with a normal cervix at the apex. A left inguinal hernia was palpable, with a 1-cm gonadal structure. Laparotomy showed a Fallopian tube and ovotestis in the left inguinal hernia. The uterus had a suggestion of bicornuate configuration and the right gonad was also an ovotestis. Both gonads and the left Fallopian tube were removed. The urogenital sinus was opened and the clitoris partially amputated during another hospitalization at 1 year of age, which provided normal appearing external genitalia.

This case demonstrates the work-up of infants with ambiguous genitalia and chromatin-positive nuclear pattern. When the history or hormonal studies do not suggest female pseudohermaphroditism, it is necessary to define the internal genitalia and gonads by endoscopy and laparotomy to make the diagnosis and to remove contradictory gonadal elements.

14. Male pseudohermaphroditism. Male pseudohermaphrodites are individuals with a testis and XY sex chromosomes who have some failure in virilization. The most common condition seen in this group is the testicular feminization syndrome. These patients are phenotypic females whose breasts may be large but the vagina is usually small or obliterated.

A. Gonad. The gonad is a testis and is usually located in a hernia. Microscopic examination of the testis reveals it to be immature and without spermatogenesis.

B. Genitalia. The internal genitalia are rudimentary and may include a uterus, Fallopian tubes, or spermatic ducts.

C. Hormones. The hormonal studies show normal male urinary 17-ketosteroids and normal male plasma testosterone levels. The pathogenesis of testicular feminization is believed to be a lack of end organ response to androgen.

Other descriptions of patients with testes and varying degrees of inadequacy of virilization have been reported by Lubs, Gilbert-Dreyfus, and Reifenstein.

15. Female pseudohermaphroditism. Female pseudohermaphroditism is seen in patients whose gonads are ovaries and who have various degrees of masculinization. The most common cause of this disorder is the adrenogenital syndrome due to congenital adrenocortical hyperplasia. Masculinization of the female fetus also is seen after maternal administration of androgens, certain progesterones, and even estrogens, and is also seen with maternal arrhenoblastoma.

The adrenogenital syndrome is caused by adrenal cortical hyperplasia secondary to an inheritable inborn error of metabolism. The incidence suggests that an autosomal recessive genetic factor is responsible. The basic defect is a congenital partial or complete absence of one or several adrenal enzymes necessary for hydrocortisone production with the resultant accumulation of androgenic steroidal precursors.

Three types of enzymatic defects that cause virilization and three rare enzymatic defects that cause little virilization have been described in congenital adrenal hyperplasia.

A. 21-Hydroxylase. The most common enzymatic defect is that of the 21-hydroxylase. This defect may be partial, with clinical manifestation of virilism and normal sodium conservation. A complete block in the 21-hydroxylase has been proposed as a cause of salt and water loss as well as virilization.

B. 11-Hydroxylase. The uncommon 11-hydroxylase enzyme defect produces virilization and hypertension.

C. 3-β-Hydroxysteroid dehydrogenase. The rare 3-β-hydroxysteroid dehydrogenase defect causes disturbance in the early stages of hormonal synthesis in both the gonad and adrenal glands. In the male fetus, there are varying degrees of feminization of the external genitalia and urogenital sinus. The female fetus has less virilization than with the two preceding enzymatic defects. Most patients with this disorder have a tendency to lose salt.

D. 17-Hydroxylase. The rare 17-hydroxylase defects produce sexual infantilism, hypertension, and hypokalemic alkalosis.

E. 20-Hydroxylase. The 20-hydroxylase defect, which is also rare, prevents the conversion of cholesterol to the active steroids and has been called "congenital lipoid adrenal hyperplasia." This uncommon condition usually involves the gonads as well as the adrenal gland; in most cases, it is fatal. Females show little virilization. Males exhibit varying degrees of male pseudohermaphroditism with female external genitalia because of the absence of androgen.

Adrenal hyperplasia is secondary to increased adrenocorticotropic hormone production by the pituitary because of deficient hydrocortisone production disrupting the adrenal-hypothalmic pituitary feedback mechanisms. The virilization is due to overproduction of adrenal androgens. Thirty percent of these patients have a sufficient decrease in hydrocortisone and aldosterone to be threatened by an addisonian crisis.

The following case history (U.V.H. #35 75 49) is of interest. This patient, born in 1949, appeared to be a normal, Negro male infant when seen at the age of 4 months except for poor nutritional development and bilateral cryptorchidism. During his 1st year he had repeated respiratory infections and gastroenteritis, weighing only 10 pounds at the age of 10 months. There was a sudden improvement in his health and growth at 1 year of age. At 15 months of age he weighed 25 pounds and was 30 inches tall. When he was 4 years old, he was much larger than his 8-year-old sister; he weighed 80 pounds and was 50 inches tall. He had heavy muscular development, a deep voice, a beard, pubic hair, large male genitalia and mild hypertension (150/90 mm Hg). The patient developed pubic hair at 1 year of age, a deepening voice and large phallus by 1 ½ years, and at the age of 3 ½ he had begun to grow a beard. X-rays of his wrists revealed a bone age of 13 years. The 24-hour urinary 17-ketosteroid secretion was 68 mg/24 hours. He was referred to The University of Virginia Hospital for evaluation with a diagnosis of adrenogenital syndrome.

Studies here in 1953 of the 4-year-old patient revealed him to have facial, pubic, and axillary hair (Fig. 3). He had a large penis with a normal urethral opening. The urinary ketosteroid secretion ranged between 56 and 76 mg/24 hours and was suppressed to 4 mg/24 hours on cortisone. Blood pressure was 150/90 mm Hg. The intravenous urogram and skull x-rays were normal. A skin biopsy specimen was interpreted as chromatin-negative with no Barr bodies, and it was compatible with a male pattern. The patient was treated with cortisone.

He was readmitted in March of 1956 at the age of 7 years because of intermittent hematuria. Physical examination showed adult male hair distribution, some enlargement of the breasts, bilateral undescended testes, and an adult-sized phallus with the urethral opening at the end of the glans penis. Urinalysis confirmed the intermittent hematuria. The intravenous urogram was normal, and the bone age was found to be 14 years. Cystoendoscopy was interpreted as showing a normal bladder and congestion of the "prostatic urethra and verumontanum." The patient was operated upon for the cryptorchidism through a left Gibson incision, and the retroperitoneal area from the bladder to the kidney was explored without locating a vas deferens or testis. The incision was enlarged and the peritoneal cavity opened; enlarged adrenals were found but no testis could be located. The patient continued to have intermittent hematuria.

In August of 1959, the patient was re-evaluated. Cystoendoscopy revealed a complete penile urethra and a blood-filled vagina opening into the posterior urethra. This finding was confirmed by urethrograms. With bimanual pelvic examination, a uterus and gonads were palpated. Buccal mucosal smears and review of the patient's old skin biopsy specimen revealed a chromatin-positive pattern. The patient was evaluated by the psychiatrists and was found to have a definitely male gender role. Abdominal exploration revealed a uterus and two normal ovaries. A hysterectomy and bilateral oophorectomy were performed. He has continued on cortisone treatment and has had some problems with recurrent backache and emotional adjustment.

16. Differential diagnosis of intersexuality. The intersex states usually are suspected when ambiguity of the external genitalia is noted. Hypospadias, a small phallus, cryptorchidism, or the presence of palpable masses in the groin or labia of an infant with female genitalia should suggest a sexual

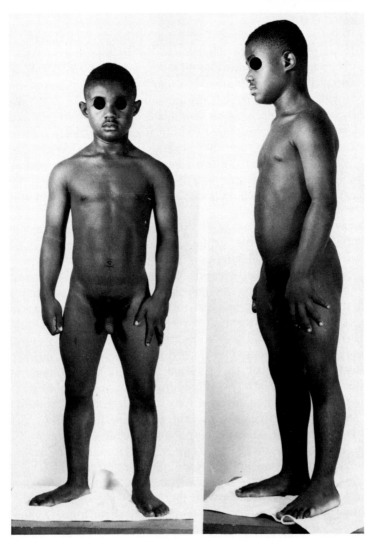

Fig. 3. Patient with adrenogenital syndrome at 4 years of age with masculinization and increased growth.

abnormality. A history of siblings with an intersex state, the phenotype of Turner's syndrome with a short stature or webbed neck, or small testes in an infertile male may be the first clues to an abnormal sexual development.

When the question of intersexuality arises, it can be diagnosed easily by defining the five morphological criteria of sex.

1) Chromosomal sex.
2) Gonadal structure.
3) Morphology of internal genitalia.
4) External genital appearance.

5) Hormonal status.

Table I shows a scheme modified from Wilkins[11] and Bunge.[2] The sex chromatin pattern should be determined by the buccal or vaginal smear. This test is obtained easily and should be the first performed, taking care to obtain good staining and fixation in order to compare the specimen with known controls that are done simultaneously. If the test is interpreted incorrectly, it can certainly result in a misdirected diagnosis, as in our case of adrenogenital syndrome. The newborn female may have lower nuclear chromatin counts during her first several days of life. When there is a positive chromatin nuclear pattern in an individual with a sexual abnormality, the differential diagnosis will be one of the following: 1) female pseudohermaphroditism, 2) true hermaphroditism, 3) Klinefelter's syndrome, or 4) gonadal aplasia.

If there is no history of maternal androgen exposure from drugs or tumor during pregnancy, then the urinary 17-ketosteroid excretion should be determined. In congenital adrenal hyperplasia there is elevation in the 24-hour excretion of 17-ketosteroids, pregnanetriol, 11-ketopregnanetriol, and 17-ketogenic steroids (the last are elevated because they include pregnanetriol and 11-ketopregnanetriol). Occasionally the 17-ketosteroids are elevated normally during the 1st week of life, and it may be necessary to repeat the measurement at 2 or 3 weeks of age.

With normal ketosteroids and no history of exposure to androgens, the morphological features of the internal genitalia and gonads must be determined to differentiate true hermaphroditism from nonadrenal female pseudohermaphroditism. Urethrography and urethroscopy should be performed initially to define the internal genitalia. Laparotomy usually is necessary to define the gonadal morphological characteristics and internal genitalia. If cystogenic study reveals an XX/XY mosaic, the patient should have a laparotomy to rule out true hermaphroditism. All female pseudohermaphrodites are chromatin-positive and 46/XX. In the classic case of congenital adrenal hyperplasia with increased 17-ketosteroids, the female sex chromatin 46/XX, and internal female genitalia, surgical exploration is unnecessary, and the patient should be reared as a female.

Patients having ambiguous external genitalia with a chromatin-negative nuclear pattern can be true hermaphrodites, male pseudohermaphrodites, or have mixed gonadal dysgenesis. These patients should be given careful urethroscopic and urethrographic examination to rule out a communicating sinus or uterine canal. If bilateral scrotal gonads are palpable, the individual is most likely a male pseudohermaphrodite. In this group, laparotomy usually is necessary to establish the diagnosis.

17. Management of intersex states. The management of patients with intersex problems must be individualized. The ideal goal is the achievement of fertility, coital function, and normal psychological adjustment. When an intersex problem is suspected in an infant, it is important that an accurate and orderly examination be accomplished so the correct gender role will be assigned. This procedure can be carried out more effectively at a

TABLE I

Workup of Infants with Ambiguous Genitalia

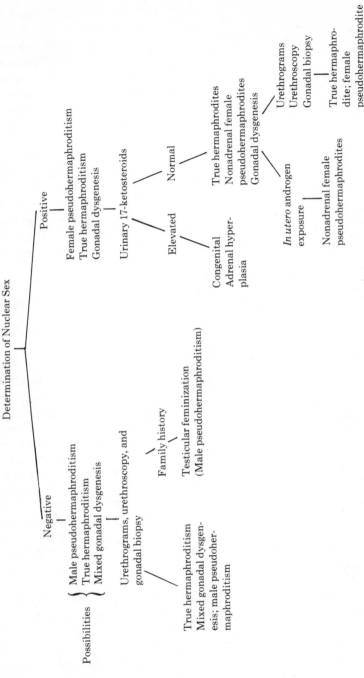

Determination of Nuclear Sex

Possibilities

Negative

Male pseudohermaphroditism
True hermaphroditism
Mixed gonadal dysgenesis

Urethrograms, urethroscopy, and gonadal biopsy

Family history

Testicular feminization
(Male pseudohermaphroditism)

True hermaphroditism
Mixed gonadal dysgenesis; male pseudohermaphroditism

Positive

Female pseudohermaphroditism
True hermaphroditism
Gonadal dysgenesis

Urinary 17-ketosteroids

Elevated

Congenital Adrenal hyperplasia

Normal

True hermaphrodites
Nonadrenal female pseudohermaphrodites
Gonadal dysgenesis

In utero androgen exposure

Nonadrenal female pseudohermaphrodites

Urethrograms
Urethroscopy
Gonadal biopsy

True hermaphrodite; female pseudohermaphrodite
Gonadal dysgenesis
(Klinefelter)

medical center because of the availability of laboratory facilities and greater clinical experience. It is important that the parents of a child with intersex problems understand that there is a possibility of incomplete sexual development which can usually be completed surgically. Parents should not be told that the child is "half-boy and half-girl." Money, Hampson, and Hampson[7] have shown that the psychological sex of an individual is not governed by the gonadal or anatomical state, but by many environmental factors. Thus, it is vital that the child receive the complete series of examinations and tests necessary to obtain an accurate diagnosis and a sexual assignment corresponding with the most appropriate sexual function.

A. Female pseudohermaphroditism. Female pseudohermaphrodites are capable of maturing as fertile women and should be raised as females if the diagnosis is made early. The patients with adrenal hyperplasia usually will need some steroid replacement, since 30% will develop adrenal insufficiency. Plastic surgical procedures may be necessary to externalize the vagina.

B. Male pseudohermaphroditism. Male pseudohermaphrodites usually should be reared according to the function of the external genitalia, since all are infertile. The external genitalia may vary from normal male to male with hypospadias. In patients with testicular feminization, most authorities believe that the testes should be removed, since one-third of the reported patients over age 30 had a gonadal tumor. Many physicians allow the testes to remain until puberty to permit a "normal" puberty. When the testes are removed, substitute estrogen therapy is essential to maintain feminization. The female siblings of patients should have nuclear chromatin pattern studies performed since testicular feminization is familial. In patients with a male phenotype and hypospadias, the hypospadias can be repaired before school years begin.

C. True hermaphroditism. The true hermaphrodite should be reared in the gender role most appropriate to the function of the external genitalia. The intra-abdominal testes should be removed to prevent malignancy. Certainly any gonadal element which would conflict with external genitalia should be removed. Since it is not possible to separate surgically most ovotestes, they should be removed. Thus, the only gonadal structure that should not be removed in the true hermaphrodite is a remaining, normal, unilateral ovary in the phenotypic female.

Infants with bilateral cryptorchidism and hypospadias should have a nuclear chromatin pattern study performed while in the nursery to rule out intersexuality. The high incidence of upper urinary tract abnormalities also warrants an intravenous urogram at this time.

REFERENCES AND SUGGESTED FURTHER READING

1. Barr, M. S. and Betram, E. G. The morphological distinction between neurone of the male and female, and the behavior of the nucleolar satellite during accelerated nucleoprotein synthesis. Nature 163:676, 1949.
2. Bunge, R. G. Intersexuality. In *Urology*, edited by W. F. Campbell and W. H. Harrison. W.

B. Saunders, Philadelphia, 1970.
3. Federman, D. D. *Abnormal Sexual Development.* W. B. Saunders, Philadelphia, 1968.
4. Gillenwater, J. Y., Wyker, A. W., Birdsong, M., and Thornton, W. N. Adrenogenital syndrome producing female pseudohermaphroditism with a phallic urethra. J. Urol. 103:500, 1970.
5. Jost, A. Embryonic sexual differentiation. In *Hermaphroditism, Genital Anomalies and Related Endocrine Disorders*, edited by H. W. Jones, Jr. and W. W. Scott. Williams & Wilkins, Baltimore, 1958.
6. Klinefelter, H. F., Reifenstein, E. C., and Albright, F. Syndrome characterized by gynecomastia, aspermatogenesis without A-Leydigism, and increased excretion of follicle-stimulating hormone. J. Clin. Endocrinol. Metab. 2:615, 1942.
7. Money, J., Hampson, J. G., and Hampson, J. L. Hermaphroditism: recommendations concerning assignment of sex, change of sex, and psychological management. Bull. Johns Hopkins Hosp. 97:284, 1955.
8. Overzier, C. Induzierter pseudohermaphroditism. In *Die Intersexualitat*, edited by C. Overzier, p. 394. Georg Thieme, Stuttgart, 1961.
9. Prader, V. A. Volkommen mannliche aubere genitalentwicklung und salzverlust und salzverlustsyndrom be: Madchen mit kongenitalem andronogenitalem syndrom. Helv. Paediatr. Acta 13:5, 1958.
10. Tijo, J. H. and Levan, A. The chromosome number of man. Hereditas 42:1, 1956.
11. Wilkins, L. *The Diagnosis and Treatment of Endocrine Disorders in Childhood and Adolescence.* Charles C Thomas, Srpingfield, Ill., 1966.

21

Tuberculosis and Other Specific Infections

ARTHUR W. WYKER, JR.

TUBERCULOSIS

Tuberculosis is a generalized infectious disease that may affect nearly every organ of the body, but since the tubercle bacilli usually enter via the respiratory tract, pulmonary disease predominates. During the initial pulmonary infection, blood-borne tubercle bacilli reach the kidneys and eventually cause renal tuberculosis 4 to 40 years later. Four percent of patients with pulmonary tuberculosis will eventually develop renal tuberculosis.

The introduction of effective antituberculous drugs over 20 years ago has markedly reduced the incidence, morbidity, and mortality from all forms of tuberculosis resulting in the current low new case rate of 20 per 100,000 (42,000 per year) and death rate of 3 per 100,000 (6,000 per year). This means that in the United States 7 new cases are reported each year for every death. Because of the time lag of 4 to 40 years between the primary pulmonary infection and the appearance of urinary tuberculosis, it is not surprising that the incidence of genitourinary tuberculosis has only declined within the past 5 years.

Formerly, tuberculosis was chiefly a disease of young adults in the 15 to 40 age group, but most of the cases now occur in older persons with a ratio of male to female cases of 2:1. At the present time, half of the patients with genitourinary tuberculosis are 15 to 40; half are over 40 years of age.

GENITOURINARY TUBERCULOSIS

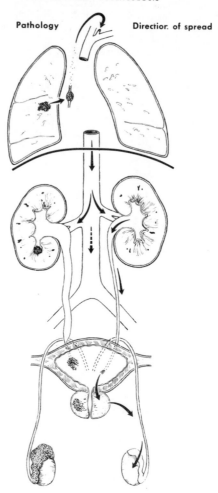

Fig. 1.

Pathogenesis and Pathology

There are three phases in the development of genitourinary tuberculosis. 1. Primary pulmonary infection, at which time blood-borne tubercle bacilli reach the kidney.

2. Latent period, lasting 4 to 40 years.

3. Endogenous reactivation of dormant renal foci with resultant clinically manifest renal tuberculosis.

Primary Pulmonary Infection

1. Preallergic phase.

A. Air-borne tubercle bacilli previously coughed into the air by someone with active pulmonary tuberculosis are inhaled and then deposited deep in the airway of the respiratory tract, producing a minute focus of tuberculous pneumonia.

B. These tubercle bacilli invoke only a nonspecific foreign body reaction and the patient is clinically asymptomatic.

C. Lymphatic spread.

1) Almost as soon as infection takes place, bacilli begin to leave the primary focus and are carried through the lymphatics to the hilar lymph nodes.

2) Most of the tubercle bacilli remain trapped here, but a few pass through the lymph nodes to reach the blood stream via lymphatic venous communication and are then disseminated throughout the body.

3) Small numbers of tubercle bacilli reach many areas of the body via this *lymphohematogenous dissemination*, but the most common sites of embolic seeding are the apices of the lungs, spleen, and the *renal cortices*.

D. The fate of these metastatic foci in the renal cortex depends upon the number of bacilli implanted and the degree of immunity present.

1) They may develop directly into active renal tuberculosis (rare), they may regress and heal completely (common), or *they may remain dormant but still harbor living tubercle bacilli.*

2. Allergic phase.

A. The body does not significantly react to the presence of tubercle bacilli until sufficient antigen is released by dead bacilli to sensitize the host to tuberculoprotein.

1) This hypersensitivity develops after 3 to 5 weeks and initiates the allergic phase.

B. With onset of the allergic phase, the tuberculin test becomes positive and the patient may become mildly symptomatic.

C. The host responds by forming a fibrous tissue capsule around all the lesions—lung and metastatic foci—and destroying the blood vessels with resultant caseation necrosis.

1) This effectively seals off the foci in the renal cortex but viable tubercle bacilli may remain within them indefinitely.

D. In most cases, the primary lesions and all of the metastatic foci regress and heal, leaving only two marks of their presence.

1) Tiny scars, often calcified.

2) Positive tuberculin test.

Latent Period

1. This interval between the primary pulmonary infection and the appearance of active tuberculosis may last 4 to 40 years, and during this time the dormant foci in the renal cortex contain *walled-off, viable tubercle bacilli.*
2. Tubercle bacilli may escape destruction because of the peculiar and unique form of tissue necrosis they induce—caseation.

   A. The tissue does not liquify but has the consistency and appearance of cheese.

   1) This *arrested autolysis* of the necrotic area inhibits reabsorption, organization, and sloughing.

   2) In other bacterial infections of the lung, autolysis of the necrotic area goes on to completion, leaving no residual bacteria.

Reactivation of Renal Foci Harboring Tubercle Bacilli

1. The blood-borne tubercle bacilli carried to the kidneys during the primary pulmonary infection lodge in the small blood vessels of the renal cortex.

   A. Experimental studies have shown that the initial lesion is in the vas efferens of the glomerulus.

   B. Most of these tiny cortical foci heal completely, but those that do not, harbor viable tubercle bacilli.
2. Reactivation with escape of these organisms occurs when *body resistance is lowered*, and 75% of the time only one kidney appears to be involved.

   A. Causes of decreased host resistance.

   1) Chronic or debilitating diseases—cancer, alcoholism, diabetes.

   2) Diminished immune response—during treatment with immunosuppressive drugs such as cortisone and Imuran.
3. The tubercle bacilli within these cortical foci erode into the tubules and are carried within the nephron lumen to the medulla where they tend to produce paracalyceal areas of necrosis.

   A. Clinically manifest renal tuberculosis now exists.

   B. These necrotizing lesions may slowly and silently expand within the kidney, gradually destroying it, or they may erode into the calyx allowing tubercle bacilli in the urine to secondarily infect the mucous membrane of the other calyces and renal pelvis, ureter, bladder and prostate.

Tuberculosis of the Ureter

1. Wherever the ureter is involved, a *stricture results* owing to fibrosis.

   A. A single stricture at the ureterovesical junction is the most common lesion and occurs 6 times as often as a stricture at the ureteropelvic junction.

   B. Multiple strictures occasionally occur and are virtually diagnostic of tuberculosis.

   C. Diffuse involvement results in a short, straight, narrow ureter.

Tuberculosis of the Bladder

1. Bladder involvement is usually in the form of *patchy areas of cystitis*, especially around the ureteral orifice draining the infected kidney.
2. Reflux may result if the inflammatory process involves the ureterovesical junction.
3. Diffuse involvement of the bladder over a long period of time results in a contracted bladder often holding less than 60 ml.

   A. Approximately 10% of all patients with genitourinary tuberculosis have contracted bladders.

Genital Tuberculosis in the Male

1. The genital tract in the male is involved in over half of all cases of renal tuberculosis owing to the direct communication between the urinary and genital tracts.

   A. Contaminated urine in the posterior urethra initiates prostatic infection with subsequent involvement of the seminal vesicles and epididymides via canalicular spread.

   B. Occasionally, genital tuberculosis appears to be blood-borne in origin.
2. Prostate.

   A. With tuberculous prostatitis, caseous areas are often sloughed out, leaving a small indurated prostate with resultant low semen volume.
3. Epididymis.

   A. Disease of the epididymis usually results from spread via the lumen of the vas deferens so that early lesions involve only the globus minor, whereas late lesions involve the entire epididymis.

   B. The vas is often thickened and scrotal sinuses are common.

Clinical Findings

Prior to 1950, any patient with severe dysuria and hematuria would immediately have been suspected of having urinary tuberculosis, but if the same patient presented today, this diagnosis would rarely be considered owing to the drastic reduction in recent years of all forms of tuberculosis. This decreased awareness may be harmful to the patient, for *undetected or unrecognized renal tuberculosis can destroy a kidney in as short a period as 3 years*.

Signs and Symptoms

The most common symptoms of genitourinary (GU) tuberculosis—painful urination, urinary frequency, and hematuria—occur only when renal tuberculosis has spread to the bladder. When the infection is limited to the kidney, the patient is *usually asymptomatic*, so that it is not unusual for a kidney to be silently destroyed by slowly progressive parenchymal disease. Renal pain and renal hematuria occur infrequently.

Signs and Symptoms Leading to Diagnosis of GU Tuberculosis

1. Painful urination, urinary frequency, and hematuria—60%.
2. Epididymitis—20%.
3. Renal pain or renal hematuria—10%.
4. No symptoms, but urological work-up performed—10%.
   A. Albuminuria.
   B. Pyuria.
   C. Microscopic hematuria.
   D. Presence of another focus of tuberculosis.
   E. Evidence of calcification in the kidney on x-ray.

Genital tuberculosis usually causes no symptoms until the epididymis is involved, although disease of the prostate and seminal vesicles may cause low semen volume or bloody ejaculate.

Physical Findings

These are often meager and nonspecific! Tuberculous involvement of the kidney, prostate, seminal vesicle, or epididymis usually causes little or no tenderness, but when the bladder is involved it is exquisitely tender to palpation. The prostate may be small and firm with a bumpy surface. The involved vas is often thicker than normal but beading is rare. The epididymis is enlarged, indurated, and slightly tender, and it may be adherent to the scrotal wall forming a sinus tract.

Diagnostic Studies for Tuberculosis

1. Urinalysis.
   A. In early cases, the only findings may be unexplained pyuria, albuminuria, or hematuria.
   B. In the usual case, the urinary sediment contains variable numbers of both white cells and red cells, but *no bacteria.*
2. Demonstration of tubercle bacilli in the urine.
   A. Two or three consecutive overnight urine specimens should be obtained and the entire urinary sediment used for smear and culture.
   B. Direct smear.
      1) Tubercle bacilli are acid-fast and may be demonstrated by special staining techniques such as the Ziehl-Neelsen method.
      2) This examination is used less frequently today for two reasons.
         a. The small number of organisms present in the urine of most patients with urinary tuberculosis necessitates a tedious, time-consuming, often unrewarding search by the microscopist.
         b. Nonpathogenic acid-fast bacteria may occasionally be present in the urine, and so the finding of acid-fast bacilli *does not give absolute diagnosis of tuberculosis.*
   C. Culture.
      1) Tubercle bacilli do not grow on ordinary media but will grow on special media.

2) Current media of choice—Middlebrook oleic acid-agar 7H-11 and Lowenstein-Jensen buffered egg-potato.

3) Incubation in an atmosphere of 5 to 10% CO_2 enhances the growth of tubercle bacilli and gives a greater yield of positive culture.

4) *The diagnosis of genitourinary tuberculosis should not be made until tubercle bacilli are cultured from the urine.*

5) The chief disadvantage of the urine culture is the time required to grow out the organisms—a *minimum of 3 weeks.*

3. Niacin test. This test should be performed on all mycobacteria cultured, for it differentiates human bacilli from all the other mycobacteria, including bovine and avian.

1) Human tubercle bacilli are niacin positive; all the others are niacin-negative.

4. Semen culture.

A. This examination is occasionally helpful in making the diagnosis when urine cultures are negative and intravenous urograms appear normal.

5. X-ray studies—intravenous urogram.

A. The first x-ray evidence of urinary tuberculosis is often a *ragged, single calyx or an obstructed single calyx.*

B. Findings suggesting tuberculosis.

1) A nonfunctioning kidney with stippled calcification in many areas.

2) Calyectasis not involving all of the calyces.

3) Calcification anywhere along the urinary or genital tract.

4) Ureter.

a. Unusually straight and narrow or grossly deformed.

b. Stricture at ureterovesical or ureteropelvic junction.

5) Bladder.

a. Small capacity plus or minus reflux.

6. Tuberculin test.

A. This skin test is based on the fact that infection with tubercle bacilli produces a specific sensitivity to the protein portion of the organism.

1) It becomes positive 3 to 7 weeks after tubercle bacilli invade the human body and remains positive as long as they survive.

B. The standard dose for differential diagnosis is 5 TU (tuberculin units).

1) Less than 10% of the U.S. population has a positive tuberculin.

2) Eighty percent of patients with genitourinary tuberculosis have a positive tuberculin test when initially tested.

a. If the negative reactors are retested with the same dose 1 to 2 weeks later, most of them become positive, raising the percentage of positive reactors to over 95%.

C. If a patient suspected of tuberculosis has two negative tests with the 5 TU dose, he should be tested with 250 TU.

1) If he has a negative reaction to 250 TU and he is not critically ill, the *patient does not have tuberculosis.*

2) If he has a negative reaction to 5 TU but a positive one to 250 TU, he

probably has been infected with mycobacteria other than tuberculosis.
7. Cystoendoscopy.
   A. Findings suggestive of tuberculosis.
      1) Dilated prostatic ducts.
      2) Patchy areas of cystitis, particularly adjacent to the ureteral orifice draining the infected kidney.
      3) Red, patulous retracted ureteral orifice.
      4) Very sensitive bladder with small capacity.
8. Tissue examination.
   A. Biopsy of bladder, prostate, or epididymal lesions occasionally helps in establishing the diagnosis of genitourinary tuberculosis.

Treatment

The combination of effective chemotherapy and surgical correction of urinary tract obstruction has decreased the mortality rate from genitourinary tuberculosis to less than 1%.

Chemotherapy

1. Antituberculous drugs, *appropriately prescribed and actually ingested*, can arrest nearly all cases of tuberculosis.
2. Drug susceptibility studies should always be performed prior to the institution of chemotherapy.
3. There are two chief causes of treatment failure.
   A. Noningestion of medication by the patient.
   B. Formation of drug-resistant strains.
4. Drug resistance.
   A. Primary.
      1) Five percent of all strains isolated prior to institution of chemotherapy are resistant to one or more of the antituberculous drugs.
      2) These can be detected by pretreatment drug susceptibility tests.
   B. Secondary or acquired.
      1) Mycobacterium tuberculosis will produce a mutant resistant to one drug once in every 100,000 to 1,000,000 cell divisions (10^{5-6}), a mutant resistant to two drugs once in every 10^{10-12} cell divisions, and so forth, so that *it is impossible to kill all the bacilli with a single drug.*
      2) Combined therapy with two drugs permits the mutants resistant to one drug to be destroyed by the other drug.
5. Current regimen of choice.
   A. Isoniazid, 300 mg/day given in a single dose by mouth, and Rifampin, 600 mg/day given in a single dose on an empty stomach.
   B. These two antituberculous drugs are odorless and tasteless, and most importantly, they are the *most potent* ones available today.
   C. These two drugs must be taken *every day for 2 years.*
      1) The patient must be indoctrinated with the importance of taking these drugs continuously.

6. Management of drug-resistant urinary tuberculosis.

A. Determine all antituberculous drugs previously taken.

B. Perform fresh drug susceptibility studies, testing the organisms against all the available antituberculous drugs.

C. An intensive triple drug regimen should be instituted based on demonstrated susceptibility of the organism to selected drugs.

Surgery

Tuberculosis may destroy functioning nephrons directly via necrotizing pyelonephritis or indirectly via obstruction secondary to tuberculous strictures at the ureterovesical or ureteropelvic junctions. These obstructing strictures, which may develop before, during, or after chemotherapy, damage the entire kidney via back-pressure effect and decreased renal blood flow.

Surgery today is largely confined to counteracting this obstruction, either by ureteral dilation or by resection of the stricture. The resultant improved drainage protects the intact renal parenchyma from further destruction, and the increased blood flow allows more antituberculous drug to reach the tuberculous foci. Nephrectomy is rarely necessary now but is indicated in a few selected patients with clinically unilateral disease.

1. Pyonephrosis with little or no renal function.

2. Persistent severe pain or hypertension secondary to an obstructing, uncorrectable stricture at the ureteropelvic junction. Nephrectomy should always be preceded by at least 3 weeks of effective chemotherapy.

When the bladder capacity remains around 30 to 60 ml after appropriate chemotherapy, surgical enlargement may be accomplished by joining a loop of intestine to the bladder. If this is not feasible, urinary diversion via ileal conduit may be necessary.

Genital tuberculosis usually requires no surgery, but occasionally an infected epididymis with a scrotal fistula may require excision.

Other Measures

1. Hospitalization.

A. This is required for diagnosis, institution of appropriate chemotherapy, and education of the patient to the nature of his disease and the importance of taking the prescribed medication.

B. It is *not* necessary for the patient to remain in the hospital until urine cultures are negative for tubercle bacilli.

C. Ambulatory treatment on an outpatient basis has replaced prolonged stays in tuberculosis sanitariums.

2. Urinary precautions.

A. To show his patients the infection potential of this disease, Belt gave them methylene blue by mouth and told them that everything that turned blue was contaminated with tubercle bacilli.

B. During the early phase of chemotherapy when viable tubercle bacilli are still present in the urine, some simple precautions seem in order even though the chance of transmitting infection via infected urine is remote.

1) The patient should sit to void, carefully cleansing toilet seat with Clorox after each voiding.

2) To minimize soiling of underclothing, remaining drops in urethra should be expressed onto toilet paper.

3) Hands should be washed after urination.

URINARY SCHISTOSOMIASIS

Schistosoma haematobium is a blood fluke with a predilection for the veins of the bladder and lower ureters, but it may affect any organ of the body. It cannot complete its life cycle without the presence of *appropriate fresh water snails*, so it survives and causes disease in man only in areas harboring these particular snails. Most of the cases occur in Egypt and other areas in Africa, primarily in the Nile Valley region. Man as the primary host and the snail as the intermediate host team together to perpetuate this parasitic disease currently affecting 40,000,000 Africans.

Life Cycle

The tiny adult worms normally live within the pelvic veins of man. Ova extruded by the female reach the bladder lumen and are evacuated in the urine. If they reach fresh warm water, the ova break open and the escaping miracidia (larval form) swim about until they are able to penetrate an appropriate snail. Within the snail, each miracidium undergoes asexual multiplication and 4 to 5 weeks later, thousands of fork-tailed cercariae break out of the snail into the water. *Man is infected when he comes in contact with these free-swimming cercariae*, most commonly while wading, swimming, or working in slow-moving fresh water.

The cercariae penetrate the skin, shed their tails, and burrow into the nearest capillary or lymphatic. These immature worms soon reach the heart and from there they are carried as blood-borne emboli throughout the body, but only those worms reaching the liver survive. These worms mature within the liver and then, swimming against the current of the portal vein, they eventually lodge in the tiny venules of the bladder and other pelvic organs. During this trip from the liver to the bladder, copulation takes place, so when the bladder is reached, the female extrudes her eggs and the cycle starts all over again.

Three factors must exist before man can become infected with *Schistosoma haematobium*.

1. The appropriate fresh water snails must inhabit the nearby waters.

2. The inhabitants must urinate or defecate in or near these snail-infested waters (children are most accomodating).

3. Man must wade, bathe, or work in these same waters, now infested with the cercariae of *Schistosoma haematobium*.

Pathogenesis and Pathology

The pathological changes seen in vesical schistosomiasis result from the *irritative effect of the eggs*, not from the intravascular adult worms. Each female worm produces 1,000 to 10,000 eggs per day, so the severity of an infection depends upon the number of viable worms present. These eggs are deposited in large numbers in the *submucosa* and their fate determines the pathological reaction.

1. Eggs retained in the tissues cause *closed lesions* which account for most of the tissue injury.

A. They mechanically and chemically irritate the local tissues and also serve as effective antibody stimulators.

1) Live eggs cause more reaction than dead ones, since the chemical irritants are elaborated by the living miracidia within the egg.

B. The retained eggs act as foreign bodies inducing a granulomatous reaction which heals with dense fibrosis.

1) When this process involves the intravesical ureter or the bladder neck, it causes obstruction.

C. Submucosal eggs may induce proliferative changes in the overlying mucosa and these may progress to squamous cell carcinoma.

D. Bladder muscle may be involved and this is particularly prone to occur in the trigone area.

1) Here, trigonal muscle is interposed between the retained eggs and the overlying mucosa, so it is damaged more commonly and more extensively.

2). Damage to the trigone muscle interferes with opening of the bladder neck contributing to bladder outlet obstruction.

E. Some eggs may move into the deeper viscera causing similar foreign body type reaction.

F. Eggs usually die in about 12 days and are then calcified, and this rim of millions of calcified eggs in the submucosa gives a characteristic x-ray picture.

2. Eggs may pass through the mucosa into the bladder lumen.

A. These eggs cause only a slight tissue reaction, but when they are evacuated in the urine, they may infect the appropriate vector snails and through them other individuals.

1) *These eggs spread the disease.*

B. All forms of inflammatory lesions may occur including ulceration.

3. Eggs may be carried back in the venous blood to the lungs, liver, or other organs.

Vesical Schistosomiasis and Cancer of the Bladder

The incidence of bladder cancer is 10 times as frequent in patients with *chronic* vesical schistosomiasis as it is in uninfected groups, and schistosomal bladders show malignant change in 6 to 7%. There are two ways in which this parasitic disease may contribute to the development of a bladder cancer.

1. Schistosomal irritation induces squamous metaplasia which may progress to squamous cell carcinoma, sometimes referred to as "Egyptian irritation cancer."

A. Sixty percent of schistosomal carcinomas are squamous cell type, 12 times the usual frequency in nonschistosomal bladder cancers (5%).

2. Vesical schistosomiasis is accompanied by increased amounts of carcinogenic substances in the urine.

A. Bladder outlet obstruction may be present if the trigone muscle and bladder neck are involved, and the resultant retention of urine enhances the effect of these urinary carcinogens by exposing the already unstable mucosa to longer and more concentrated action.

Clinical

In endemic areas, infection occurs early in life reaching maximal incidence in the 15 to 30 age group, but no age is exempt. Many patients have only mild symptoms which they often ignore. In heavy infections, symptoms may be severe and may appear as early as 1 month after infection.

Signs and Symptoms

There are two stages in this disease.

1. Developmental stage—immature worms penetrate man's skin, mature within the liver, and then go to the bladder.

A. Cercarial penetration of the skin *initiates* infection in man.

1) Native Africans usually experience no symptoms at this time, but others often note severe itching and a rash at the site of penetration.

B. Invasion of the tissues by the immature worm.

1) These worms cause a local inflammatory reaction wherever they land and they also induce an allergic body response.

2) Flu-like syndrome often results with general malaise, headache, cough, abdominal pains, and fever.

3) Allergic response may be manifest by urticaria and eosinophilia in up to 50 to 60%.

2. Oviposition stage—eggs are deposited in the submucosa and mucosa of the bladder causing bladder symptoms.

A. Hematuria is the most characteristic symptom.

1) When a patient with hematuria gives a history of residence in a country where vesical schistosomiasis is endemic (*e.g.*, Africa), include this disease in your differential diagnosis.

B. Painful urination and urinary frequency are other common symptoms.

Diagnostic Studies

1. Urinalysis.

A. In the usual case, the urinary sediment contains variable numbers of red blood cells, white blood cells, and the characteristic *terminal-spined eggs of Schistosoma haematobium.*

B. More eggs are passed around mid-day, so the sediment should be examined from urine collected between 10 A.M. and 2 P.M., but if only a few eggs are likely to be present, the sediment from a 24-hour collection should be used.

1) Add warm water to this sediment and wait 30 min so that viable eggs present can release their miracidia.

2) If miracidia are identified, the diagnosis of *active vesical schistosomiasis is established.*

3) Dead eggs may be passed for a long period after worms have died, either from natural causes or after a course of treatment.

2. Intravenous urogram.

A. Calcification of the bladder, lower ureters, and seminal vesicles is *pathognomonic* of chronic vesical schistosomiasis.

1) The bladder wall is outlined by a thin rim of calcium due to calcification of millions of dead eggs in the submucosa.

B. Hydroureter and hydronephrosis occur when the intravesical ureter is involved in the inflammatory process.

1) The ureterovesical junction may become incompetent with resultant reflux or it may become stenosed with resultant obstruction.

3. Cystoscopy.

A. Earliest finding is area of erythema and edema of the periureteric mucosa.

B. Later there are patchy areas of cystitis with shiny, gray tubercles most commonly found on the floor of the bladder in the vicinity of the ureteral orifices.

C. Sandy patches looking like "sand under water" are typical of chronic vesical schistosomiasis.

1) Appearance is due to presence of calcified eggs beneath the thinned out mucosa.

D. Proliferative nodules and ulcers may be present in the far advanced cases.

E. Carcinoma is frequently associated with *chronic* vesical schistosomiasis so that all suspicious areas should be biopsied.

1) This rarely occurs without evidence of bladder calcification on x-ray.

F. *Bladder biopsy may reveal schistosomal eggs when urine examination is negative.*

1) Mucosal snips, unfixed and unstained, should be pressed between

two glass slides and examined for eggs via microscopy.

4. Cystograms.

A. Reflux occurs commonly in the long standing cases owing to schistosomal inflammation of the intravesical ureter rendering it rigid, pipelike, and incompressible.

B. Bladder capacity usually remains close to normal even when there is extensive calcification of the bladder wall, but in some long standing cases, the extensive fibrosis results in a small capacity bladder.

5. Blood count.

A. Leukocytosis with eosinophilia is common and eosinophil count is usually 10 to 60%.

B. Anemia usually is present.

6. Schistosomal skin test and serological tests.

A. These tests are positive in over 90% of patients with past or present vesical schistosomiasis and may become positive in the developmental stage *before* the eggs are deposited in the bladder wall.

1) Early diagnosis may permit curative treatment before any bladder damage has been sustained.

Treatment

Antischistosomal drugs should not be prescribed unless the patient is passing viable eggs or miracidia in the urine. These drugs damage the worm's enzyme system so that he is carried back to the lungs via venous system and there he eventually dies.

The drug of choice is niridazole which cures over 90% of *Schistosoma haematobial* infections. It is administered orally, 25 mg/kg, in divided doses for 5 to 7 days.

Surgery occasionally is necessary because of massive reflux, ureterovesical obstruction, or schistosomally induced carcinoma of the bladder.

URINARY CANDIDIASIS (MONILIASIS)

Candida albicans is a fungus which is normally found in only three sites—mouth, intestinal tract, and vagina. In these three locations, Candida organisms are saprophytes coexisting with gram-negative bacteria in a happy balance. If this delicate balance is upset, as by antibiotic destruction of competing bacteria, the normally harmless fungi gain the upper hand and may become pathogens causing fungal infections.

Candida organisms are not normally present in the urinary tract, so when detected there, they are usually pathogens. They are *opportunistic fungi causing infection only when the host resistance is lowered.*

Causes of Reduced Host Resistance

1. Antimicrobial therapy.

A. When the normal bacterial flora are knocked out, there is more available nourishment for the fungi.

B. Virtually 100% of patients with systemic candidiasis have been treated with antibiotics.
2. Diabetes mellitus.
A. The increased sugar content in blood and urine facilitates the growth and proliferation of fungi.
3. Cortisone therapy.
A. Hypercortisolism inhibits the cellular host response to bacterial or fungal invasion.
4. Immunosuppressive drug therapy.
A. Renal transplant patients on Imuran are vulnerable because their cellular mediated immunity is reduced.
5. Malignancy and other chronic debilitating diseases such as leukemia.
A. Host resistance is reduced.
6. Prolonged intravenous catheterization.
A. This catheter often serves as a portal of entry for the candidal organisms.

Clinical

Urinary tract candidiasis may take the following forms.
1. Candidal cystitis.
A. This is the most *common form* of urinary tract candidiasis.
B. Symptoms are similar to those accompanying bacterial cystitis, but urine smears and cultures confirm the presence of candidal organisms.
C. Cystoscopy often reveals a white membrane adherent to reddened, friable bladder wall.
2. Candidal pyelonephritis.
A. This relatively rare form occurs in the absence of blood stream invasion or other organ involvement.
B. Most patients have diabetes mellitus and bacterial pyelonephritis and have been treated aggressively with powerful antibiotics.
C. The inflammatory process seems to be a necrotizing one and papillary necrosis is not uncommon.
D. Ureteral obstruction may be caused by fungus balls (candidal organisms plus necrotic debris) or sloughed papillae.
3. Systemic candidiasis.
A. These patients all have *candidemia* with widespread candidiasis, and the urinary tract is one of many organ systems involved.
B. The extensive renal destruction usually leads to renal failure and death.

Diagnosis

1. Urinary tract candidiasis must be considered in any patient with urinary symptoms and proven candidal infection elsewhere.
2. Urinalysis.
A. Demonstration of the budding yeast or mycelial form of *Candida*

albicans in fresh urine obtained by catheter or aspiration from the bladder indicates probable candidal infection.

3. Urine culture.

A. Organisms are readily cultured on Sabouraud's dextrose agar.

B. Finding greater than 1,000 Candida colonies per ml of urine is diagnostic of urinary tract candidiasis.

1) If the blood culture also grows out Candida organisms, the patient has systemic candidiasis, not candidal cystitis or pyelonephritis.

4. Intravenous urogram.

A. Calyectasis is common with candidal pyelonephritis.

B. Radiolucent filling defects may be present in the kidney, ureter, or bladder due to fungus balls or necrotic papillae.

5. Cystoendoscopy.

A. The bladder is usually reddened, edematous, and irritable. Adherent grayish white patches may be present.

6. Serodiagnosis via serum precipitin or agglutinin titer.

A. Detection of serum antibodies against candidal antigen is an excellent way of detecting deep seated infection.

1) Candidal cystitis→no serum antibodies.

2) Candidal pyelonephritis without parenchymal involvement→no serum antibodies.

3) Candidal pyelonephritis with parenchymal involvement→positive for serum antibodies.

Treatment

1. Eliminate factors that reduce host resistance or encourage infection *if feasible*.

A. Stop antibiotics, steroid, or immunosuppressive therapy.

B. Remove catheters.

2. Mild infections which induce no serum antibody production may be treated with *contact antibiotics*.

A. Bladder or renal pelvis may be lavaged 2 or 3 times each day for 7 to 10 days with amphotericin B solution (5 mg/100 ml of 5% dextrose in water) with high probability of eradicating the candidal infection.

3. Deep seated infections which induce a serum antibody response require systemic treatment with amphotericin B.

A. This relatively toxic drug has recently been shown to be clinically effective in low doses.

1) The small dose regimen causes no significant toxicity.

REFERENCES AND SUGGESTED FURTHER READING
Tuberculosis

1. Beck, A. D. and Marshall, V. F. Is nephrectomy obsolete for unilateral renal tuberculosis? J. Urol. 98:65, 1967.
2. Borthwick, W. M. Genito-urinary tuberculosis. Tubercle 37:120, 1956.

3. Canetti, G. Present aspects of bacterial resistance in tuberculosis. Am. Rev. Respir. Dis. 92:687, 1965.
4. Hanley, H. G. Conservative surgery in renal tuberculosis. Br. J. Surg. 48:415, 1961.
5. Kaufman, J. J. and Goodwin, W. E. Renal hypertension secondary to renal tuberculosis. Am. J. Med. 38:337, 1965.
6. Lattimer, J. K. Current concepts—renal tuberculosis. N. Engl. J. Med. 273:208, 1965.
7. Lattimer, J. K. Renal tuberculosis in children. Postgrad. Med. 28:336, 1960.
8. Lattimer, J. K., Wechsler, H., Ehrlich, R. M., and Fukushima, K. Current treatment for renal tuberculosis. J. Urol. 102:2, 1969.
9. Lester, W. Treatment of drug-resistant tuberculosis. Disease-a-Month, April, 1971.
10. Medlar, E. M. Cases of renal infection in pulmonary tuberculosis—evidence of healed tuberculous lesions. Am. J. Pathol. 2:401, 1926.
11. Medlar, E. M., Spain, D. M., and Holliday, R. W. Post-mortem compared with clinical diagnosis of genitourinary tuberculosis in adult males. J. Urol. 61:1,078, 1949.
12. Mitchell, R. S. Control of tuberculosis. N. Engl. J. Med. 276:842, 905, 1967.
13. National Tuberculosis and Respiratory Disease Association. Diagnostic standards and classification of tuberculosis. The Association, New York, 1969).
14. Stead, W. W. The new face of tuberculosis. Hosp. Prac. 4:62, 1969.
15. Veenema, R. J. and Lattimer, J. K. Genital tuberculosis in the male: clinical pathology and effect on fertility. J. Urol. 78:65, 1957.
16. Wechsler, H., Westfall, M., and Lattimer, J. K. The earliest signs and symptoms in 127 male patients with genitourinary tuberculosis. J. Urol. 83:801, 1960.

Schistosomiasis

1. Chapman, D. S. The surgical importance of bilharziasis in South Africa. Br. J. Surg. 53:544, 1966.
2. Makar, N. Some clinicopathological aspects of urinary bilharziasis. In *Bilharziasis*, edited by F. K. Mostofi, p. 45. Springer-Verlag, New York, 1967.
3. Marks, C. Schistosomiasis and its surgical sequelae. Am. J. III: 805, 1966.
4. Mofty, A. E. Clinical aspects of bilharziasis. Bilharziasis Ciba Foundation Symposium, p. 174. Little Brown, Boston, 1962.
5. Tarabulcy, E. Z. The radiographic aspect of urogenital schistosomiasis (bilharziasis). J. Urol. 90:470, 1963.

Candidiasis

1. Harbach, L. B., Burkholder, C. V., and Goodwin, W. E. Renal candidiasis—a cause of anuria. Br. J. Urol. 42:258, 1970.
2. Kozinn, P. J. and Taschdjian, C. L. *Candida albicans:* saprophyte or pathogen? J.A.M.A. 198:170, 1966.
3. Medoff, G., Dismukes, W. E., Meade, R. H., and Moses, J. M. A new therapeutic approach to Candida infections —a preliminary report. Arch. Intern. Med. 130: 241, 1972.
4. Price, W. E., Webb, E. A., and Smith, B. A. Urinary tract candidiasis treated with Amphotericin B. J. Urol. 98:523, 1967.
5. Tennant, F. S., Jr., Remmers, A. R., Jr., and Perry, J. E. Primary renal candidiasis—associated perinephric abscess and passage of fungus balls in the urine. Arch. Intern. Med. 122:435, 1968.
6. Wise, G. J., Ray, B., and Kozinn, P. J. The serodiagnosis of significant genitourinary candidiasis. J. Urol. 107:1,043, 1972.
7. Wise, G. J., Wamstein, S., Goldberg, P., and Kozinn, P. J. Candidal cystitis—management by continuous bladder irrigation with Amphotericin B. J.A.M.A. 224:1,636, 1973.

22

Venereal Disease in Males

ARTHUR W. WYKER, JR.

The Public Health Service officially recognizes five venereal or genito-infectious diseases—gonorrhea, syphilis, chancroid, lymphogranuloma venereum, and granuloma inguinale. Gonorrhea and syphilis are the major ones accounting for over 99% of the total venereal cases reported. To this list, I would add—herpes genitalis, *Trichomonas vaginalis* urethritis, and other forms of nongonococcic urethritis.

GONORRHEA

This is the oldest and most prevalent of all the venereal diseases. It is estimated that in 1970, between $1\frac{1}{2}$ and 2 million cases of gonorrhea occurred in the United States, the majority in the 15 to 30 age group. If this contagious disease were transmitted in any way other than by sexual intercourse, the present situation would be declared an epidemic and the public would demand an all out effort by health authorities to eradicate it.

1. Etiology. The causative agent is the gonococcus, a gram-negative, kidney shaped diplococcus transmitted *only* by sexual intercourse. The gonococcus (*Neisseria gonorrhoeae*) has the following characteristics:

A. Fragility.

1) It is easily killed by drying, sunlight, and various chemicals.

a. The organism will not survive on a swab for a long period so it must be plated immediately or placed in a transport medium that retains moisture.

B. It primarily attacks only one kind of epithelium—*columnar*.

1) The gonococcus can multiply on the surface of stratified squamous or transitional cell epithelium, but *it cannot penetrate through the layers of cells* to reach the subepithelial tissue.

a. Only the *single layer*, columnar epithelium, is vulnerable.

b. Intact skin is not vulnerable.

2) Tissues which may be involved in males.

a. Portion of urethra surrounded by corpus spongiosum.

b. Prostatic ducts and glands.

c. Epididymis.

d. Rectum and pharynx.

C. *Endotoxin* is responsible for inflammatory reaction.

1) Living organism is harmless but when it dies, endotoxin is released and this produces the inflammatory reaction.

2. Pathology. The male urethral meatus is the usual portal of entry for the gonococcus since intact skin resists penetration. The organisms can only establish a foothold when they have passed beyond the protective collar of stratified squamous epithelium in the fossa navicularis to reach the susceptible columnar epithelium of the spongy urethra. Here they penetrate to the subepithelial tissue and, when they die, a potent endotoxin is released causing anterior urethritis and a purulent urethral discharge. The time from inoculation to the appearance of this urethral discharge is 2 to 5 days. If adequate treatment is given at this point, the infection is eradicated and there are no complications or sequelae. However, if the infection is untreated or inadequately treated, it extends to the underlying corpus spongiosum, and may spread to the prostatic ducts and epididymis via lymphatics and surface extension.

When the acute changes have subsided, the resultant scar in the corpus spongiosum may cause a downward curvature of the penis with erections (chordee) or a urethral stricture. Involvement of the epididymides may cause infertility.

Infrequently, gonococci may enter the general circulation via the lymphatics and blood vessels producing metastatic lesions of the joints, skin, or endocardium.

3. Clinical findings.

A. Signs and symptoms. The usual presenting symptoms of gonorrhea —*painful urination and a purulent urethral discharge*—are due to anterior urethritis and most commonly appear 2 to 5 days after sexual intercourse. Less than 5% of men with gonorrhea are asymptomatic carriers.

Physical examination usually reveals a thick, yellow-green discharge bathing the red and swollen urethral meatal lips. If the infection has extended to the prostatic urethra, the prostate and epididymis may be swollen and tender.

4. Laboratory findings. Diagnosis usually is easily made by demonstrating typical gram-negative *intracellular* diplococci on a methylene blue or gram stain of the purulent exudate. If the smear is not diagnostic but gonorrhea is still suspected, culture the exudate directly onto Thayer-Martin VCN media. This excellent culture media for the gonococcus incorporates antibiotics which inhibit the growth of nongonococcal organisms, facilitating the demonstration of pathogenic gonococci. If laboratory facilities are not immediately available, the specimen should be placed on *Transgrow*, a new *culture and transport medium* that permits the organisms to grow while in transit to the nearest bacteriological laboratory. Whenever the gonococcus is cultured, it is necessary to have an atmosphere of 2 to 10% CO_2. This may be accomplished by placing the culture plate into a candle jar or special CO_2 incubator, or by pumping CO_2 into the culture tube and sealing the top (Transgrow). The diagnosis can also be made with

almost equal facility by culturing *urinary sediment*. This technique is particularly useful when the patient has little or no urethral discharge.

An immunofluorescent method is available for the detection and identification of gonococci in exudate, and it is *faster* and *more sensitive* than cultures. The exudate is fixed on a slide, covered with fluorescent labeled gonococcal antiserum, and subsequently examined under a special microscope equipped with mercury arc lamp and appropriate filters. This FA (fluorescent antibody) technique is currently used only by the larger laboratories because of the high cost of the equipment.

5. Treatment.

A. Penicillin is the drug of choice.

1) Gonorrhea requires high blood levels for a short period of time, so intramuscular injection of 4.8 million units of aqueous procaine penicillin G is recommended, preceded by 1 g of oral probenecid taken 20 min prior to the injection.

a. Oral penicillin or long acting, low blood level benzathine penicillin G is *not* recommended.

2) Virtually all gonococci are susceptible to penicillin, but 10% are relatively resistant to the usual dosage.

a. These *relatively* resistant strains originate in the Far East and Mexico owing to the practice there of treating "hostesses" with long acting penicillin to prevent syphilis.

b. The resultant long, low blood levels do not kill all the gonococci, and the surviving strains become increasingly resistant to penicillin.

3) Give alternative drugs if the patient is allergic to penicillin.

a. Tetracycline—administer orally 1.5 g stat. followed by 500 mg 4 times a day for 4 days.

b. Spectinomycin—give 2 g or 4 g intramuscularly stat.

B. Five percent of patients with gonorrhea (incubation period, 3 days) have coexisting incubating syphilis (incubation period, 21 days).

1) Recent studies have shown that 2.4 million units of aqueous procaine penicillin G, in addition to curing over *95% of cases of gonorrhea, is 100% effective in aborting incubating syphilis.*

a. Although the above data are reassuring, it is advisable to obtain a serological test for syphilis when the patient is first seen and again 3 to 4 months later.

C. All of the patient's contacts should be examined and treated, and the public health department notified.

If follow-up examination 3 to 5 days after initiation of treatment indicates persistence of gonorrhea, switch to oral tetracycline or intramuscular spectinomycin in previously recommended dosages.

6. Factors limiting control of gonorrhea. Despite the availability of effective antibiotics, gonorrhea is out of control with approximately 2 million cases in the United States in 1970.

A. Extremely short incubation of 3 to 5 days.

1) Epidemiologists do not have the time to trace contacts.

B. The asymptomatic female is the reservoir.

1) Ninety percent of women with gonorrhea are asymptomatic.

C. Lack of immunity.

D. Increased incidence of sexual intercourse among teenagers.

1) Most cases of gonorrhea occur in the 15 to 30 age group, and the highest rate increase is in the 15 to 19 age group.

E. Increased incidence of homosexual lesions.

1) In women with gonorrhea, 40% have positive rectal cultures and one-fifth of these have negative cervical cultures.

F. Oral contraceptives.

1) In addition to contributing to the increased frequency of sexual intercourse, the "pill" has decreased the use of the condom by the male.

G. Increasing resistance of the gonococcus to penicillin G.

7. Prevention of gonorrhea in males. Since the gonococcus cannot penetrate intact skin, proper use of the condom is *almost 100% protective*. Large doses of penicillin or tetracycline taken *before and after* sexual contact offer significant protection against both gonorrhea and syphilis.

Urination and thorough washing of the genitalia after sexual contact may offer some protection, but instillation of medications into the urethra is not recommended.

PRIMARY SYPHILIS

Syphilis is the second most common venereal disease with an estimated 25,000 cases being diagnosed and treated in the United States in 1970.

1. Etiology. The causative organism is a motile spirochete, *Treponema pallidum*. This delicate organism requires both moisture and tissue to survive, but once it penetrates into the deeper tissues, it is not destroyed by the body defenses. It is transmitted from person to person by intimate contact—lesion to lesion—but often the transmitting lesion is painless, hidden, and undetected.

2. Clinical findings.

A. Signs and symptoms. The primary lesion (chancre) is a *painless, flat ulcer* with serous discharge and a firm, smooth rim. Usually single, the chancre appears most commonly on the penis or scrotum about 21 days after sexual contact, although the incubation period range is 10 to 60 days. Occasionally it occurs in the anorectal region or in the mouth. The regional lymph nodes may be enlarged, but they are not usually painful or tender.

3. Laboratory findings.

A. Dark field examination. The serum obtained from early lesions contains *Treponema pallidum*, and in a satisfactory dark field preparation, the trained microscopist can identify these characteristic spirochetes, establishing the diagnosis of syphilis.

4. Serological tests for syphilis (STS). The serological tests are negative when the chancre first appears, but 1 to 4 weeks later, they become positive.

The VDRL test using nontreponemal antigens is *not highly specific* but is an excellent screening test. If the VDRL test is positive, it should be followed by the highly specific fluorescent treponemal antibody absorption test (FTA-Abs) test. Whereas false positives occur fairly frequently with the VDRL test, they are rare with the FTA-Abs test.

5. Treatment.

A. Penicillin is the drug of choice.

1) Despite extensive use of penicillin for over 25 years, the *Treponema pallidum* has developed no measurable resistance to penicillin.

2) Primary syphilis requires long, low blood levels; therefore, a single intramuscular injection of 2.4 million units of long acting benzathine penicillin G is recommended.

3) The altermative drug if the patient is allergic to penicillin is tetracycline. Administer orally 500 mg 4 times a day for 2 weeks.

B. All cases of infectious syphilis should be reported *immediately* to the local health department.

1) Trained public health investigators locate all sexual contacts who have been exposed within the preceding 90 days, and they are treated with the same dose of benzathine penicillin G as used in the treatment of primary syphilis.

CHANCROID (SOFT CHANCRE)

This is the third most common of the *officially* recognized venereal diseases.

1. Etiology. The causative organism is a gram-negative, nonmotile, short plump bacillus, *Hemophilus ducreyi*. It is transmitted by sexual contact and is fostered by poor genital hygiene.

2. Clinical findings.

A. Signs and symptoms. The typical lesion is a *dirty, painful ulcer* on the penis, appearing 1 to 7 days after sexual contact. In about 50% of the cases, the inguinal nodes are enlarged and tender, and fluctuation is often present.

3. Laboratory findings. Although the diagnosis is often made on clinical grounds only, serous exudate from the undermined border of the ulcer often will demonstrate *H. ducreyi* on a gram stain. Borchardt and Hoke[2] were able to culture *H. ducreyi* in almost all of their cases of chancroid by employing the patient's blood as a culture medium and serous fluid from the lesion as an inoculum. In all patients, dark field and serological examinations for syphilis should be performed prior to treatment.

4. Treatment.

A. A sulfonamide is the drug of choice.

1) Sulfasoxazole—administer orally 1 g 4 times day for 10 days.

2) Alternate drug—tetracycline. Administer orally 1 g initially, then 500 mg 4 times a day for 7 days.

B. Cleanse the ulcer gently with bland soap and warm water and pat dry.

1) Apply wet compresses (Burow's solution) 3 times a day followed by

gentamicin sulfate cream, 0.1%.

C. Aspirate fluctuant inguinal lymph nodes to prevent rupture.

LYMPHOGRANULOMA VENEREUM

This is a relatively rare venereal disease seen in scattered areas throughout the United States.

1. Etiology. The causative agent is a large *lymphotropic virus* of the psittacosis group.

2. Clinical findings.

A. Signs and symptoms. The primary lesion is a small papule appearing on the glans penis or prepuce, or in the anterior urethra, usually 1 to 4 weeks after sexual contact. This penile lesion is often painless and transient and may go undetected. One to 2 weeks later, the lymphotropism of the virus results in the characteristic lesion of lymphogranuloma venereum—the *bubo*. The inguinal nodes are matted, tender, and often fluctuant. Systemic symptoms such as fever and muscle pains may be present.

In the female, primary involvement of the vagina may result in a rectal stricture, since the vaginal lymphatics drain to the perirectal lymph nodes. In both sexes, extensive involvement of the lymphatics may cause genital elephantiasis.

3. Laboratory findings. The diagnosis is most commonly made by a serum complement-fixation test, using LGV antigen, and by a specific skin test (Frei). These tests are positive in 80 to 90% of all patients with lymphogranuloma venereum.

4. Treatment.

A. A sulfonamide is the drug of choice.

1) Sulfasoxasole—administer orally 1 g 4 times a day for 14 to 21 days.

2) Alternate drug—tetracycline. Administer orally 500 mg 4 times a day for 14 to 21 days.

B. Aspirate fluctuant buboes to prevent rupture.

GRANULOMA INGUINALE (DONOVANOSIS)

This relatively rare venereal disease is more common in Negroes and particularly in homosexuals.

1. Etiology. The causative organism is a gram-negative, encapsulated, nonmotile bacillus, *Calymmatobacterium granulomatis* (Donovan body).

2. Clinical findings.

A. Signs and symptoms. After an indefinite incubation period of 3 days to 6 months, a small papule appears on the perineum or genitalia and soon progresses to a painless ulcer covered by bright red, velvety granulation tissue. Untreated, the ulcer extends peripherally with accompanying scarring. The lymph nodes are not primarily involved, and the inguinal region is involved in 10 to 25% of cases.

3. Laboratory findings. The diagnosis may be made. by demonstrating

Donovan bodies in crushed tissue preparations stained with Wright-Giemsa stain.

4. Treatment.

A. Tetracycline is the drug of choice, administered orally, 500 mg 4 times a day for 2 to 3 weeks or until the lesions are completely healed.

GENITAL HERPES SIMPLEX

This is the third most common venereal disease behind gonorrhea (first) and syphilis (second).

1. Etiology. The causative agent is a herpes simplex virus with special predilection for the genitalia.

2. Clinical findings.

A. Signs and symptoms. After an indefinite incubation period, single or multiple erosive or vesicular lesions appear on the penis. A sensation of burning and pain often *precedes* the appearance of the lesion.

3. Laboratory findings. A presumptive diagnosis may be made if the biopsy shows viral acantholysis, intranuclear inclusions, and multinucleated giant cells. A final diagnosis can be made if the virus is isolated in tissue culture and identified by serological methods. Dark field examination and serological tests for syphilis should always be done.

4. Treatment. The lesions require no specific treatment, healing up spontaneously in 5 to 10 days. Efforts should be directed at avoiding secondary infection of the lesions.

TRICHOMONAS VAGINALIS URETHRITIS

This form of urethritis in the male always results from sexual intercourse with an infected partner.

1. Etiology. The causative organism is *Trichomonas vaginalis*, a motile, 1-cell protozoan with a flagellum.

2. Signs and symptoms. The presence of trichomonads in the male urethra and prostate *may or may not* cause local inflammation. Symptomatic male patients complain of an itching sensation in the urethra and a small amount of grayish white, watery urethral discharge coming on 3 to 21 days after sexual contact.

3. Laboratory findings. The characteristic motile *Trichomonas vaginalis* may be identified in wet preparations of the urethral discharge or in the urinary sediment. If discharge is absent and *Trichomonas vaginalis* urethritis is still suspected, 2 or 3 drops of saline should be instilled into the anterior urethra. Pinch the urethral meatus closed, and after 2 min, massage the anterior urethra and examine the escaping fluid for tri-chomonads.

4. Treatment.

A. The drug of choice is Flagyl. The patient and his sexual partner both must be treated simultaneously with 250 mg 3 times a day for 10 to 14 days.

NONGONOCOCCAL URETHRITIS

Many cases of urethritis, often labeled nonspecific urethritis, due to nongonococcal bacteria and viruses, result from sexual contact with an infected individual. Smears and cultures of the urethral discharge and urinary sediment should be obtained and appropriate treatment instituted. If no bacteria are seen on the smear and cultures are negative, viral etiology is probable, and in most cases, the urethritis will subside spontaneously after 1 to 2 weeks.

REFERENCES AND SUGGESTED FURTHER READING

1. Abrams, A. J. Lymphogranuloma venereum. J.A.M.A. 205:199, 1968.
2. Borchardt, K. A. and Hoke, A. W. Simplified laboratory technique for diagnosis of chancroid. Arch. Dermatol. 102:189, 1970.
3. Brown, W. J., Lucas, J. B., Olansky, S., and Norins, L. C. Roundtable: Venereal Disease. Med. Aspects Human Sexuality 5:74, 1971.
4. Davis, C. M. Granuloma inguinale. A clinical, histological and ultrastructural study. J.A.M.A. 211:632, 1970.
5. Deacon, W. E., Peacock, W. L., Jr., Freeman, E. M., and Harris, A. Identification of Neisseria gonorrhoeae by means of fluorescent antibodies. Proc. Soc. Exp. Biol. Med. 101:322, 1959.
6. Fiumara, N. J. The diagnosis and treatment of gonorrhea. Med. Clin. North Am. 56:1105, 1972.
7. Fiumara, N. J. Veneral disease. Pediatr. Clin. North Am. 16:333, 1969.
8. Harkness, A. H. The pathology of gonorrhoeae. Br. J. Vener. Dis. 24:137, 1948.
9. Lucas, C. T., Chandler, F., Jr., Martin, J. E., Jr., and Schmale, J. D. Transfer of gonococcal urethritis from man to chimpanzee. J.A.M.A. 216:1612, 1971.
10. Nahmias, A. J., Dowdle, W. R., Naib, Z. M., Jorey, W. E., McLone, D., and Domescik, G. Genital infection with type 2 herpes virus hominis: commonly occurring venereal disease Br. J. Vener. Dis. 45:294, 1969.
11. Pariser, H. Infectious syphilis. Med. Clin. North Am. 48:625, 1964.
12. Schroeter, A. L., Turner, R. H., Lucas, J. B., and Brown, W. J. Therapy for incubating syphilis. Effectiveness of gonorrhea treatment. J.A.M.A. 218:711, 1971.
13. Thayer, J. D. and Moore, M. B., Jr. Gonorrhea: present knowledge, research and control efforts. Med. Clin. North Am. 48:755, 1964.

23

Sexual Problems in the Male

STUART S. HOWARDS

INTRODUCTION

The topics of male infertility and impotency are often neglected in medical education. There are multiple reasons for this underemphasis, including the following: 1) These functions are taken for granted by the majority of physicians; 2) infertility and impotency do not affect life expectancy; and 3) psychosexual taboos inhibit candid discussion of these problems. Nevertheless, hypogonadism is a relatively common disease which is extremely important to the affected individuals. The impact of impotency on the sexually mature male hardly needs emphasis. Infertility can devastate either partner in an infertile union and often threatens the marriage itself. Indeed, this is a field in which the competent, interested physician can provide a vital, critically needed service.

INFERTILITY

1. Definition and incidence. A couple that does not conceive after engaging in intercourse for 1 year without practicing any form of birth control is arbitrarily defined as infertile. It is estimated that approximately 10 to 15% of all unions are barren by this definition. In 30 to 45% of these couples, the male contributes to the infertility. It should be emphasized that infertility is always a problem involving two people, and that either or both partners may be responsible for this state.

2. Growth and development of the testis. At 3 to 5 weeks of gestation, an indifferent gonad appears. It is composed of coelomic epithelial cells, primordial germ cells and mesenchymal cells. Chromosomal factors determine whether the indifferent gonad develops into an ovary or testis. In general, if a Y chromosome is present, a testis develops, and if there is no Y chromosome, an ovary evolves. However, recent evidence indicates that the X chromosome and autosomal chromosomes also play a role in gonadal differentiation.

By the 8th week, if the gonad is to become a testis, the medulla becomes dominant and the cortex regresses. As demonstrated beautifully in the classic studies of Jost, the testis releases a substance (Mullerian inhibiting factor) which is distinct from fetal androgen; this causes regression of the Mullerian ducts and, along with androgen, effects differentiation of the Wolffian duct structures into the male internal genitalia (see the chapter on

344

intersex). Fetal androgen is necessary at this stage for normal development of the external genitalia.

In summary, chromosomes determine gonadal development, Mullerian inhibiting factor and androgen control the internal genitalia, and androgens effect the evolution of male external genitalia.

3. Testicular descent. The testis usually descends into the scrotum *in utero* or shortly after birth. In one study, 1.8% of full term infants and 17.2% of premature infants had undescended testicles. Seventy-five percent of these testicles reached the scrotum by the age of 1 year, at which time the incidence of undescended testicles was 0.8%. Undescended testicles may be incompletely descended and halted somewhere along their normal route of descent or ectopically located after having traversed the inguinal canal. The undescended and ectopic testicle must be distinguished from the retractile testis which is withdrawn from the scrotum by the cremasteric reflex. If the testis is not in the cool environment of the scrotum, normal spermatogenesis cannot occur.

4. Testicular Maturation.

A. Early. Between the ages of 4 and 10, the seminiferous tubules mature, some spermatogonia mature into primary and secondary spermatocytes and spermatids, while the undifferentiated cells develop into Sertoli cells.

B. Pubertal. After 12 years of age, there is an increase in plasma luteinizing and follicle-stimulating hormones (LH and FSH), and the Leydig cells mature and release testosterone, which helps to maintain spermatogenesis and initiate puberty. The testes enlarge approximately 2 years before the other signs of puberty are evident. Thus, if the testicles have enlarged, the physician can reassure the patient with delayed puberty that within 2 years he will go through a normal puberty.

5. Spermatogenesis.

A. Initiation. The initiation of spermatogenesis requires FSH and high local testosterone concentration.

B. Maintenance. Testosterone is necessary to maintain spermatogenesis. It is not clear whether FSH is also required to sustain spermatogenesis.

C. Duration. Maturation from a spermatogonia to a mature spermatozoon takes approximately 74 days.

6. Endocrine function. The androgen production of the testes is carried out in the Leydig cells under the control of LH. LH-releasing factor is synthesized in the hypothalamus and releases both LH and FSH. Testosterone is the principal feedback regulator for LH. Destruction of the germinal cells will result in an elevation of FSH. However, the factor (often called "Inhibin") responsible for the feedback control of FSH has not been isolated.

7. Sperm maturation and transport.

A. Transport. After the mature spermatozoa are released from the seminiferous tubules, they must travel 6 to 8 m through the rete testes, ductuli efferentes, and the epididymis.

B. Maturation. This takes approximately 2 weeks, so that the total time from the initiation of spermatogenesis to the ejaculation of a mature spermatozoon is 3 months. During the several weeks they reside in the epididymis, the sperm mature, acquiring motility and fertility which they did not have at the time they left the testis. Also while sojourning through the caput and corpus of the epididymis, the sperm undergo innumerable additional alterations in their metabolism and physiology. Currently, little is known of the physiology of the epididymis. In the future, when it is better understood, clinicians will be more successful in reversing male infertility.

8. Emission, ejaculation, and capacitation.

A. Emission and ejaculation. At the time of emission and ejaculation, mature spermatozoa from the cauda epididymis, vas deferens, and ampulla of the vas are released into the posterior urethra and are forcefully ejaculated through the urethral meatus.

B. Capacitation. The ejaculated sperm are not fertile. In the female reproductive tract, under the influence of several factors the sperm acquire the capacity to fertilize. This process is called capacitation and involves alterations in the metabolic and membrane characteristics of the sperm as well as release of enzymes from the acrosome of the sperm head. These acrosomal enzymes facilitate the sperm's penetration of the vestments of the ovum.

9. Classification and etiology of fertility disorders. Appropriate treatment of male infertility must be based on accurate diagnosis of the underlying defect.

A. Congenital and genetic diseases.

1. Cryptorchism (see above).

2. Hypospadias. In this condition, the urethral meatus is located on the ventral surface of the penis somewhere proximal to the glans penis. If the urethral meatus is not located distal enough to allow the ejaculated sperm to be deposited into the vagina, the patient will be infertile.

3. Reifenstein syndrome. Hereditary male pseudohermaphroditism with ambiguous genitalia or hypospadias, gynecomastia, and seminiferous tubular sclerosis. Chromosomes normal. Androgen replacement often is necessary because of Leydig cell hypofunction.

4. Klinefelter's syndrome (see the chapter on intersex). Secondary sexual development is usually initiated at the appropriate time, but complete sexual maturation is not achieved. Hyalinization of the testicles begins in puberty, and the adult usually has small, firm testes. Gynecomastia is often present. The most common karyotype is 47/XXY, but others occur. Urinary gonadotropins and serum FSH are markedly elevated.

5. Mosaicism. Some patients with features of Klinefelter's syndrome have more than one cell line in their karyotype.

6. Anorchia. Absent testicles. Male internal and external genitalia. 46/XY karotype.

B. Endocrine disease.

1. Panhypopituitarism. Characterized by deficient thyroid, adrenal, and gonadal function as well as growth retardation.

2. Hypogonadotropism. Hypogonadotropism usually becomes evident when the patient fails to mature sexually. Kallman's syndrome is hypogonadotropic eunuchoidism associated with anosmia. Anosmia and small testicles help to distinguish Kallman's syndrome from physiological delayed puberty. A few patients have been described with an isolated LH deficiency and normal FSH secretion. In the adult male, hypogonadotropism presents with decreased libido and potency and may be secondary to a pituitary tumor.

3. Adrenal. Congenital adrenal hyperplasia is a rare entity which causes precocious puberty without maturation of the germinal epithelium. Replacement of cortisone results in maturation of the germinal epithelium, presumably by decreasing adrenocorticotropic hormone (ACTH) secretion, which reduces adrenal androgen production; this in turn allows normal secretion of pituitary gonadotropins.

4. Thyroid. In spite of the larger literature to the contrary, hypothyroidism is an extraordinarily rare cause of infertility.

C. Drugs and x-ray. Alkylating agents, antimetabolites, nitrofurantoins, Methotrexate, antidepressants, amebicides, and many additional compounds interfere with spermatogenesis. X-radiation also destroys the germinal epithelium.

D. Ductal obstruction. Congenital absence of the seminal vesicle, vas deferens, and part of the epididymis results in infertility. Most patients with cystic fibrosis also have azoospermia secondary to absent vasa. Acquired ductal obstruction can be the result of tuberculous, bacterial or "nonspecific" epididymitis, gonorrhea, and surgical ligation of the vas during herniorrhaphy, or planned vasectomy.

E. Retrograde ejaculation. Retrograde ejaculation can occur after surgery to the bladder neck or after surgical or medical sympathectomy. The sympathetic nervous system plays a role in the contraction of the bladder neck which prevents retrograde passage of semen at the time of ejaculation.

F. Varicocele. A varicocele is a group of dilated veins in the scrotum which is usually best demonstrated with the patient in the standing position. A Valsalva maneuver brings out a varicocele, and assuming the supine position results in dissipation of the varicocele. It is classically described as feeling like "a bag of worms." Ninety-eight percent of varicoceles are on the left side because the left spermatic vein joins the left renal vein directly and is often deficient of valves. Most men with varicoceles are fertile. However, after surgical repair, sperm count and paternity rate increase in the infertile man. The mechanism of the effect of varicocelectomy on semen quality is not known.

G. Immune disorders. Several investigators have reported a high incidence of sperm antibodies in infertile men. The significance of these findings is presently unclear.

H. Infectious disease. There is some evidence to suggest that infection of the urine or prostate with trichomonas, bacteria, or mycoplasm may cause infertility.

I. Testicular failure. In addition to those states listed above, there are several disorders of spermatogenesis which cause infertility. Biopsy of the testes in these patients may reveal germinal cell aplasia (Sertoli only syndrome), spermatogenic arrest, or hyalinization of the seminiferous tubules.

Table I lists the etiology of infertility in 1,294 men reported by Dubin and Amelar.[2] They claimed to have made a definite diagnosis in 95% of the patients. However, a clear causal relationship between the listed etiology and the infertility was not established in all cases.

10. Evaluation of the infertile male. While evaluating the infertile male, the physician should keep in mind the various etiologies of male infertility in order to focus his inquiry.

A. History. The following areas should be included in the history.

    1. Present.

        a. Duration of sexual relations without birth control.

        b. Sexual technique; use of lubricants (some spermatocidal).

        c. Pattern and frequency of intercourse.

    2) Past.

        a. Developmental—age of testicular descent, age of puberty.

        b. Surgical—undescended testicle, pelvic or retroperitoneal surgery, herniorrhaphy, sympathectomy, vasectomy.

        c. Medical—urinary infections, venereal disease, mumps, renal disease, diabetes, radiotherapy, recent febrile or viral illness, epididymitis, tuberculosis.

TABLE I
Causes of Male Subfertility—1,294 Cases[a]

Cause	Number	Percent
Varicocele	512	39.0
Testicular failure	176	14.0
Ductal obstruction	96	7.4
Pituitary abnormality	92	7.1
Sexual problems	64	5.1
Cryptorchidism	56	4.4
Ejaculatory disturbance	24	2.0
Necrospermia	15	1.3
Adrenal abnormality	11	0.9
Thyroid abnormality	8	0.6
Miscellaneous associated findings in-cluding variations in semen volume	170	12.9
Unknown	70	5.4

[a] Dubin, L. and Amelar, R. D. Etiologic factors in 1,294 consecutive cases of male infertility. Fertil. Steril. 22:469, 1971.

    d. Drugs—complete list of all past and present medications.

    e. Occupation and habits—exposure to chemicals and heat, hot baths, steam baths.

    f. Past marital history of both partners.

  B. Physical examination.

    1) General. Habitus, hair distribution, breasts, secondary sexual development, height and span, upper and lower proportions.

    2) Neurological. Check for visual field defects and anosmia, evaluate rectal tone, perineal sensation, and deep tendon reflexes.

    3) Genital tract. All of the following should be palpated—penis, urethra, meatus, testes, prostate, epididymides, vasa. Check for varicocele in the upright and supine positions after Valsalva maneuver.

  C. Laboratory evaluation.

    1) All patients should have the following laboratory studies.

      a. Urinalysis.

      b. Semen analysis.

      (1) Reliability. The results of semen analysis are variable and therefore multiple analyses are indicated in any equivocal or difficult situation. Repeat studies may have to be done over a duration as long as 6 months because viral and febrile illnesses can affect the semen quality for months after the acute episode.

      (2) Collection.

        a) Timing. The semen specimen should be collected after 1 to 2 days of sexual abstinence. Shorter or longer periods of continence may alter the character of the semen.

        b) Technique. The specimen is usually collected by masturbation into a clean, dry wide-mouth container.

      (3) Physical characteristics—general. The freshly ejaculated semen is a mixture of a coagulum and liquid which completely liquifies within 20 min.

        a) Coagulation. The constituents of the semen responsible for coagulation arise in the seminal vesicles. Therefore, in patients with congenital bilateral absence of the vas deferens and seminal vesicles, coagulation does not occur.

        b) Liquification. The enzyme responsible for liquification comes from the prostate, and therefore lack of liquification implies absence of prostatic secretions.

        c) Viscosity. Semen of normal viscosity flows freely and can be poured drop by drop, whereas hyperviscous semen does not flow drop by drop. There is a debate as to whether or not hyperviscosity is a cause of infertility.

        d) Volume. The usual range of semen volume in man is 2 to 6 ml. There is no agreement as to whether or not small and large volumes cause infertility. The prostate and seminal vesicles provide more than 90% of the total volume of the ejaculate.

(4) Sperm count. The sperm count is performed using a white blood cell pipette counting in the red blood cell field at a 1:20 dilution. Healthy young men generally have a sperm concentration of greater than 40 to 60 million per cc. However, the count is quite variable and poorly correlated with fertility. Thus, men with counts as low as 5 to 10 million per cc have fathered children, and it is not unusual for a man with a count of between 15 to 40 million to become a father. Total sperm count may be more important than count per cc.

(5) Motility. Within 2 to 3 hours after ejaculation, the motility of the spermatozoa should be observed under the microscope, recording the percentage of motile sperm and the quality of their motility. A healthy semen usually has greater than 60% motility.

(6) Morphology. A portion of the semen should be stained and viewed under the compound microscope to evaluate morphology. The number of immature and abnormal forms is recorded. A "normal" semen contains 60% or more normal forms and may have 2 to 3% immature forms.

(7) Additional parameters. There are innumerable other components of the normal semen which are not monitored in a routine analysis. Fructose is secreted by the seminal vesicles and its absence in a semen implies absence of the seminal vesicles.

2) Selected patients.

a. Endocrine evaluation. The best single test to detect hypogonadotropism is the serum testosterone. The serum LH and FSH will be low in these patients, but there is overlap with the normal values. Patients with germinal cell failure will have a high serum FSH. There is currently no treatment available for these individuals.

b. Biopsy. All patients with normal sized testicles and azoospermia should have a testicular biopsy since they may have a ductal obstruction which is a potentially reversible lesion. In practice, many additional patients with poor semen quality receive biopsies to document their pathology.

c. Vasography. Patients with azoospermia and normal spermatogenesis require vasography to pinpoint the site of obstruction.

d. Chromosome karyotype determination aids in establishing the diagnosis in patients with Klinefelter's syndrome and other abnormal forms of sexual development.

11. Medical treatment of male infertility. There are innumerable nonspecific remedies for male infertility. Most of these treatments are of doubtful value. It is difficult to document a response to therapy without a properly controlled clinical study because reassurance and time alone will result in pregnancies for a significant percentage of infertile couples.

A. Infection.

1) Bacterial. Men with urinary or prostatic infection should be treated with the appropriate drug. Men with white blood cells in their semen and positive bacterial cultures should be treated with the antibiotic indicated

by the sensitivities. Erythromycin and trimethoprim are possibly the only antibacterials which attain effective levels in the prostatic fluid.

2) Others. If cultures are negative but pyospermia persists, trials with tetracycline and metronidazole are indicated to eliminate possible mycoplasm and trichomonas infections. Both partners should be treated. It is often difficult to distinguish immature forms from leukocytes in the semen.

B. Hypogonadotropism. Initiate virilization with human chorionic gonadotropin (LH). When androgenization is apparent, add Pergonal (FSH).

C. Congenital adrenal hyperplasia. This is the only disease in which cortisone therapy is clearly indicated.

D. Hypothroidism. The only documented benefit of thyroid treatment for male infertility is in the exceedingly unusual case due to hypothyroidism.

E. Immune states. Recent, thus far unsubstantiated, reports suggest that the glucocorticoids may be helpful in the treatment of infertile patients with sperm antibodies.

F. "Idiopathic" infertility.

1) Testosterone rebound. Administration of 100 to 200 mg of testosterone weekly suppressed gonadotropin secretion resulting in decreased androgen production by the Leydig cells. This decreases the level of testicular androgen which is normally 100 times the serum concentration and causes azoospermia. Cessation of treatment is followed in 6 to 12 months by significant increases above pretreatment values in sperm count in two-thirds of the patients. Pregnancy rates of 40% have been claimed after the treatment. Proof of efficacy is lacking, but the initial experience is encouraging.

2) Split ejaculate. The initial part of the ejaculate has more sperm of better quality than the terminal portion in 85 to 90% of men. Therefore, use of the first fraction has been suggested for men with low sperm concentration or high volume ejaculates. Artificial insemination or withdrawal coitus can accomplish this. Efficacy is not proven.

G. Retrograde ejaculation.

1) After ejaculation, semen can be withdrawn with a catheter from men with retrograde ejaculation and inseminated into the cervix of the spouse.

2) Ephedrine has been reported to correct retrograde ejaculation.

H. Heat withdrawal. Men who regularly take hot baths or steam baths should desist since heat interferes with spermatogenesis.

12. Surgical treatment of male infertility.

A. Varicocele ligation. All infertile men with a varicocele should undergo high ligation of the internal spermatic vein. The size of the varicocele or the level of the sperm count does not matter. Many authors have reported 55 to 75% improvement in semen quality and a 35 to 40% pregnancy rate.

B. Ductal obstruction. All ductal obstructions should be repaired. This may require a vasostomy or an epididymovasostomy. Patency rates are reported from 40 to 90% and pregnancy rates from 25 to 40%.

C. Undescended testicle. All cryptorchid testes should be placed in the scrotum before the age of 8 years.

D. Hypospadias. The urethral meatus should be advanced to a site distal enough to allow sperm to be deposited in the vagina.

MALE SEXUAL INADEQUACY

1. Introduction. Sexual problems in men are very common and often unrecognized by the physician. The patient may present to his doctor with complaints unrelated to sexual function. The physician should be alerted by such nonspecific maladies to obtain a sexual history. In order to accomplish this, the practitioner must resolve his own sexual anxieties and be frank, confident, and straight-forward in his discussion with the patient. He should not impose his morals on the patient.

A. Adolescent. The adolescent requires education and reassurance concerning his genitalia, masturbation, homosexuality, intercourse, female genitalia, venereal disease, and contraception.

B. Premarital patient. This patient needs information regarding contraception and sexual technique as well as reassurance that any behavior which is mutually acceptable is normal.

C. Young adult. Same as A and B.

D. Aging adult. The older adult should be educated as to the changes in sexual function that occur with age (see Section 5-F below).

2. Definitions and incidence.

A. Premature ejaculator.* A man who cannot control his ejaculatory process for a sufficient time to satisfy an orgasmic female partner 50% of the time.

B. Ejaculatory incompetent.* A man who cannot ejaculate during intercourse.

C. Primary impotent. A male who has never been able to maintain an erection sufficient to achieve a successful coital connection.

D. Secondary impotent.* A man who was potent and subsequently has become unsuccessful in 25% or more of his coital opportunities.

E. Decreased libido. It is difficult to give a precise definition of decreased libido. An individual may have adequate libido to be compatible with one partner and not another. Frequency of intercourse varies greatly from individual to individual. Nevertheless, if a man feels his libido is inadequate, the physician should help him to increase his libido or to modify his expectations.

F. Miscellaneous. A discussion of homosexuality, fetishism, voyeurism, etc., is beyond the scope of this chapter.

G. Cotherapy.* This is a form of treatment during which a male professional and a female professional work as a pair to give therapy to a sexually inadequate couple. Joint sessions are conducted as well as sessions

---

* Adapted from Masters and Johnson.

during which the male therapist works with the male partner while the female therapist treats the female. Thus the term cotherapist refers to the therapist of the opposite sex who works with the partner of his or her sex. The term has nothing to do with surrogate sexual partners.

H. Incidence of impotency. The reported incidence of impotency increases with age (Table II).

3. Evaluation of sexually inadequate male.

A. History. The patient and his partner must be interviewed to obtain a complete, accurate history. Discrepancies in the two histories may provide insight into the problem and must be resolved.

1) General history should include developmental, surgical, medical, drug, and occupational history as outlined in the section on infertility.

2) Specific history.

a. Chief complaint. What is the problem and what is its effect on the man, the woman, and their relationship?

b. Childhood history. Including religious training, relationship with family members, and sexual education.

c. Sexual history.

(1) Early—masturbation, dating, petting, homosexual experience.

(2) Premarital—first and subsequent coital experiences, foreplay, number of partners.

(3) Marital—pattern of sexual behavior in previous and current marriages.

If impotency is the problem, the physician should inquire as to whether the patient is potent with other partners, whether he masturbates, has nocturnal emissions, morning erections, or erections during dreams or fantasies. A careful history of drug and alcohol consumption is essential.

B. Physical examination. This should be similar to the examination of the infertile male.

TABLE II

Incidence of Impotency

Age	Impotency
	%
A. From Kinsey—1948 (4,108 men)	
40	1.9
50	6.7
60	18.4
70	27.0
80	75.0
B. From Pearlman and Kobashi—1972 (2,801 men)	
40–49	5.0
50–59	11.3
60–69	35.6
70–79	59.0
80+	85.0

C. Laboratory examination. Complete blood count, urinalysis, serum creatinine, fasting blood sugar, serum testosterone are indicated for all patients. Any additional tests suggested by the history or physical examination should be obtained.

4. Etiology.

A. Psychological. The vast majority of cases of male sexual inadequacy have a psychological basis and should be treated accordingly.

B. Organic. Occasionally impotency has an organic basis. Table III outlines the more common organic causes of impotence. Many men with organic disease who are impotent have an additional psychological reason for their impotence.

5. Treatment of male sexual inadequacy.

A. Introduction. The therapy for all forms of male sexual inadequacy begins with a careful history by a concerned therapist. In most instances, the female partner must be interviewed and should cooperate in the treatment. Any reversible organic disease should be treated.

There are four levels of treatment.

1) An interested primary physician (family physician, urologist, gynecologist).

2) A physician with a special interest in sexual inadequacy.

3) Sexual inadequacy clinic with cotherapists.

4) Psychiatrist.

Therapists in category 1 can aid many affected individuals. The difficult problems must be referred to practitioners in group 2, 3, or 4, depending on the nature of the problem and the availability of the services. The primary

TABLE III
Common Organic Causes of Impotence

I. Endocrine
  A. Diabetes mellitus
  B. Hypogonadotropism[a]
  C. Testicular failure[a]
II. Drugs
  A. Alcohol
  B. Addictive drugs
  C. Antihypertensive drugs
  D. Drugs used to treat emotional disorders
  E. Estrogen and anti-androgens[a]
III. Surgery
  A. Perineal prostatectomy (almost always)
  B. Abdominal perineal colon resection (occasionally)
  C. Castration[a] (frequently)
  D. Sympathectomy (usually interferes with emission and ejaculation)

IV. Neurological
  A. Demyelinating diseases
  B. Central nervous system tumors
  C. Traumatic or neoplastic spinal cord disease
  D. Temporal lobe epilepsy
V. Vascular disease
  A. Priapism
  B. Atherosclerotic disease
  C. Aortic aneurysm
  D. Leriche syndrome
VI. Miscellaneous
  A. Pelvic fracture
  B. Peyronie's disease
  C. Any severely debilitating condition

[a] Presents with decreased libido, with or without impotence.

physician *should never state that the situation is hopeless.*

B. Decreased libido.

1) If the patient's serum androgens are low, treatment should be initiated with parenteral androgens. Subsequently, oral preparations may be substituted. Because the intestinal absorption of oral androgens is unpredictable, the patient may require parenteral treatment indefinitely.

2) If serum androgens are normal, reassurance and psychotherapy by a therapist as outlined in section A1-4 is indicated.

C. Premature ejaculation. The patient should be reassured that he is normal and that his problem can be resolved. The support and understanding of his partner are vital.

1) Less severe.

a. Inhibit psychic stimuli to orgasm by:

(1) Occupying the mind with nonsexual fantasy until the female achieves orgasm.

(2) Pinching the skin, biting the tongue, etc.

(3) Judiciously employing depressants such as alcohol.

b. Reduce tactile stimuli with variations in foreplay or use of a condom.

c. Repeat coitus after refractory period. The second or third erection may be maintained for a longer period than the first and result in orgasm for the female partner.

2) More severe.

a. Semans' technique.

(1) Extravaginal penile stimulation until ejaculation is imminent.

(2) Stop stimulation and squeeze the penis with the thumb at the frenulum and two fingers on the ventral surface of the coronal sulcus.

(3) Brief rest period.

(4) Restart cycle.

b. Masters and Johnson adapted Semans' technique with emphasis on the following:

(1) Cotherapy with a female therapist for the wife.

(2) Follow Semans' technique as outlined above for several days. Then initiate a period of nondemanding intromission with the female superior. Finally more vigorous coitus is allowed. The entire progression takes 3 to 4 weeks.

c. Results. Masters and Johnson claim 97.8% cure.

d. Complications. Some men experience a period of secondary impotence after treatment, possibly because of the psychic effect of increased demand for performance.

D. Ejaculatory incompetent.

1) Charney has reported return of ejaculatory competence after massage of the seminal vesicles. He stated that these patients had ejaculatory ducts which were plugged with viscous secretions that could be expressed by massage.

2) Masters and Johnson feel that cotherapy is essential to treat this problem. Their method is analogous to that used to treat premature ejaculation. Initially the wife forces an ejaculation with extravaginal penile manipulation. The couple then proceeds to coitus with emphasis on vigorous pelvic thrusting by the female.

3) Psychotherapy may aid in resolving underlying emotional conflicts and thus effect a cure.

4) Results. Masters and Johnson report 86.4% success in treating this uncommon disorder.

E. Impotence (primary and secondary).

1. General.

a. Role of the partner and cotherapist. Again, interviewing and working with the patient's mate, with or without a cotherapist, is usually necessary. The presence of a cotherapist avoids a triangle and eliminates the feeling that the therapist is taking sides. This facilitates a cooperative effort by all parties.

b. Fear of failure. Many secondarily impotent men have a history of premature ejaculation. Regardless of the underlying psychological etiology, the impotent male has developed a *fear of failure* which generates *tremendous anxiety* that in turn *reinforces* his impotence. His partner must understand that a demanding and critical attitude will increase the fear of performance and thus be counterproductive.

c. Alcohol and drugs. A history of heavy alcohol intake or drug abuse is very common in secondarily impotent men. The consumption of alcohol and drugs should be controlled and stopped if possible.

2) Specific.

a. Simple problems. The primary physician can:

(1) Reassure the patient that he is normal and that his impotence can be reversed.

(2) Control alcohol and drug abuse.

(3) Discuss the problem with both partners and encourage a period of noncoital, nondemanding sexual contact during which the patient can overcome his fear of performance, and the partner can express genuine concern and willingness to cooperate. Then encourage the couple to progress to nondemanding coitus and eventually to normal intercourse.

b. Complex problems.

(1) *Sexual clinics.* Modeled after the methods of Masters and Johnson, these clinics employ cotherapists to achieve the same ends outlined above. Masters and Johnson emphasize resolving the fear of performance and eliminating the "spectator role" of the impotent man. They report 59.4% and 74.8% success in primary and secondary impotence, respectively. *Warning.* There are many bogus sex clinics. The physician should carefully check the credentials of any therapist before referring patients to these clinics.

(2) Psychiatry. Psychotherapy may be indicated to resolve under-

lying emotional conflicts which contribute to the impotency.

F. Impotency in the aging male.

1) Education. The aging male should be informed of the changes in the physiology of erection and ejaculation which occur in later years. These include the following, as outlined by Masters and Johnson.

a) Erection comes after a longer period of stimulation.

b) The plateau (pre-ejaculatory) phase of erection lasts longer.

c) Ejaculation may be of shorter duration.

d) Ejaculated seminal fluid volume diminishes.

f) The expulsive force which propels the ejaculate decreases.

g) The refractory period is prolonged.

h) There is increased ejaculatory control and decreased ejaculatory demand. The aging man *may not wish to ejaculate* each time he has intercourse.

2) Further treatment.

a) After the man and his wife have been educated, they should then be reassured that the above listed alterations do not in any way preclude satisfactory sexual activity. Eliminating the fear of performance which these changes may engender will often resolve the problem. Manipulation of the penis will often evoke a reflex erection even when a psychic stimulus fails to induce an erection.

b) If this is unsuccessful, the measures discussed for the treatment of impotency in the younger male should be employed.

G. Surgical treatment for impotency. For men with organic impotency or selected patients with intractable psychological impotency, a Silastic penile implant is available. These Silastic implants are placed below Buck's fascia on the dorsal aspect of the penis or into the corpora cavernosa. This allows the male to achieve intromission. Results have been generally satisfactory, although failures and complications do occur.

REFERENCES AND SUGGESTED FURTHER READING
Infertility

1. Amelar, R. D. and Dubin, L. Male infertility. Urology 1:1, 1973.
2. Dubin, L. and Amelar, R. D. Etiologic factors in 1,294 consecutive cases of male infertility. Fertil. Steril. 22:469, 1971.
3. Federman, D. D. *Abnormal Sexual Development.* W. B. Saunders, Philadelphia, 1967.
4. Hotchkiss, R. S. *Infertility in Urology,* edited by Campbell and Harrison, W. B. Saunders, Philadelphia and London, 1970.
5. Walsh, P. C., Howards, S. S., and Sherins, R. J. Management of the infertile male. American Fertility Society, Postgraduate Course Syllabus, Course VI, 1974

Sexual Inadequacy

1. Hastings, D. W. *Impotence and Frigidity.* Little, Brown and Company, Boston, 1963.
2. Masters, W. H. and Johnson, V. E. *Human Sexual Inadequacy.* Little, Brown and Company, Boston, 1970.
3. Pearlman, C. K. and Kobashi, L. I. Frequency of intercourse in men. J. Urol. 107:298, 1972.
4. Semans, J. H. Premature ejaculation: a new approach. South. Med. J. 49:353, 1956.